THE CASE FORMULATION APPROACH
TO COGNITIVE-BEHAVIOR THERAPY

Guides to Individualized Evidence-Based Treatment

Jacqueline B. Persons, *Series Editor*

Providing road maps for managing real-world cases, volumes in this series help the clinician develop treatment plans using interventions of proven effectiveness. With an emphasis on systematic yet flexible case formulation, these hands-on guides provide powerful alternatives to one-size-fits-all approaches. Each book addresses a particular disorder or presents cutting-edge intervention strategies that can be used across a range of clinical problems.

Cognitive Therapy of Schizophrenia
David G. Kingdon and Douglas Turkington

Treating Bipolar Disorder:
A Clinician's Guide to Interpersonal and Social Rhythm Therapy
Ellen Frank

Modular Cognitive-Behavioral Therapy for Childhood Anxiety Disorders
Bruce F. Chorpita

Cognitive-Behavioral Therapy for PTSD:
A Case Formulation Approach
Claudia Zayfert and Carolyn Black Becker

Cognitive-Behavioral Therapy for Adult Asperger Syndrome
Valerie L. Gaus

Cognitive-Behavioral Therapy for Anxiety Disorders:
Mastering Clinical Challenges
Gillian Butler, Melanie Fennell, and Ann Hackmann

The Case Formulation Approach to Cognitive-Behavior Therapy
Jacqueline B. Persons

Mindfulness- and Acceptance-Based Behavioral Therapies in Practice
Lizabeth Roemer and Susan M. Orsillo

The Case Formulation Approach to Cognitive-Behavior Therapy

Jacqueline B. Persons

THE GUILFORD PRESS
New York   London

Library of Congress Cataloging-in-Publication Data

Persons, Jacqueline B.
   The case formulation approach to cognitive-behavior therapy / Jacqueline B. Persons.
      p. ; cm. — (Guides to individualized evidence-based treatment)
   Includes bibliographical references and index.
   ISBN 978-1-59385-875-9 (hardcover : alk. paper)
   ISBN 978-1-4625-0948-5 (paperback : alk. paper)
   1. Cognitive therapy. 2. Psychiatry—Case formulation. I. Title. II. Series.
   [DNLM: 1. Cognitive Therapy—methods. 2. Psychological Theory. 3. Treatment Outcome.
WM 425.5.C6 P467c 2008]
   RC489.C63P468 2008
   616.89′1425—dc22

                                                                        2008023695

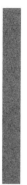

About the Author

Jacqueline B. Persons, PhD, is Director of the San Francisco Bay Area Center for Cognitive Therapy and Clinical Professor in the Department of Psychology at the University of California, Berkeley. She is a clinician, teacher, researcher, writer, and scientist-practitioner. She maintains an active clinical practice, providing cognitive-behavior therapy for mood and anxiety disorders and related problems, and teaches and provides clinical supervision to students and professionals in many settings. Dr. Persons conducts research on the mechanisms underpinning symptoms of depression and anxiety and on the process and outcome of cognitive-behavior therapy, especially as it is implemented in routine clinical practice. Her first book, *Cognitive Therapy in Practice: A Case Formulation Approach*, published by W. W. Norton in 1989, is widely considered a classic. She is past president of the Association for Advancement of Behavior Therapy (now the Association for Behavioral and Cognitive Therapies) and of the Society for a Science of Clinical Psychology, a section of the Society of Clinical Psychology of the American Psychological Association.

Preface

My struggles, as a young therapist, to respond to the rich and constantly surprising variety of situations I encountered daily in my clinical work led me to discover the way a case formulation can guide clear thinking and good decision making. That discovery led to my first book, *Cognitive Therapy in Practice: A Case Formulation Approach* (Persons, 1989).

In this volume I expand and elaborate on that book and my other writings on case formulation. The most significant advance over my earlier work is that I now embed the case formulation in a larger framework of clinical hypothesis testing. The formulation (or, more accurately, formulations—the clinician develops multiple formulations at multiple levels to guide work for each patient) is a hypothesis. The clinician collects data at every therapy session to test it and to evaluate the effectiveness of the treatment plan based on it. The chapter on progress monitoring (Chapter 9) is a centerpiece of this volume.

I struggle in this book to rely on the empirically supported therapies (ESTs). This is an awkward business. Most EST protocols consist of a list of interventions that are to be carried out in order to treat the disorder targeted by the EST. The EST protocol assumes that the mechanisms causing and maintaining the symptoms of the patient who is being treated at that moment match the mechanisms that underpin the design of protocol. The protocol also assumes that the patient's goal is to treat the DSM disorder targeted by the protocol. These assumptions often appear to be incorrect.

My solution to these problems, described in detail in this book, is to recommend that clinicians examine the EST protocols to understand the formulations that underpin them and how the interventions in the protocol flow out of the formulations. Then they can use that information (not the step-by-step procedures of the protocol itself) to guide their work. To facilitate those tasks, this book includes three chapters that lay out in detail the principles of the three major groups of models that underpin most ESTs: cognitive models (especially Beck's theory), learning theories, and basic models of emotion.

The approach to cognitive-behavior therapy described here is difficult to implement. However, it is rewarding. My goal is to help clinicians do effective work that is responsive to the situation at hand, guided by clear thinking, and evidence based.

Acknowledgments

My first thanks go to my husband, Jeffrey M. Perloff, for his unfailing support of all my personal and professional efforts.

I owe a major debt of gratitude to my patients, who have been generous and forgiving teachers for more than 25 years. They permitted me to present many examples of my work with them here. I have modified details that would identify them. An especially generous and talented patient gave comments that improved the monitoring chapter (Chapter 9) considerably.

I was fortunate to receive outstanding training as a graduate student in clinical psychology at the University of Pennsylvania and as a postgraduate student at the Behavior Therapy Unit at the Eastern Pennsylvania Psychiatric Institute. My teachers included Aaron T. Beck, David D. Burns, Edna B. Foa, Martin E. P. Seligman, and the late Joseph Wolpe. My dissertation supervisor, Jonathan Baron, gave generous and thoughtful support of my research and thinking.

I thank my colleagues at the San Francisco Bay Area Center for Cognitive Therapy, especially Michael A. Tompkins, who helped me integrate the empirically supported treatment protocols into my thinking, and Joan Davidson, who provided steady and enduring support.

Cannon Thomas provided stimulating and thought-provoking interactions throughout the years I spent writing this book that contributed greatly to my thinking. Kelly Koerner provided skillful consultation that helped me learn dialectical behavior therapy and, more generally, wise and balanced judgment in the trenches of tough clinical situations. She also read the learning theory chapter (Chapter 3) to be sure I did not make any stupid mistakes. Ann Kring read every chapter and offered useful feedback, especially on the emotion chapter (Chapter 4). Many students and trainees, including Janie Hong, Judy Glinder, Lisa Talbot, and Colleen Cowperthwait, provided useful comments.

Many of my ideas about case formulation had their origins in my experiences providing training at Ricardo Muñoz's stimulating Depression Clinic at San Francisco General Hospital at the University of California, San Francisco. There I also met Jeanne Miranda, who was my student and later research collaborator for several wonderful years.

I have been greatly influenced by Marsha M. Linehan's work and personal support and encouragement. Other important influences include David H. Barlow, Gerald C. Davison, Steven C. Hayes, James P. McCullough, Zindel V. Segal, Ira Turkat, and G. Terrence Wilson. Neil Jacobson supported my professional development in many small but significant ways, and I miss him very much.

The Association for Advancement of Behavior Therapy (now the ABCT, the Association for Behavioral and Cognitive Therapies) has provided me with a professional home since my postdoctoral fellowship days that has played a vital and sustaining role in my work and development. Many ABCT colleagues, too numerous to mention here, have contributed to my thinking, and I hope they will see their influence in these pages.

At The Guilford Press, Kitty Moore has been a dear friend and encouraging editor for more years than she planned. Developmental editor Barbara Watkins reviewed and gave comments on three versions of the manuscript. This book is far better for her talent and hard work. The ideas in this book led to a Guilford series, Guides to Individualized Evidence-Based Treatment. I am indebted to the authors of the books in the series for their creative efforts to flesh out what it means to do individualized evidence-based therapy.

I thank my friends Polly Bloomberg and Hanna Levenson for their friendship and personal and professional support, and my mother-in-law, Mimi, and my daughter, Lisa, for their encouragement and patience.

Finally, I thank Corey A. Pallatto for her amazing work ethic and editorial assistance. I could not have gotten this book out the door without her help.

Contents

THE CASE FORMULATION APPROACH
TO COGNITIVE-BEHAVIOR THERAPY

ONE

What Is the Case Formulation Approach to Cognitive-Behavior Therapy?

The case formulation approach to cognitive-behavior therapy is a framework for providing cognitive-behavior therapy (CBT) that flexibly meets the unique needs of the patient at hand, guides the therapist's decision making, and is evidence based. Case formulation-driven CBT is not a new therapy. It is a method for applying empirically supported CBTs and theories in routine clinical practice. The elements of the case formulation approach to CBT are depicted in Figure 1.1. The therapist begins by collecting assessment data to obtain a diagnosis and develop an individualized formulation of

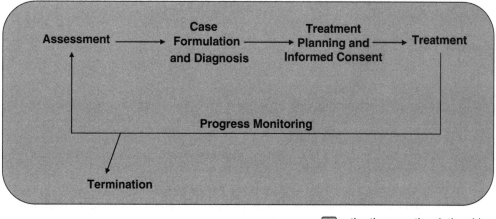

FIGURE 1.1. The case formulation approach to CBT. Copyright 2008 by the San Francisco Bay Area Center for Cognitive Therapy. Reprinted by permission in Jacqueline B. Persons (2008). Permission to photocopy this figure is granted to purchasers of this book for personal use only (see copyright page for details).

the case. The therapist uses the formulation to aid the work of developing a treatment plan and obtaining the patient's consent to it. As treatment proceeds, the therapist uses the formulation to guide decision making and works with the patient to collect data to monitor the progress of therapy and make adjustments as needed. All this happens in the context of a collaborative therapeutic relationship.

WHY IS A CASE FORMULATION APPROACH TO CBT NEEDED?

The development of empirically supported treatments (ESTs) for psychiatric disorders and psychological problems is an important positive development in our field and a boon to psychotherapists who strive to provide evidence-based treatment. Nevertheless, the EST protocols do not provide guidance to the evidence-based clinician in many challenging situations. These situations include: the patient who has multiple disorders and problems, the patient who has multiple providers, a need for the therapist to make decisions that are not referenced in the EST protocols, the patient who has disorders and problems for which no ESTs are available, the patient who does not adhere to the EST protocol, the patient who cannot establish the collaborative therapeutic relationship that is needed to implement the EST protocol, the patient who fails to respond to the EST protocol, or the ever-burgeoning number of ESTs the therapist is called upon to master.

I elaborate on each of these challenging situations briefly in the next section. Then I describe the case formulation approach to CBT and show how it addresses those situations. I conclude the chapter with a review of the intellectual foundations and empirical underpinnings of a case formulation approach to CBT. The remainder of the book describes in detail how to use the case formulation approach to provide CBT to the heterogeneous group of adult patients typically seen in outpatient practice. These patients generally present with chief complaints of anxiety and/or depression and all the problems that go with them.

Multiple Disorders and Problems

ESTs typically target single disorders, but patients typically have multiple disorders and problems. To treat these patients, the therapist must answer several questions, including the following: Which disorders and problems are interfering most with the patient's quality of life? Is it best to treat the multiple disorders and problems in sequence or simultaneously? If I use a sequential strategy, which problem ought I to target first? Might treating some problems lead to improvements or setbacks in other problems? The ESTs themselves do not (nor can they) answer these questions.

Another challenge posed by the multiple-problem patient is that sometimes the patient's various problems all seem to be caused by many of the same psychological mechanisms, as in the case of the depressed socially phobic grocery store checker whose depression and social anxiety can both be conceptualized as driven by schemas of himself as inadequate and defective and of others as critical and rejecting. An EST approach to treating this person seems to suggest that the therapist carry out two EST protocols in sequence—one for depression, one for social phobia. But this strategy feels cumbersome and inefficient, particularly when the two protocols are both founded on the same cognitive-behavior model and rely on many of the same interventions.

Multiple Providers

EST protocols describe a single psychosocial therapy. They do not provide any guidance to help the therapist with the common situation in which a patient is simultaneously receiving treatment from other clinicians. Examples include the woman seeking treatment for panic disorder who is already receiving benzodiazepine therapy from her primary care physician and the young man with obsessive–compulsive disorder who also consults a spiritual advisor (Bell, 2007). These adjunctive treatments may undermine— or facilitate—the treatment the cognitive-behavior therapist is providing.

Situations Not Referenced in the EST Protocols

Clinicians make large and small decisions dozens of times each day that are not referenced in the EST protocols. For example, is Susan's wish to reduce her academic course load this term an example of avoidance behavior or healthy limit setting? An EST protocol cannot answer questions at this level of detail. The EST protocol is based on a nomothetic (general) formulation that describes classes of target behaviors (e.g., in the case of Beck's cognitive therapy for depression, distorted cognitions and maladaptive behaviors) but does not identify *which specific* cognitions and behaviors are problematic for a particular patient. Without a systematic way to determine whether a particular behavior is adaptive or maladaptive, the therapist may shoot from the hip or be guided by convenience when making these decisions. The available evidence indicates that psychotherapists are not very skilled at decision making (Garb, 1998; Wilson, 1996a).

No EST Is Available

People often seek treatment for problems for which no EST is available, such as a somatization disorder, Asperger syndrome, a dissociative disorder, or distress about a husband's affair. And sometimes people have a disorder for which an EST is available but treating that disorder is not their goal. A common example is the depressed socially phobic man who wants to begin dating and marry. Although the man's DSM disorders interfere with his ability to date and marry, he does not wish to treat the DSM disorders to remission (as the ESTs assume).

Nonadherence

Nonadherence, including treatment refusal, homework noncompliance, and premature termination, are common. This is not surprising. Many cognitive-behavior therapies, such as exposure treatments for anxiety disorders, impose a substantial workload on patients and require them to tolerate significant distress. The effective cognitive-behavior therapist needs strategies to promote adherence with taxing and distressing interventions. Although a creative therapist can often generate good ideas for promoting adherence (Kendall, Chu, Gifford, Hayes, & Nauta, 1998), the EST protocol itself does not usually provide any explicit assistance.

Difficulty Establishing a Collaborative Therapeutic Relationship

The EST protocols require patient and therapist to work closely and collaboratively on demanding and sensitive tasks. Many patients have presenting problems that interfere with their ability to establish the collaborative therapeutic relationship that is needed to carry out the interventions described in the ESTs. Tension, disagreement, failure to collaborate, and ruptures in the therapeutic relationship can interfere with the smooth progress of treatment. The EST protocols themselves are not able to provide the therapist with much guidance in this situation.

Treatment Failure

Many patients do not respond to the ESTs. For example, 40 to 50% of patients who receive CBT for depression in the randomized controlled trials fail to make a full recovery by the end of treatment (Westen & Morrison, 2001). The only guidance the ESTs provide in this situation is the suggestion to attempt another EST. However, they do not offer any guidance about which EST is most likely to be helpful.

A related difficulty is that the EST protocol does not help the therapist effectively manage early failure. The therapist following an EST protocol who carries out the protocol as written will, in the case of Beck's cognitive therapy for depression, for example, complete a full trial of 18 to 20 sessions before declaring the treatment to be a success or failure. This strategy is inconsistent with data from Ilardi and Craighead (1994) indicating that after as few as four to six sessions it is possible to make a good prediction about the patient's ultimate treatment outcome.

Multiple ESTs

A final challenge is the proliferation of ESTs. Of course, the availability of a large number of ESTs is good news. In fact, our field needs even more effective therapies. At the same time, the ever-increasing number of ESTs poses a very real burden to the evidence-based psychotherapist. The EST protocols are often large tomes. As clinicians struggle to find time to read these tomes, it is frustrating to discover that many of them overlap considerably. Cognitive-behavior conceptualizations and ESTs for many disorders and problems are based on the same models and describe many of the same interventions (Chorpita, 2006; Zayfert & Becker, 2007).

Therapists who succeed in learning multiple protocols are faced with making decisions about which treatment is most likely to be helpful to the patient who is in the therapist's office at that moment. But the ESTs themselves do not provide any answers to that question.

The case formulation approach to CBT provides a framework to guide clinicians' handling of these challenges as they strive to use ESTs. In the next section I offer an overview of the case formulation approach to CBT and show how it addresses these issues.

ELEMENTS OF THE CASE FORMULATION APPROACH TO CBT

Assessment to Obtain a Diagnosis and Initial Case Formulation

The therapist begins by collecting assessment data in order to obtain a diagnosis and an initial case formulation that are used to guide treatment planning and clinical decision making (see Figure 1.1). The therapist collects data from multiple sources, including the clinical interview, self-report scales, self-monitoring data provided by the patient, structured diagnostic interviews, and reports from the patient's family members and other treatment providers.

Diagnosis is important for several reasons, including that the EST and other scientific literatures are tied to diagnosis, and diagnosis can aid in formulation, treatment planning, and intervention decision making.

But diagnosis is not enough to guide treatment; a case formulation is needed. A case formulation is a hypothesis about the psychological mechanisms and other factors that are causing and maintaining all of a particular patient's disorders and problems.

Elements of a Case Formulation

A complete case formulation ties all of the following parts together into a logically coherent whole:

1. It describes all of the patient's *symptoms, disorders, and problems.*
2. It proposes hypotheses about the *mechanisms* causing the disorders and problems.
3. It proposes the recent *precipitants* of the current disorders and problems, and
4. The *origins* of the mechanisms.

So, for example, a case formulation for Jon, a patient with depression, based on Beck's theory, reads as follows. The elements of the formulation are identified with CAPITAL LETTERS.

In childhood and adolescence, Jon was brutally teased and humiliated by his father (ORIGINS). As a result, Jon learned the schemas "I'm inadequate, a loser," and "Others are critical, attacking, and unsupportive of me" (MECHANISMS). These schemas were activated recently by a poor performance evaluation at work (PRECIPITANT). As a result, Jon began having many automatic thoughts (MECHANISMS), including, "I can't handle this job," and experienced anxiety and depression (SYMPTOMS, PROBLEMS), with which he coped by avoiding (MECHANISM) important work projects and withdrawing from collegial interactions with both peers and superiors (PROBLEMS). The avoidance caused Jon to miss some deadlines (PROBLEM), which resulted in criticism from his colleagues and boss (PROBLEM) and led to increased sadness, feelings of worthlessness, self-criticism and self-blame, low energy, and loss of interest in others (SYMPTOMS, PROBLEMS). Jon's low energy and hopelessness (PROBLEM) caused him to stop his regular program of exercise, which exacerbated his prediabetic medical condition (PROBLEM).

As this example illustrates, a good cognitive-behavior formulation is *internally coherent*. Its elements cohere to tell a compelling story that pulls together many aspects of the patient's history and functioning (Persons, 1989). The formulation of Jon's case ties together all of his problems, including his depression, alcohol use, and medical condition. A case formulation helps the therapist understand how apparently diverse problems are related and develop an efficient treatment plan to address them.

A simple example is the case of Jane, who sought help for what she described as "compulsive shopping." A comprehensive assessment revealed that she also had panic and some agoraphobic symptoms. Careful monitoring of all these symptoms revealed that Jane's urges to shop were triggered by anxiety and panic symptoms that, in turn, were triggered by catastrophic cognitions about unpleasant somatic sensations. Shopping was negatively reinforced by its anxiolytic effects. Based on this formulation, Jane's therapist developed a plan that treated *all of Jane's problems simultaneously* by teaching Jane to monitor her somatic experiences, catastrophic cognitions, and urges to shop, and to use strategies other than shopping (e.g., cognitive restructuring, present-moment mindfulness) to manage uncomfortable somatic sensations and the anxiety they provoked.

The Process of Developing an Initial Case Formulation

Early in treatment the therapist develops an initial working case formulation that guides initial treatment planning, gives the patient enough information to provide informed consent to treatment, and helps the patient engage in treatment. However, a complete and fully elaborated case formulation typically is available only after treatment has begun and further information is collected, including information from progress monitoring, described later. In fact, the formulation is a hypothesis and is subject to constant testing and revision as information gathering and treatment go forward.

The task of case formulation begins with developing a comprehensive list of all of the patient's problems. The therapist assesses all domains of the patient's life, including housing, finances, and other arenas, in order to develop a Problem List. The formulation accounts for all of the patient's problems, disorders, and symptoms and offers hypotheses about how they are related and what mechanisms are causing and maintaining them.

Developing a Mechanism Hypothesis

The heart of the formulation is the mechanism hypothesis. To develop a mechanism hypothesis, the therapist begins with a *nomothetic* theory and individualizes it to account for the case at hand. A *nomothetic* formulation is a general one. An example of a nomothetic formulation is Beck's cognitive theory that depressive symptoms result when schemas are activated by life events to produce dysfunctional automatic thoughts, maladaptive behaviors, and problematic emotions. The therapist's task is to translate a *nomothetic* formulation to an *idiographic* one. An *idiographic* formulation describes the particular symptoms, the schemas, and the automatic thoughts, maladaptive behaviors, and emotions experienced by a *particular individual.*

To develop an idiographic mechanism hypothesis for any particular patient, the therapist can use one of two strategies. The first is to identify a nomothetic formulation that underpins an EST (e.g., behavioral activation for depression) and then individualize and extrapolate that formulation to account for all of the problems of the particular patient who is in the therapist's office at that moment.

The second strategy is to base the formulation on a more general evidence-based psychological theory (e.g., operant conditioning theory) and then individualize and extrapolate that formulation to account for the details of the case at hand. To aid in this process, Chapters 2, 3, and 4 describe the basic principles and clinical implications of the main cognitive, learning, and emotion theories that underpin large numbers of ESTs.

Learning these theories helps the therapist address the problem of the proliferation of protocols. Most ESTs are based on these theories. Instead of learning the details of each and every EST, the clinician learns one or two of the ESTs that target problems and disorders he or she commonly treats, and relies heavily on the basic principles that underpin those and many other ESTs to guide formulation, treatment planning, and clinical decision making.

Levels of Formulation

Formulations are developed at three levels: *case, disorder or problem,* and *symptom.* The three levels are nested. A *case* consists of one or more *disorders/problems,* and a *disorder* consists of *symptoms.* Thus, a case-level formulation generally consists of an extrapolation or extension of one or more disorder- and symptom-level formulations.

Formulations at the various levels guide different aspects of treatment. The case-level formulation guides the process of treatment planning, especially the process of setting goals and making decisions about which problems to tackle first. It also frequently guides agenda setting in the therapy session.

Most intervention happens at the level of the symptom and is guided by a symptom-level formulation. However, the interventions used to treat a symptom do not just depend on the symptom-level formulation. The symptom of rumination illustrates how the disorder-level formulation guides the formulation for a symptom. Behavioral activation (Martell, Addis, & Jacobson, 2001) identifies the symptom of rumination as avoidance behavior and uses interventions to promote behavioral approach and reengagement with one's environment. In contrast, Beck's cognitive model views ruminations as consisting of distorted thoughts and intervenes to help patients change the content of their thoughts.

Treatment Planning

The function of the formulation is to guide effective treatment (S. C. Hayes, Nelson, & Jarrett, 1987). A key way the formulation guides treatment is by identifying the targets of treatment, which are generally the mechanisms that the formulation proposes are causing the symptoms. In the case of a formulation like the one above for Jon, which is based on Beck's cognitive theory, the treatment targets are the schemas, automatic thoughts, and maladaptive behaviors that the cognitive model views as mechanisms causing and maintaining patients' symptoms. In contrast, a formulation based on Lewinsohn's behavioral theory (Lewinsohn, Hoberman, & Hautzinger, 1985) identifies deficits in social skills and a dearth of pleasant activities as treatment targets.

Treatment Planning When Multiple Providers Are Needed

Treatment planning in the case formulation approach to CBT happens at the level of the case. That is, it considers *all* of the therapies the patient is receiving, not just the one that the cognitive-behavior therapist is providing. A case formulation approach to CBT also focuses the therapist's attention on mechanism, not just the procedures of the interventions. For example, in the case of Mary, the patient with panic symptoms who was receiving both exposure therapy and a benzodiazepine, a case formulation-driven approach helped the therapist realize that the cognitive-behavior and benzodiazepine components of Mary's treatment conflicted with one another. The CBT was designed to help Mary expose herself to and learn to tolerate her anxiety symptoms to learn they were not dangerous, whereas the benzodiazepine treated the anxiety symptoms by abolishing them. In this particular case, the problem was easily solved. When Mary's cognitive-behavior therapist explained the conflict between the two therapies, Mary proposed that after she learned some anxiety management strategies she would ask her primary care physician to begin tapering the benzodiazepine.

Preventing Nonadherence

The use of an idiographic formulation to guide treatment helps the therapist prevent nonadherence by selecting a conceptualization and treatment plan that best fits the case at hand. For example, the case of a patient with depression can be conceptualized using any of several evidence-based nomothetic formulations, including Beck's cognitive model (A. T. Beck, Rush, Shaw, & Emery, 1979), Lewinsohn's behavioral model (Lewinsohn & Gotlib, 1995), behavioral activation (Martell et al., 2001), problem-solving therapy (Nezu & Perri, 1989), or Cognitive Behavioral Analysis System of Psychotherapy (CBASP; McCullough, 2000). The therapist can carry out an idiographic assessment of the case at hand and select the model that best fits the case (Haynes, Kaholokula, & Nelson, 1999) or is most acceptable to the patient.

This approach to treatment can prevent and reduce nonadherence because the therapist works to adapt to the patient rather than the other way around. For example, Jackie reported that she had successfully overcome a previous depressive episode by increasing her exercise and social contacts. Thus, she wanted to use that strategy again. Her strategy seemed to be based on a conceptualization of her depression that was similar to Lewinsohn's (1974) view of depression as due to a loss of positive reinforcers. Because the interventions Jackie described had helped her in the past and were consistent with an EST-based formulation and intervention plan, I was happy to support them. I worked with Jackie on using exercise and activity scheduling to overcome her current depressive episode rather than requiring her to learn a new set of cognitive or problem-solving skills (Rude, 1986).

This approach to treatment is reminiscent of Acocella's (2003) description of the approach of George Balanchine, the choreographer of the New York City Ballet.

> He was convinced that you could not really change a dancer. All you could do was develop what she already had. In choreographing a ballet, he would often say to the people he had assembled, "Well, what can you do?" Then, if he liked what they showed him, he would work it up, and put it in, and let the dancers complete it. ... When the cast of a ballet changed, he often changed the choreography to fit the new performers. As a result, many of his ballets exist in a number of versions. (p. 53)

Thus, the therapist can select different formulations for different patients, depending on which appears most acceptable or helpful to the patient who is in his or her office at that time. In fact, the therapist can use different formulations at different moments in time for a single patient. For example, if a patient who generally benefits from behavioral activation to treat depressive symptoms balks at it one day, I might shift to Socratic dialogue to identify and address distorted cognitions instead. The rationale for this strategy is that the behavioral activation and cognitive models, although different, do not conflict with one another. In fact, both might be valid, even for a single patient!

The strategy of using multiple conceptualizations simultaneously is risky. It is especially risky when models conflict because then the interventions driven by the different formulations may work at cross-purposes. However, this risk is small, because most CBT models do not conflict. Another risk is that the therapist's use of multiple formulations can contribute to fuzzy thinking or no thinking, just a random going back and forth from one intervention to another without any rationale. So this strategy must be used with care. In fact, whether the benefits of this strategy outweigh the risks is a fascinating empirical question. Nevertheless, it allows the therapist a high degree of flexibility that can help him or her flexibly respond to the patient to keep him or her engaged in treatment.

Treatment Planning When No EST Is Available

When patients seek treatment for problems and disorders for which no EST is available, evidence-based practitioners face a dilemma. Ought they refuse to provide treatment? This option is not very appealing. The case formulation approach to CBT offers several alternatives.

One is to adopt the strategy used by Opdyke and Rothbaum (1998). They used the empirically supported formulations and interventions for one impulse control disorder (trichotillomania) as templates to develop formulations and interventions for other impulse control disorders (e.g., kleptomania and pyromania) for which no empirically supported formulations and therapies are available. This strategy is particularly useful when patients do not meet full criteria for a DSM disorder for which an EST is available or when the patient has the disorder but has goals other than to treat the disorder. These patients can be offered a treatment based on the EST even though the patient does not meet full criteria for the disorder targeted by the EST.

Another strategy is to develop an idiographic formulation based on one of the basic theories that underpin many of the ESTs, such as Beck's cognitive theory, theories of respondent and operant conditioning, and Lang's (1979) bioinformational theory of emotional processing (described in Chapters 2, 3, and 4) and use the formulation to develop a treatment plan. This strategy is a transdiagnostic one (Harvey, Watkins, Mansell, & Shafran, 2004). That is, it is not tied to diagnosis. It allows the clinician to draw on basic science to guide conceptualization and treatment.

Thus, a case formulation-driven mode of treatment allows the therapist to offer treatment to patients who have disorders or problems that are not targeted by an EST. Of course, because the therapist treating these patients is not using an EST, the therapist must obtain the patient's informed consent before embarking on what is essentially an experimental treatment.

Obtaining Informed Consent for Treatment

The initial case formulation, diagnosis, and treatment plan are developed in the context of a collaborative relationship with the patient and are shared with the patient.

Ideally this happens gradually as a process of mutual discovery. But before beginning treatment, the therapist reviews the key information in a formal process to obtain the patient's informed consent to proceed with the proposed treatment.

The case formulation aids in the process of obtaining informed consent because most patients are not willing to go forward in treatment unless they have confidence that the therapist truly understands their difficulties and will provide treatment that addresses them—that is, that patient and therapist have a shared formulation about the nature and causes of the patient's problems and what is needed to treat them effectively. The formal process of obtaining the patient's informed consent before going forward also helps prevent nonadherence by getting the patient's agreement to the goals and interventions of treatment before beginning it.

All of the elements of therapy described so far (initial assessment, diagnosis, case formulation, treatment planning, and informed consent for treatment) make up the pretreatment phase of the therapy. This phase of therapy lasts one to two or four sessions. The activities of the pretreatment phase are described in detail in Chapters 5, 6, and 7. If these elements are successfully accomplished and patient and therapist can agree on a treatment plan, treatment begins.

Treatment

Treatment is guided by the formulation (or more accurately, by multiple formulations, because, as already described, the therapist develops formulations at multiple levels). In Chapters 10 and 12, I discuss how the therapist uses the various levels of formulation to guide decision making and intervention. I do not say much in this book about the details of the interventions themselves for two reasons. First, those details are provided in many other places and I assume the reader is familiar with them. Second, in my experience, carrying out the intervention is the easy part of clinical work. The hard parts are collecting and sorting through all of the information that comes the clinician's way in order to determine when to intervene and what treatment target to address at that moment, and therefore I focus my attention on those decision-making tasks.

Using the Formulation to Guide Idiographic Decision Making

The case-level, disorder-level, and symptom-level formulations guide the therapist's decision making in situations that are too unique to be addressed by the EST protocols. The case formulation translates the nomothetic (general) protocol into an idiographic (individualized) one for the case at hand. The idiographic formulations guide the clinician's decision making, for example, in the case of Susan, mentioned above, who wanted to reduce her course load for the upcoming semester. The therapist needed to work with Susan to determine whether her wish to reduce her course load was adaptive coping or maladaptive avoidance.

Susan's therapist had earlier worked with Susan to develop the formulation that she held the self-schema that she was weak, fragile, and helpless. This formulation suggested that Susan's wish to reduce her course load was a maladaptive one driven by that schema. However, rather than simply assuming that this was true, the therapist worked with Susan to test it. They carried out a Thought Record in which Susan examined the automatic thoughts that arose when she reviewed her course plan (which was a very typical one, not unduly heavy or light) for the semester. Consistent with the formulation hypothesis, Susan's automatic thoughts included "I won't be able to complete the work" and "I'll fall apart and get depressed again and my life will be ruined." Susan and her therapist identified these thoughts and were able to agree that these predictions, although they felt emotionally compelling to Susan, were not consistent with how well she was functioning.

Another student, Erik, also felt anxious about his course load. His anxiety occurred in the context of returning to school after a long illness and was driven by thoughts like "If I make any accommodation at all to my illness, my life will be ruined," a line of thinking that stemmed from a self-schema of "I am ruined, defective, and doomed because of my illness." In Erik's case, the formulation suggested that reducing his course load might allow him to test his belief that if he accommodates to his illness his life will be ruined.

In both Susan's and Erik's cases, the idiographic case formulation gave the therapist an initial hypothesis about what line of intervention to take to help the student evaluate his or her course load. And in both cases, the therapist worked collaboratively with the patient to flesh out and test the formulation hypothesis. Next, patient and therapist will collect data to monitor the patient's adherence to the interventions flowing out of the formulation and their helpfulness.

The case formulation also provides a guide to clinical decision making in situations involving scheduling and business aspects of therapy that are typically not addressed in the ESTs. Leonora called and left a phone message saying that she was facing a major deadline at work and wanted to cancel the session we had scheduled for the next week and reschedule her session to meet with me after the deadline passed. What answer do I give? I consulted my formulation of her case. Leonora suffered from worry and she and I had recently developed the conceptualization that her worry behavior (especially the worry thought "I made a mistake; I shouldn't have married my husband") functioned to promote her avoidance of acknowledging and taking action to solve her marital problem. Based on this conceptualization, I hypothesized that Leonora's request to postpone the therapy session might be an instance of one of the treatment targets (avoidance behavior) described in her case formulation. I called Leonora and explained, referring to our previous collaborative conceptualization, why I recommended that she keep her appointment. She accepted my rationale and we met and had a productive session that helped her move forward to take some action to solve her marital problem.

Using the Formulation to Handle Nonadherence

The individualized case formulation helps the therapist understand and manage nonadherence behavior effectively. For example, my formulation of my patient Chie's case proposed that one of her major strategies for coping with stressful situations was to "shut down and give up." In fact, often she simply went to bed. If Chie was scheduled to meet with me for a therapy session during one of her "shut down" phases, she'd leave a phone message canceling her session and sometimes even quitting the therapy altogether.

My formulation of her case helped me by reminding me that Chie's "shut down and give up" mode was a key problem behavior that was common to all of her symptoms and problems. Therefore it was completely expectable and in fact *good news* that it appeared in therapy, where I could get a detailed assessment of it and intervene with it directly. That is, the formulation helped me increase my empathy and reduce my frustration when Chie's problem behavior appeared in therapy. The formulation also helped me prioritize and target this behavior for intervention when it occurred and reminded me that interventions that addressed this behavior could not only increase Chie's compliance in therapy but help her solve many other problems.

Monitoring and Hypothesis Testing

As treatment proceeds, the patient and therapist collect data to test the formulation and monitor the process and outcome of therapy. Chapter 9 describes this part of therapy in detail. Data collection allows patient and therapist to answer questions like the following:

> Is the patient accepting and adhering to the interventions the therapist provides?
> Are the mechanisms changing as expected?
> Do the mechanisms (e.g., cognitive distortions) and symptoms (e.g., hopelessness) covary as expected?
> Are the symptoms remitting?
> Are problems in the therapeutic relationship interfering?

If process (mechanism change, the therapeutic alliance, or adherence) and/or outcome are poor, the therapist works with the patient to collect more assessment data to get more information about what is interfering with progress and to evaluate whether a different formulation might lead to a different intervention plan that produces better results. Thus, therapy is an idiographic hypothesis-testing process, where the treatment of each case is like an experiment, where the formulation is the hypothesis and the therapist can carry out assessments or even experiments to directly test the formulation (e.g., see Iwata, Duncan, Zarcone, Lerman, & Shore, 1994, and Turkat & Maisto, 1985). More commonly, the therapist tests the formulation indirectly by monitoring the degree to which the treatment plan based on the formulation leads to the expected changes in processes and outcomes.

Progress monitoring strengthens the patient–therapist alliance by building an ongoing evidence-based process of work that patient and therapist share. It also helps the therapist address nonadherence and failure. These topics are addressed in detail in Chapter 11. The case formulation approach to CBT calls for the therapist to monitor adherence carefully at every step in order to identify and address early signs of nonadherence before they worsen and destroy the therapy altogether.

The case formulation approach to treatment helps address treatment failure in several ways. First, progress monitoring identifies failure early so the therapist can begin problem solving promptly.

Second, the model provides the therapist with a systematic decision-making strategy to manage treatment failure. When treatment fails or appears likely to fail, the therapist using a case formulation-driven approach works collaboratively with the patient on the problem. One piece of the work is to gather more assessment data to consider whether a different formulation of the case might lead to a different treatment plan that might be more effective. Thus, for example, if monitoring shows that a patient with depression is not responding to therapy driven by a cognitive formulation and in fact that cognitive restructuring interventions appear to promote suppression (Beevers, Wenzlaff, Hayes, & Scott, 1999), the therapist can shift to a formulation and interventions based on mindfulness-based cognitive therapy (Segal, Williams, & Teasdale, 2002) or behavioral activation.

The Therapeutic Relationship

The therapeutic relationship supports all of the other parts of the therapy. That fact is reflected in its depiction in Figure 1.1 as a background shading that encompasses all of the other stages of case formulation-driven CBT.

The therapeutic relationship is essential to the process at every stage. In fact, the therapist begins working to develop the relationship with the initial telephone call from the potential patient. Throughout pretreatment and treatment, the therapist works to build a trusting, collaborative therapeutic relationship. He or she works to strengthen the patient's motivation for change and willingness to carry out the proposed therapy by working collaboratively with the patient to develop a shared formulation, set treatment goals that are emotionally meaningful to the patient, and clearly tie the interventions to the patient's goals.

The case formulation approach to CBT relies on a dual view of the relationship that is described in detail in Chapter 8. One part of the relationship is the necessary-but-not-sufficient (NBNS) view. In this view, the trusting collaborative relationship is the foundation upon which the technical interventions of CBT rest. The other view of the relationship is as an assessment and intervention tool itself, as illustrated in the case of Chie, above. In that example, Chie's behavior with me, her therapist, exemplified behavior she also exhibited with others in her life. I was able to use that fact to guide my conceptualization of her case and to intervene to address the problems in our relationship and other aspects of her life.

The case of Adrienne offers another example of how the therapist uses the relationship in case formulation-driven CBT. Adrienne called for help coping with a stressful meeting she was scheduled to lead. When I was unable to return her call before the meeting, she flew into a rage and attacked me for being not supportive when she needed it. My formulation of her case helped me by guiding me to think about her problematic behavior as an example of the behavior for which Adrienne sought treatment. That meant that I could use the case formulation to understand her behavior and guide intervention to address it. In Adrienne's case, assessment revealed that her anger resulted from her feeling abandoned and tricked by me. We had a good discussion in which we were able to agree that her feelings of rage toward me and the belief that I was tricking her were caused by and consistent with how her abusive parents had treated her but were not valid in her relationship with me. This discussion resolved the problem in our relationship and gave Adrienne some useful tools to address other situations in which she felt enraged and tricked by others.

The case formulation approach to CBT also helps the therapist establish a good relationship at the beginning of therapy by adapting the formulation and treatment plan to the needs and mode of working of the patient, as was described in the discussion of adherence above, and by constantly monitoring the quality of the relationship so that glitches and ruptures can be identified and addressed early.

The case formulation approach to CBT also helps the therapist anticipate potential problems in the alliance. For example, when the case formulation proposes that the patient tends to view authority figures as attacking and critical, the therapist can expect that the patient might feel attacked and criticized in therapy and can use that expectation to try to head off relationship problems before they develop.

To summarize, the case formulation approach to CBT is a framework for using the ESTs in clinical practice that helps the therapist address many issues and difficulties that are not addressed by the EST protocols themselves. One way case formulation-driven CBT does this is by focusing on the whole patient and all the therapies the patient is receiving, not just on a single disorder or treatment protocol.

The case formulation approach to CBT also addresses flexibly difficulties the clinician encounters because it is a principle-driven approach to treatment rather than a protocol-driven approach. One way to capture this notion is via the analogy of a trip. The protocol-driven approach and formulation-driven approaches to treatment are analogous to two approaches to determining the route on a road trip—say, a trip from San Francisco to New York. The protocol-driven approach is analogous to following a list of directions that specifies, in order, what turns to make to get from San Francisco to New York. The formulation-driven approach is analogous to using a map. If, on the way to New York, you encounter a roadblock, a list of instructions gives no guidance on what to do next. In contrast, a map allows you to find an alternate route. Case formulation-driven CBT is like a map. Patient and therapist select the destination, choose a route, monitor progress at every step of the way, and make adjustments as needed to overcome the obstacles and roadblocks that inevitably arise along the way.

INTELLECTUAL FOUNDATIONS
OF CASE FORMULATION-DRIVEN CBT

The case formulation approach to CBT has multiple origins within and outside of CBT. Within CBT, case formulation-driven CBT borrows heavily from functional analysis (Haynes & O'Brien, 2000; Turkat & Maisto, 1985) and paradigmatic behavior therapy (Eifert, Evans, & McKendrick, 1990). Probably the main difference between the functional analysts and the model I present here is that the functional analysts focus exclusively on case conceptualizations that are based on operant conditioning, whereas case formulation-driven CBT also permits case conceptualizations based on Beck's and other cognitive theories (described in Chapter 2) and on emotion theories (described in Chapter 4).

The material presented here relies on work by other cognitive-behavior therapists who have written about case formulation, including J. S. Beck (1995); Freeman (1992); Koerner & Linehan (1997); Nezu, Nezu, and Lombardo (2004); Padesky (1996); Turkat (1985); Hersen (1981); and Tarrier (2006). The approach to treatment described here also rests heavily on the long-standing tradition in behavior therapy—indeed, in psychology—of the value of observing the single organism (Kazdin, 1982; Morgan & Morgan, 2001).

The EST movement underpins case formulation-driven CBT as described in this book (Kendall & Chambless, 1998). Other underpinnings include the field of program evaluation (cf. Bloom, Fischer, & Orme, 1995); recent writings about outcome evaluation in clinical practice (Woody, Detweiler-Bedell, Teachman, & O'Hearn, 2003); the scientist-practitioner tradition in clinical psychology (Barlow, Hayes, & Nelson, 1984; Peterson, 1991; Stricker & Trierweiler, 1995), medicine (Sackett, Richardson, Rosenberg, & Haynes, 1997), and social work (Gibbs & Gambrill, 1999); and even the scientific method itself (Cone, 2001).

The case formulation approach to CBT also draws on earlier discussions of the need for modularized (Wilson, 2000) and principle-driven protocols (Castonguay & Beutler, 2006; G. M. Rosen & Davison, 2003) and protocols in which interventions are guided by idiographic assessment (Persons, 1991). Evidence-based protocols of this sort that are already available include multisystemic therapy (MST; Henggeler, Schoenwald, Borduin, Rowland, & Cunningham, 1998), dialectical behavior therapy (DBT; Linehan, 1993a), acceptance and commitment therapy (ACT; S. C. Hayes, Strosahl, & Wilson, 1999), the modular therapy for depressed adolescents developed by Curry and Reinecke (2003), Blanchard's (Greene & Blanchard, 1994) cognitive-behavior protocol for treating irritable bowel syndrome, and Chorpita's (2006) protocol for treating childhood anxiety disorders. Others that are currently being developed include protocols for treating substance abuse (McCrady & Epstein, 2003), depression in adolescents (Albano, 2003), and eating disorders (Fairburn, Cooper, & Shafran, 2003).

EMPIRICAL SUPPORT FOR CASE FORMULATION-DRIVEN CBT

Has the case formulation approach to CBT been shown in controlled studies to be effective? In one sense, this is not a sensible question, because the method described here is not a new treatment. It is a simply a systematic method for adapting empirically supported treatments to meet the needs of the case at hand (Sackett et al., 1997). From this idiographic vantage point, the method itself provides a way to answer the effectiveness question because it calls for the therapist and patient to collect data to evaluate the effectiveness of the therapy for each case.

However, the question of whether CBT guided by a case formulation has been shown to be effective can also be posed from a more general, nomothetic point of view. The evidence on this question is sparse. A handful of randomized trials comparing outcomes of case formulation-driven and standardized CBT shows that formulation-driven treatment produces outcomes that are not different from and sometimes a bit better than standardized treatment (Jacobson et al., 1989; Schneider & Byrne, 1987; Schulte, Kunzel, Pepping, & Schulte-Bahrenberg, 1992).

Although the Schulte et al. (1992) study is frequently described as showing that patients who received individualized treatment had worse outcomes than those who received standardized treatment, a careful review of the findings suggests that the study fails to show a difference between individualized and standardized treatment. Schulte et al. (1992) randomly assigned 120 persons with phobia to standardized exposure treatment, individualized treatment, or yoked control treatment (patients in the yoked control group received an individualized treatment that had been developed for a patient in the individualized treatment condition). Although a multivariate analysis of variance (MANOVA) showed that the three treatment conditions differed significantly at the $p < .05$ level for three of nine outcome measures at posttreatment, these results faded over time (appearing on only two measures at 6-month follow-up, and on none at 2-year follow-up). Furthermore, no statistical tests were conducted to directly compare the patients in the standardized condition with those in each of the other conditions.

Three uncontrolled trials that I and my colleagues conducted of the methods described in this book have shown that treatment of patients with depression (Persons, Bostrom, & Bertagnolli, 1999; Persons, Burns, & Perloff, 1988) and both depression and anxiety (Persons, Roberts, Zalecki, & Brechwald, 2006) guided by a cognitive-behavioral case formulation and weekly progress monitoring has outcomes similar to outcomes of patients receiving cognitive-behavior therapy or cognitive-behavior therapy plus pharmacotherapy in the randomized controlled trials. An uncontrolled trial showed that patients with bulimia nervosa who received individualized treatment guided by a functional analysis had better outcomes than patients who received standardized treatment on some measures (abstinence from bulimic episodes, eating concerns, and body shape dissatisfaction) but not others (self-esteem, perceived social support from friends, and depression) (Ghaderi, 2006).

Another relevant literature is the literature on the treatment utility of idiographic assessment, as the main role of the idiographic case formulation is to aid in the treatment process. Nelson-Gray (2003) and Haynes, Leisen, and Blaine (1997) reported that functional analysis (one of the methods of case formulation described in of this book; see Chapter 3) had good treatment utility in the treatment of individuals with severe behavioral problems, such as self-injurious behavior. The treatment utility of functional analysis and other idiographic assessment methods for the types of outpatient cases described in this book has unfortunately rarely been studied.

The case formulation approach to treatment requires frequent monitoring of the process and outcome of the therapy. Surprisingly, the effects of monitoring on outcome have rarely been studied. One exception is the work of Michael Lambert and his colleagues, who have conducted several studies showing that patients treated by therapists who received feedback through monitoring data had better outcomes than patients treated by therapists who did not receive feedback. In particular, patients who had poor outcomes early in treatment improved after the therapist was alerted to the patient's poor progress (Lambert, Hansen, & Finch, 2001; Lambert, Harmon, Slade, Whipple, & Hawkins, 2005; Whipple et al., 2003).

The studies reviewed here converge to provide support for the assertion that reliance on a cognitive-behavioral case formulation can contribute to treatment outcome. However, few studies have examined this question directly. For that reason, it is probably fair to say that the strongest empirical support for the treatment utility of a cognitive-behavioral case formulation currently comes from the method's reliance on evidence-based nomothetic formulations as templates for the idiographic formulation and from the idiographic data that the therapist collects to monitor each patient's progress.

* * *

This chapter describes the essential elements of the case formulation approach to CBT, which are presented in Figure 1.1. Central to case formulation-driven CBT is a solid understanding of the theories of cognition, learning, and emotion that underpin the currently available empirically supported cognitive-behavioral protocols. These theories are described in the next three chapters, beginning with cognitive theories and therapies.

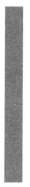

TWO

Cognitive Theories and Their Clinical Implications

This chapter describes cognitive theories that underpin evidence-based protocols for treating mood, anxiety, and related disorders and spells out clinical implications of those theories. I focus in detail on the cognitive theory developed by Aaron T. Beck because it underpins a large number of ESTs. The therapist will want to understand Beck's theory thoroughly in order to be able to use it flexibly to guide case conceptualization, treatment planning, intervention, and other clinical decision making. The chapter also provides brief accounts of other cognitive theories and therapies. It ends with an overview of the use of cognitive theories, especially Beck's theory, to guide formulation and intervention.

BECK'S COGNITIVE THEORY AND THERAPY

Beck's cognitive theory (A. T. Beck, 1976) proposes that we all have deep cognitive structures called schemas that enable us to process incoming information and interpret our experiences in a meaningful way (A. T. Beck et al., 1979). Symptoms of psychopathology (*emotions, cognitions,* and *behaviors*) result when pathological *schemas* are activated by *stressful events* (see Figure 2.1).

Beck (1976; A. T. Beck et al., 1979) first proposed his cognitive theory as an account of depression, and he and others have since adapted it to account for a wide variety of disorders and problems, including anxiety (A. T. Beck, Emery, & Greenberg, 1985); schizophrenia (Kingdon & Turkington, 2005); bipolar disorder (Basco & Rush, 1996; Newman, Leahy, Beck, Reilly-Harrington, & Gyulai, 2002); chronic pain (Morley, Eccleston, & Williams, 1999); irritable bowel syndrome (Greene & Blanchard, 1994); somatoform disorder (Looper & Kirmayer, 2002); personality disorders (A. T. Beck, Freeman, Davis, & Associates, 2004); bulimia nervosa (Whittal, Agras, & Gould, 1999); anger (R. Beck & Fernandez, 1998); suicide (G. K. Brown et al., 2005); marital distress (Dunn & Schwebel, 1995); and substance abuse (A. T. Beck, Wright, Newman, & Liese, 1993).

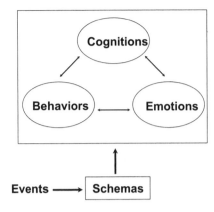

FIGURE 2.1. Beck's cognitive theory of psychopathology. From Persons, Davidson, and Tompkins (2001). Copyright 2001 by the American Psychological Association. Reprinted by permission.

Flowing directly from his theory, Beck developed a therapy that treats psychopathology by intervening to change the automatic thoughts, behaviors, and schemas that cause unpleasant emotions and to change the relationships among them. Some interventions also target the events and situations that trigger schemas to cause symptoms. Because automatic thoughts, behaviors, and emotion are reciprocally causal, changes in automatic thoughts or behaviors are expected to lead to changes in emotion. Changes in schemas are expected to reduce the number, likelihood, and intensity of future episodes of illness.

EMPIRICAL SUPPORT FOR BECK'S THEORY AND THERAPY

An exhaustive review of the evidence base underpinning Beck's theory and therapy is not possible here. Instead, I provide a brief overview of the literature and I highlight some important and illustrative studies.

Studies conducted to test Beck's theory have produced results that are by and large supportive of the theory (Haaga, Dyck, & Ernst, 1991; Garratt, Ingram, Rand, & Sawalani, 2007; Whisman, 1993). However, most tests of the theory provide only correlational data (e.g., demonstrating that negative emotions and distorted thinking occur together). Relatively few studies have been conducted to test the causal hypotheses of the theory largely because these studies are so difficult to conduct. One such hypothesis is that schemas, when activated by life events, lead to the development of symptoms (Gotlib & Krasnoperova, 1998). Support is strongest for depression (Scher, Ingram, & Segal, 2005) and anxiety, which have been more extensively researched than other problems.

Efficacy data from randomized controlled trials (RCTs) for many of the disorders and problems listed above generally show that Beck's cognitive therapy (CT) is superior to wait list and equal but not superior to pharmacotherapy and other active treatments (see recent reviews by A. C. Butler, Chapman, Forman, & Beck, 2006; Hollon & Beck, 2004). Emerging evidence shows that for depression and some anxiety disorders, cognitive therapy provides better protection from relapse than pharmacotherapy (A. C. Butler et al., 2006; Hollon et al., 2005). For several disorders, cognitive therapy has best outcomes when it is paired with pharmacotherapy (e.g., schizophrenia, bipolar disorder, and perhaps severe major depressive disorder) (DeRubeis et al., 2005; Friedman et al., 2004). Effectiveness data show that with some exceptions (Organista, Muñoz, & Gonzalez, 1994), cognitive therapy, at least for depression and anxiety, and for the treatment of adults, can be successfully transported from research settings to clinical practice (Haaga, DeRubeis, Stewart, & Beck, 1991; Merrill, Tolbert, & Wade, 2003; Persons, Bostrom, & Bertagnolli, 1999; Persons, Burns, & Perloff, 1988; Persons, Roberts, Zalecki, & Brechwald, 2006). At the time of this writing, Beck's cognitive therapy has more empirical support from randomized controlled trials and other controlled studies than any other psychosocial therapy.

Disappointingly little is known about the mechanisms of action of cognitive therapy (Garratt et al., 2007; Whisman, 1993). Studies that support the model's predictions that the therapy is effective because it produces cognitive change include the demonstration by DeRubeis & Feeley (1990) that cognitive change is more predictive of symptom change in patients receiving cognitive therapy than in patients not receiving it; the report by Segal, Gemar, and Williams (1999) that cognitive therapy produces schema change but pharmacotherapy does not; and the demonstration (Segal et al., 2006) that patients who have recovered from depression and who received cognitive therapy are less reactive to a sad mood provocation than patients who received antidepressant medication, and that reactivity to a sad mood provocation predicted relapse. These findings provide impressive support for the notion that cognitive therapy produces a cognitive change that protects patients from relapse. Other supportive studies include the demonstration that self-reported mood change during a session of cognitive therapy was a function of cognitive change during the session and the quality of the therapeutic relationship (Persons & Burns, 1985); that depressed patients who were more skillful at completing the Thought Record were less depressed 6 months after group CBT than patients who were less skillful (Neimeyer & Feixas, 1990); and that treatment response in patients who receive CBT for social phobia is mediated by changes in the estimated negative consequences of certain negative social events (Hofmann, Moscovitch, Kim, & Taylor, 2004). Support for cognitive therapy's proposed mechanism of action is also provided by studies showing that patients who receive it show cognitive changes (Imber et al., 1990; Simons, Garfield, & Murphy, 1984). However, this last finding provides only weak support for the theory because, as Hollon, DeRubeis, and Evans (1987) pointed out, the demonstration that cognitive change *covaries* with symptom change is not sufficient to prove that cognitive change *causes* symptom change.

Moreover, several studies have produced findings that run contrary to the cognitive theory. Shaw et al. (1999) found that competence in implementing the specific interventions of cognitive therapy was not related to outcome of cognitive therapy for depression in the Treatment of Depression Collaborative Research Program. However, they did find that competence in implementing the skills relating to agenda setting and other structuring of the therapy *was* related to its outcome. And several studies have shown that noncognitive therapies, including pharmacotherapy, produce cognitive change (Imber et al., 1990; Jacobson et al., 1996). These studies suggest that cognitive change may be a consequence of therapeutic improvement that occurs via other mechanisms, not the direct cause of improvement. Although cognitive change occurs in cognitive therapy, it also occurs in other therapies. One account of the weak evidence supporting the mediating role of cognitive change in cognitive therapy is that common factors like the therapeutic relationship produce much of the change in all psychotherapies (Wampold, 2001). Another is the hypothesis, discussed in some detail below, that the various aspects of symptoms (cognitive, behavioral, the subjective experience of emotion), including biology (Baxter et al., 1992), are tightly linked to one another, and changes in one lead to changes in all of the others.

Finally, remember that the studies reviewed here present *nomothetic* findings (i.e., general findings that apply to groups). As discussed later (see Chapter 9), therapists will want to collect *idiographic* data for their individual patients to evaluate both the process and the outcome of the therapy they are conducting. For example, the therapist can work with his patient to collect data to test the hypothesis that spending time in the therapy session and in homework assignments on cognitive restructuring exercises appears to lead to changes in the patient's thinking and improvement in his emotions and functioning.

PROPOSITIONS OF BECK'S COGNITIVE THERAPY AND THEIR CLINICAL IMPLICATIONS

In the following discussion I highlight aspects of Beck's cognitive theory that I find to be particularly clinically useful. In the service of clinical utility, I extrapolate and extend the theory in several ways. Specifically, I propose that Beck's theory can be used not only to formulate a particular symptom or disorder but can also be extended to account for all of a patient's symptoms, disorders, and problems. In other words, I suggest using the theory as the template for a formulation of a case. Of course, whether others find these extensions to be useful and whether they contribute to good treatment outcomes are important empirical questions. The propositions discussed here are:

- Symptoms are made up of interconnected and mutually causal emotions, behaviors, and automatic thoughts.
- Schema activation triggers emotions, automatic thoughts, and behaviors, and changes in those symptom elements cause schema change.
- Schema activation can account for a symptom, a set of symptoms, and an entire case.
- Pathological schemas about the self, others, world, and future underpin symptoms of psychopathology.
- Schemas are triggered by events that "match" or support the schema.
- Schemas distort many aspects of thinking and behavior, and can do so outside of awareness.
- Schema-driven behavior can produce evidence that confirms the schemas.
- Symptom topography reflects schema content.
- Schemas are learned through childhood experiences.

- Schemas do not easily change in response to disconfirming information.
- Schema change requires schema activation.

Symptoms Are Made Up of Interconnected and Mutually Causal Emotions, Behaviors, and Automatic Thoughts

Symptoms in Beck's model are conceptualized as made up of behaviors, automatic thoughts, and emotions. Behaviors include both physiological responses (e.g., increased heart rate) and overt motor behaviors (leaving the room). "Automatic thoughts" are described by A. T. Beck (1976) as thoughts that occur automatically—that is, without effort and attention—and that we are often unaware of until we are asked to focus on them. Automatic thoughts can include images (J. S. Beck, 1995; Hackmann, 1998). Beck uses the word *emotion* to refer to subjective experience.

The double arrows linking behaviors, automatic thoughts, and emotion in Figure 2.1 reflect the theory's statement that all these elements are linked in reciprocal causal relationships. That is, change in any one of the elements is expected to produce changes in the others. Cognitive therapy strives to change emotions by changing behaviors and cognitions, often using the Activity Schedule (Figure 2.2) and the Thought Record (Figure 2.3).

The theory's proposition that changes in *either* automatic thoughts *or* behaviors can produce symptom change provides the therapist with quite a bit of flexibility. It suggests that at any particular moment, the therapist can focus on either cognitions or behaviors (or go back and forth between the two) to promote change. Thus, if the patient is so behaviorally immobilized that he is unable to make much use of cognitive interventions, or if the patient denies the presence of thoughts or doesn't "get" the concept of standing back to examine his thoughts, the therapist can focus on behaviors. If the patient is aware of and wanting to change his thoughts, the therapist can focus there, even if the patient's behaviors are quite dysfunctional. Thus, rather than simply moving in to target the patient's behaviors or cognitions, the therapist can assess each patient to determine which element (behaviors or thoughts) is most likely to facilitate change for that patient at that moment.

The Key Role of Behavior Change

The cognitive element of Beck's model tends to receive the most attention. In fact, an early version of the Daily Record of Dysfunctional Thoughts (A. T. Beck et al., 1979) does not include a column for behaviors! However, behaviors play a key role in the change process, as demonstrated by Jacobson et al. (1996), who found that patients with depression who received treatment targeting their dysfunctional behaviors had outcomes equal to those who received interventions targeting behaviors and automatic thoughts or interventions targeting behaviors, automatic thoughts, and schemas. In addition, because of their transparency, behaviors are a useful marker of change. It is easy to directly observe that the woman with agoraphobia reached her treatment goal of driving across the Bay Bridge. In contrast, it is not so easy to observe whether her schema changed.

(text continues on page 24)

	MONDAY DATE:	TUESDAY DATE:	WEDNESDAY DATE:	THURSDAY DATE:	FRIDAY DATE:	SATURDAY DATE:	SUNDAY DATE:
7–8							
8–9							
9–10							
10–11							
11–12							
12–1							
1–2							
2–3							
3–4							
4–5							
5–6							
6–7							
Evening							

FIGURE 2.2. Activity Schedule. Copyright 1999 by the San Francisco Bay Area Center for Cognitive Therapy. Reprinted by permission in Jacqueline B. Persons (2008). Permission to photocopy this figure is granted to purchasers of this book for personal use only (see copyright page for details).

DATE	SITUATION (event, memory, attempt to do something, etc.)	BEHAVIOR(S)	EMOTIONS	THOUGHTS	COPING RESPONSES

FIGURE 2.3. Thought Record. Copyright 2000 by the San Francisco Bay Area Center for Cognitive Therapy. Reprinted by permission in Jacqueline B. Persons (2008). Permission to photocopy this figure is granted to purchasers of this book for personal use only (see copyright page for details).

Schema Activation Triggers Emotions, Automatic Thoughts, and Behaviors and Changes in Those Symptom Elements Cause Schema Change

Beck's theory proposes that when schemas are triggered, they cause symptoms, as indicated by the arrow in Figure 2.1 leading from schemas to symptoms. Figure 2.1 also includes an arrow indicating that changes in automatic thoughts and behaviors and emotions (symptoms) lead to schema change. The proposal that changes in automatic thoughts and behaviors lead to schema change is not directly stated by Beck's theory. Nevertheless, I propose it here because it is consistent with quite a lot of clinical phenomena and some evidence, and it is clinically extremely useful.

The notion that change in automatic thoughts can lead to schema change is consistent with the fact that it is frequently difficult to distinguish automatic thoughts from schemas (e.g., "I'm worthless"). Furthermore, many of the interventions of CT that are designed to treat schemas target the maladaptive behaviors and automatic thoughts that are tied to those schemas (Padesky, 1994; Tompkins, Persons, & Davidson, 2000).

Clinical Implications

The proposal that changes in behaviors and automatic thoughts lead to schema change has several important clinical implications. A key one is that therapists can strengthen the power of their interventions by using schema hypotheses about the case to guide clinical decisions of all sorts. A common clinical dilemma for therapists is whether to encourage the patient to ask for more help from them or to be more self-sufficient. If the clinician has conceptualized the case as one in which the patient's schemas include a view of others as uncaring, unavailable, and unwilling to help, the therapist might encourage the patient to telephone when she needs help. In contrast, if the case conceptualization is that the patient views herself as weak and helpless, the therapist might elect to encourage the patient to be more self-sufficient. Schema hypotheses can also guide agenda-setting decisions. The therapist can get "more bang for the buck" out of therapy by choosing agenda items that are tightly tied to the patient's problematic schemas.

Another important clinical implication is that the interventions the therapist carries out to change overt behaviors and automatic thoughts produce not just symptom change, but also deeper change, at the schema level. This proposal is consistent with the fact that cognitive therapy has not been shown to lead to symptom substitution and in fact has been shown to produce long-term benefits (Hollon et al., 2005). A final clinical implication is that the therapist need not wait until later in the treatment to identify and target the schemas. In fact, the experimental work by Miranda and Persons (1988) and Miranda, Persons, and Byers (1990) showing that schemas in vulnerable individuals must be primed in some way (in their studies, by a mood activation) in order for the individuals to be able to report them points to the advantages of assessing and intervening to treat the schemas early in treatment when emotional distress makes it easier for patients to access and report information about them (Persons & Miranda, 1991).

Schema Activation Can Account for a Symptom, a Set of Symptoms, and an Entire Case

Beck's theory (Figure 2.1) states that schema activation causes disorders, which are made up of symptoms, which are themselves made up of cognitions, automatic thoughts, and behaviors. Beck's theory as depicted in Figure 2.1 was originally developed to account for a *disorder*. However, it is clinically useful to extrapolate the theory "downward" to account for a *single symptom*, and "upward" to account for *all of a patient's symptoms and disorders and problems*.

To use Beck's theory to account for a *disorder*, use Figure 2.1 to identify the automatic thoughts, behaviors, and unpleasant emotions that make up the symptoms of the disorder and the schemas and triggering life events that cause the symptoms. For example, Marla has major depressive disorder (MDD). Her symptoms include behaviors of withdrawal and passivity, automatic thoughts of "I am alone," "No one cares about me," "I don't want to see people when I feel like this," and emotions of loneliness, worthlessness, inadequacy, and sadness. These symptoms resulted when schemas of "I'm worthless and unlovable" and "No one cares about me" were triggered by her husband's threatening to leave the relationship.

To use Beck's theory to account for a symptom, use Figure 2.1 to identify the automatic thoughts, behaviors, and emotions of the symptom and the schemas and triggering life events that cause the symptom. For example, Marla engaged in suicidal behaviors (Internet research to find a fail-safe method of killing herself) and had suicidal thoughts ("I hate myself," "I should be dead," "No one would care if I were dead") and emotions (self-hate and self-loathing) that were triggered by her husband's threat to leave, which activated her schemas, as described above.

To use Beck's theory to account for all of the symptoms, disorders, and problems of a patient, use Figure 2.4 to identify all of the patient's problems, the schemas that are (directly or indirectly) causing many or all of them, and the life events that are triggering the schemas (Persons, 1989; Persons, Davidson, & Tompkins, 2001). Thus, for example, Marla had multiple problems, including MDD, suicidality, a marital problem, and an unsatisfying and low-paying job, all of which could be explained as resulting from the activation of her worthlessness schema. It was easy to account for Marla's MDD and suicidality as resulting from schema activation when her husband threatened to leave. Her chronically unsatisfying job situation resulted from multiple other schema-activating events, including critical remarks from her boss

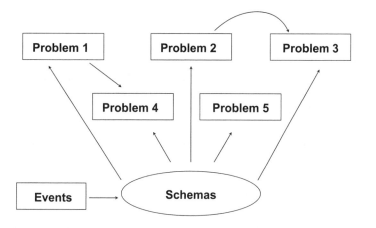

FIGURE 2.4. Using Beck's theory to conceptualize a case. From Persons, Davidson, and Tompkins (2001). Copyright 2001 by the American Psychological Association. Reprinted by permission.

that led to feelings of inadequacy that impeded her from taking action to find a better job.

Clinical Implications

The notion that Beck's theory accounts for disorders (Figure 2.1), symptoms (also Figure 2.1), and cases (Figure 2.4) has several clinical implications. The most significant one is that we treat symptoms, disorders, and cases by treating symptoms (Cohen, Gunthert, Butler, O'Neill, & Tolpin, 2005; Gunthert, Cohen, Butler, & Beck, 2005). Most intervention happens at the level of the symptom. When the therapist is using Beck's model, the format of the Thought Record is used to assess and intervene to change the details of the automatic thoughts, behaviors, and emotions that occur or are activated in a particular situation. I use the term "format of the Thought Record" because I find that even when I am not using the Thought Record itself, I am using its format to guide my conceptualization and intervention using Beck's theory.

Another clinical implication is that when the patient seeks help with an emotional reaction in a particular situation, the therapist can begin the assessment process with the hypothesis that the schemas underpinning this instance of distress are likely some of the same schemas that underpin the patient's other symptoms, problems, and disorders. Thus, if the patient has an anxiety disorder, the patient likely holds schemas of "I am vulnerable" and "the world is dangerous" (A. T. Beck et al., 1985). When the patient comes into the office highly anxious about a recent upsetting event, the therapist can begin to conceptualize the patient's current upset with the hypotheses that the "I am vulnerable" and/or "the world is dangerous" schemas have been activated.

Beck's theory also allows the therapist to work in the other direction. That is, the conceptualization about the schemas underpinning a patient's emotional distress in a particular situation can feed into the conceptualization about the schemas underpinning the disorder. Thus, the therapist can build up a disorder-level formulation, and even a case-level formulation, from emotional-event-level formulations. J. S. Beck (1995) capitalizes very elegantly on this notion in her case formulation worksheet, which guides the therapist to build up a disorder- or case-level formulation from a series of emotional-event-level formulations. Thus, Sam came to a series of therapy sessions asking, in each one, for help with a different situation that had triggered anxiety: his car battery died when he was far from home; he was appointed to lead a fractious committee; his son was diagnosed with diabetes; his book was not going well. We addressed each situation by using a Thought Record to identify and help him change the thoughts that gave rise to anxiety in that situation. Every single Thought Record included the thoughts "I can't handle this situation" and "A catastrophe will result." It was easy, by reviewing these Thought Records, to develop the formulation hypotheses that Sam's self-schema was "I am weak and helpless," and his world-schema was "Catastrophes will happen." These case-level formulation hypotheses arose from repeated symptom-level formulations. Furthermore, after developing the case-level formulation, every time Sam came in asking for help with another anxiety-provoking situation, my first hypothesis was that Sam's helplessness self-schema and his catastrophic world schema had been activated by the current situation.

Another clinical implication is that a therapist can help a patient make headway on big-ticket problems by addressing smaller-scale situations that result from activation of the same schemas that cause the big-ticket issues. So, for example, Peter resolved repeatedly to break up with his girlfriend, Hagar, but simply could not carry it off. Peter and his therapist identified schemas of "I am selfish," "I am fragile and I can't handle emotional pain," and "Others (including Hagar) are fragile" as impeding him from breaking off the relationship. The therapist addressed the breakup roadblock by helping Peter address these schemas in less threatening but nevertheless difficult situations, such as asking Hagar for her rent check and inviting her to go with him to a movie he wanted to see but she did not. He was able to accomplish these tasks, and in so doing he obtained evidence disconfirming his schemas that he was selfish and fragile. In addition, Hagar's resentful and balky responses to his requests reminded him of why he wanted to break up with her! Armed with this information and experience, Peter was finally able to break off the relationship.

The use of Beck's model to conceptualize an entire case helps the therapist see the relationships among the patient's various symptoms and problems rather than viewing the patient as simply a list of Axis I, II, III, and IV disorders and problems. Of course, not all problems can be conceptualized as resulting from activation of schemas. Medical problems, which typically have important biological causes, are a good example. However, often the patient's response to problems like medical problems *can* be understood as schema-driven behavior. An example is noncompliance with medical treatment, which can exacerbate medical problems. And because Beck's model has been used to conceptualize and develop treatments for so many disorders and problems, the notion of extrapolating the theory to guide treatment of the multiple-problem patient has some empirical foundation.

Pathological Schemas about the Self, Others, World, and Future Underpin Symptoms of Psychopathology

Beck proposed that underpinning the symptoms of psychopathology is a cognitive triad: the patient's views of *self*, his *personal world*, and his *future* (A. T. Beck et al., 1979). The notion of the triad is clinically quite useful. For example, the anxious person typically has a view of himself as weak and vulnerable and of the world as dangerous and threatening (A. T. Beck et al., 1985); the suicidal person has a view of the future as hopeless (A. T. Beck, Brown, Berchick, Stewart, & Steer, 1990). These are evidence-based proposals and can help clinicians focus their interventions to address these key issues.

In addition, it is clinically helpful to add a fourth element to the group so that instead of a cognitive trio there is a quartet. The fourth member is the patient's views of *others*. (Beck includes *others* in the *personal world* element of the triad.) Developing a distinct conceptualization of the patient's views of *others* is clinically useful for at least two reasons. One is that the patient can have very different views of the *world* and *others*. For example, a housewife and mother who had generalized anxiety disorder had a view of the *world* as dangerous (that is, bad things could happen at any moment) and a view of *others* as fragile and helpless. As a result, she was quite overprotective of and took excessive responsibility for the well-being of everyone she was close to. Second, it is particularly important to have an understanding of the patient's views of *others* because the therapist is an *other*. As a result, the conceptualization of the patient's views of others can be extremely useful to the therapist in his or her efforts to understand and manage the therapeutic relationship.

Schemas Are Triggered by Events That "Match" or Support Them

Beck's theory states that symptoms arise when schemas are triggered by external (e.g., being turned down for promotion) or internal (e.g., increased heart rate or a memory) events that "match" the schemas. Thus, a personal rejection is expected to be unduly distressing to a person who holds the schema "I am worthless unless I am loved by everyone around me," whereas being turned down for promotion is expected to be particularly distressing to a person who holds the belief "I am worthless unless I am successful at everything I do" (A. T. Beck, 1983). Increased heart rate is expected to be unduly distressing to the person who holds a view of himself as vulnerable to a medical catastrophe.

Clinical Implications

Several clinical implications flow from this part of the theory. One is that information about events that trigger symptoms yields clues about the nature of the patient's problematic schemas. For example, an attorney became quite anxious when her therapist praised her for completing a difficult therapy homework assignment. Investigation revealed that praise triggered the patient's beliefs that others would develop excessive expectations for her and abandon her when she did not meet them.

Another implication is that clinicians can help patients overcome their symptoms by helping them change the situations in which they place themselves. A change of scene can reduce the activation of problematic schemas and/or increase the activation of adaptive schemas. Many happy and successful individuals are happy and successful in part because they are skilled at seeking out environments in which they feel good and function well. Therapists can teach their patients to do this too. So, for example, the therapist can help the coed who has bipolar disorder and a seizure disorder perceive that the retail store where she works, a clothing store that has loud music and flashing lights, is likely to exacerbate her symptoms. Similarly, a husband contributes to his marital problem by repeatedly allowing himself to get pulled into unproductive discussions with his wife about her unhappiness. I worked in therapy to teach him that his marriage would improve if he participated in fewer of those interactions and instead engaged his wife in activities they both enjoyed.

Of course, avoiding situations that activate one's schemas is sometimes good coping and sometimes maladaptive avoidance and it is not always easy to determine which is which. Reference to the patient's goals and the case formulation can help patient and therapist sort this out.

Interventions targeting external events are not included in Beck's (A. T. Beck et al., 1979) protocol because they do not directly modify the essential mechanisms in the person that give rise to symptoms. Nevertheless, as I have just argued, these types of interventions can be quite useful clinically. In addition, conceptually, beliefs and situation selection are often tightly intertwined. Often maladaptive beliefs prevent individuals from selecting healthy environments. Therapeutic work to help patients select healthier environments often requires work on the cognitions that impede them from doing this on their own. For example, one of my patients stayed in an abusive and stressful work setting because she believed "I should be able to cope with any workplace, no matter how stressful it is, and if I can't there is something wrong with me." Therapeutic work on this belief and her choice of workplace proceeded in tandem.

Schemas Distort Many Aspects of Thinking and Behavior

Schemas distort multiple aspects of thinking, including perception, imagery, memory, judgment, and decision making (Ingram, 1984), and they drive behavior, including facial expression, somatic arousal, and motor behavior, and they can do so outside of awareness. Pete, whom I was treating for generalized anxiety disorder, viewed the world as full of dangers and threats. One day he very energetically alerted me to the danger posed by an area rug in the waiting room that he believed was likely to cause someone to trip and fall. This rug had been observed, without remark, by literally hundreds of other patients, students, and colleagues. However, Pete felt certain that it posed an imminent danger.

Sally, another chronic worrier, came to her session one day and reported her recent experience at an air show. She had attended a San Francisco 49ers' football game and during halftime the Blue Angels had performed an air show. In the middle of the show, one of the planes seemed to encounter a technical difficulty, peeled away, and flew off. Sally described this event as one that supported her world-view that catastrophic events happen frequently. Sally's point of view was so strong and her mode of communicating it so emotional that I found myself drawn into her interpretation of the event. It was not until 20 minutes later that it penetrated my brain that nothing bad had happened. In fact, the event at the air show was best seen as evidence *contradicting* Sally's world-view!

Clinical Implications

This proposition of Beck's theory tells the therapist not to accept at face value the patient's interpretations of his or her experiences. Instead, it is essential to find out exactly what happened—in blow-by-blow detail. And even the blow-by-blow description can be biased by schema-driven perception or recall.

Another clinical implication is that the therapist cannot accept without question the patient's proposal about what occurrences during the past week belong on the agenda for the therapy session. Because patients' perceptions and judgments are driven by their schemas, they may minimize or fail to notice altogether events that merit discussion. For example, one of my patients, a nurse, reported in passing that she had decided to resign from her job. She viewed this plan as a good one and not one that needed further discussion. In contrast, I saw this as a bad thing that merited a high priority on the therapy session agenda. My judgment of the importance of discussing this topic flowed out of my attention to the patient's problems, our schema hypotheses, and her treatment goals. The patient had a history of starting and stopping jobs and relationships repeatedly, had schemas of the world and others as "deficient, unreliable, never meeting my needs," and one of her therapy goals was to improve her ability to maintain long-term work and personal relationships. Nevertheless, the schemas driving her urge to resign her position were so powerful that she had no awareness that her behavior was problematic in any way until I suggested that her decision to quit her job merited some attention.

Schema-Driven Behavior Can Produce Evidence That Confirms the Schemas

When we or our patients (it happens to us all) experience a *situation* that activates our *schemas* to produce *irrational thinking* and *negative emotions,* we often have urges to *behave maladaptively.* When we give in to those urges, the result often provides evidence to confirm our irrational thinking. Thus, for example (thanks to Pamela Balls Organista for this example), a teacher who held the schemas "I'm not very smart" and "Others will reject me for being stupid" attempted to mitigate his fears by using long words in an attempt to convey that he was erudite and well educated. The result of his strategy was that he sounded pompous and intellectually unsophisticated. In fact, his compensatory strategy led to exactly the events he most feared: others lost respect for his intelligence and rejected him.

David Clark (Bates & Clark, 1998; Clark & Wells, 1995) shows very compellingly how this notion plays out for many persons with social phobia. The social phobic's compensatory behaviors, which Clark calls safety behaviors (e.g., poor eye contact, trying to hide), are typically the main causes of the rejection these people fear so much (see also Salkovskis, 1991). Seligman and Johnston (1973) offer a model of avoidance behavior (described in more detail in Chapter 3) that includes the proposal that behavior that produces results consistent with a belief strengthens the belief. Thus, the person with agoraphobia who avoids driving on the Bay Bridge because he believes "If I drive on the bridge, I'll panic, lose control, and cause an accident" actually produces a piece of evidence to support this belief every time he avoids driving on the Bay Bridge. His avoidance behavior thus strengthens the belief that triggers his anxiety and urge to avoid.

A fascinating illustration of this idea appears in Jane Brody's (2000) article titled "How Germ Phobia Can Lead to Illness." Brody compellingly described how germ phobia leads to the use of antibacterial agents, which itself can cause illness in several ways, such as by killing only the most susceptible bacteria so that some bacteria that might not otherwise have survived now do (competing bacteria that might have killed them were destroyed by the antibacterial) and multiply.

Analogously, therapy can produce an upward (adaptive) spiral if the patient, instead of being driven by his belief, pushes against it. Thus, if the young man pushes against his fear that "If I ask her out she'll turn me down and I won't be able to handle that" and actually asks out the woman of his dreams, he will, with a bit of luck, get a date. If he does not, he will learn that he does not fall apart. Thus, Beck's theory suggests that if the patient can change his behavior to test his irrational beliefs and disconfirm them, he will not only solve the problem at hand but will experience a positive shift in the downstream situations and events he encounters.

Symptom Topography Reflects Schema Content

Beck's theory is a *structural* theory, that is, a theory in which the topography (that is, the descriptive details) of the overt symptoms is expected to reflect the content of the underlying mechanisms (Nelson & Hayes, 1986a). This concept is conveyed by the *New Yorker* cartoon of the tourists who, visiting a massive pyramid, conclude, "It was built when the Mayans were feeling good about themselves."

Clinical Implications

This topographical aspect of Beck's theory has multiple clinical implications. One is that the content of the patient's automatic thoughts, behaviors, and emotions provides information about the content of his schemas. This proposal is quite useful because of course the schemas are not directly observable. Thus, for example, the poor eye contact of the person with social phobia can be seen as reflecting her view of herself as defective and inadequate and her view of others as attacking and critical. The self-hate, suicidal, and self-harming behaviors of the individual with borderline personality disorder or bipolar disorder can be seen as reflecting her sense of herself as loathsome, deserving of punishment, and unworthy of compassion and nurturing.

Another implication is that the content of one element of a symptom (e.g., the emotional experience of anger) yields information about the likely content of other elements (e.g., "should" statements and attacking behaviors). This concept is endlessly helpful clinically, as it allows patient and therapist to more easily capture, identify, and intervene to address the automatic thoughts and behaviors that are tied to a particular emotional experience. In support of this aspect of Beck's theory, several studies have shown that specific cognitive profiles are characteristic of particular symptoms and disorders (see review by A. T. Beck, 2005). A. T. Beck et al. (2001) showed that each personality disorder is characterized by particular beliefs.

Schemas Are Learned through Childhood Experiences

Beck's theory states that schemas are learned from early experiences, especially early experiences with significant others. This proposition is illustrated in a *New Yorker* cartoon of two butterflies; one says to the other, "You're a butterfly now, but you still think like a caterpillar," So, for example, the child who is regularly physically abused by his mentally ill parents may develop schemas of others as likely to harm or mistreat him. In support of this proposal, Barlow & Chorpita (1998) reviewed evidence showing that individuals who later develop anxiety disorders frequently have childhood experiences that lead them to develop schemas of the self as helpless and of the world as uncontrollable.

Clinical Implications

One clinical implication of this proposal is that obtaining a good family and social history (discussed further in Chapter 6) is essential to the process of developing schema hypotheses. However, careful consideration of the information obtained is needed, because the way in which early experiences lead to schemas is not always obvious. A young Hispanic woman grew up in a family in which her mother sacrificed everything so her kids would have a better life than she had had. Unfortunately, the mother's sacrifice had the unanticipated consequence that her daughter learned (from her mother's model) that "My needs don't count; to be worthwhile, I must sacrifice for others."

Another clinical implication is that people can begin to make revisions in their schemas by reviewing early childhood events in detail, examining an event and their conclusions or inferences from the event, and evaluating the accuracy and reasonableness of those conclusions in the light of later perspectives and experience (Young, 1999).

Schemas Do Not Easily Change in Response to Disconfirming Information

Schemas do not change easily, for many reasons. One is that the schemas themselves bias retrieval of information from memory, interpretation of ambiguous events (as in the examples above of the air show and the carpet in the waiting room), and other cognitive processes (Ingram, 1984; Teasdale, 1988), thus making it difficult for individuals to acquire information that disconfirms distorted schemas. In fact, Giesler, Josephs, and Swann (1996) showed that individuals with depression seek out information that confirms their negative self-schemas.

The resistance of schemas to change has multiple implications for the clinician. Bennett-Levy et al. (2004) note that the therapist cannot assume the patient who tests a key belief in a behavioral experiment will collect and process the data obtained in an unbiased way. Instead, before the experiment the therapist must carefully think through with the patient what pieces of data would most emphatically disconfirm the belief and after the experiment the therapist must review with the patient the results of the experiment and the conclusions that are best drawn from them. Padesky (1993) proposes that schemas are like prejudices—strong beliefs that we tend to hold to even in the face of disconfirming evidence. It is useful to teach this idea to patients and use it to help them override the tendency to ignore evidence that disconfirms their schemas. Probably every therapist has had the experience of treating with extra care a patient who views others as untrustworthy and hurtful in an effort to provide the patient with evidence disconfirming those schemas only to find, after months or even years, that the patient persists in her view of others—including the therapist!—as untrustworthy and hurtful. To address this issue, McCullough (2000) suggests that it is important not only for therapists to behave in a way that disconfirms the patient's schemas but also to discuss this behavior with the patient to help him learn from it.

Schema Change Requires Schema Activation

Beck proposes that effective therapy sessions involve activation of emotion (and thus presumably the schemas underpinning it; cf. A. T. Beck et al., 1979, Ch. 2). However, the notion that schema activation is needed to produce change is described most explicitly by the emotional processing model of Foa, Huppert, and Cahill (2006) and Foa and Kozak (1986), which proposed that activation of the fear network and the presentation of information that disconfirms key elements of the network is the active ingredient of behavioral treatment of pathological fears (I discuss the emotional processing model further in Chapter 4).

Clinical Implications

One way Beck's cognitive therapy addresses the need for schema activation is via the Situation column of the Thought Record (Figure 2.3). As Burns (1989a) points out, if the therapist collects negative automatic thoughts from the patient without focusing on a concrete, specific situation, the thoughts tend to be vague, there is no emotional charge present in the room, and the therapy session tends to devolve into a sterile intellectual debate. In contrast, when the therapeutic work is focused on a concrete situation, emotional charges are evoked and the work is much more productive. Other explicit strategies can be used to activate schemas in order to work on them, including *in vivo* and imaginal exposure, empty chair and other gestalt interventions (Samoilov & Goldfried, 2000), and methods to carefully re-create early events in which patients learned key schemas in an effort to rework the event and its meaning to the patient (Padesky, 1994; Young, 1999).

Because schema activation is so important in promoting change, the therapist will want to pay close attention to schema activation when it occurs and capitalize on it to promote change. For example, Jeannie was working in therapy to overcome her obsessive fears that she was homosexual. She reported that a few days earlier she had become "freaked out" because she had discovered that she had made a major mistake at work. She had flown into a panic, concluded she was completely incompetent, and nearly resigned. With help from her husband, boss, and coworkers, she had been able to regroup and get down to problem solving to determine how the mistake had been made and take action to correct her error. As I listened to her report of this event, which was no longer troubling her, I suggested we put it on the agenda to review what had happened and what she had learned. Three factors cued me to suggest this agenda item: (1) if Jeannie had been so distressed, key schemas must have been activated and I wanted to learn more about them; (2) the fact that the topography of her response to this work situation (urge to quit) was similar to the topography of her anxiety about being homosexual (urge to leave her marriage) suggested that the same schemas may underpin both concerns; and (3) we might be able to learn something from the work situation (which she had successfully mastered) about how to handle the homosexuality fear (with which she continued to struggle).

Of course, schema activation does not necessarily produce intense emotional expression. It can also lead to a dissociated emotional state, or to avoidance or minimization (as with the nurse described above who planned to resign from her job).

Similarly, taking advantage of schema activation to promote change does not always mean making the schema activation the focus of the therapy session. For example, Amy had schemas of herself as helpless and of others as not meeting her needs. She frequently found these were activated in the therapy session when I did not agree with her or did not immediately give her the empathy she wanted at that moment. In several sessions our agenda was completely derailed by attention to Amy's emotional distress in these situations. We then conceptualized these moments as opportunities for Amy to practice her skills for managing emotional distress without diverting from the therapy session agenda. These skills stood her in good stead outside the therapy session as well, where frequent derailments due to emotional dysregulation impeded her from accomplishing important goals.

Summary of Formulation and Treatment Based on Beck's Theory

Beck's theory proposes that schemas are learned from early experiences, activated by "matching" events, and lead to symptoms that reflect the content of the schemas. Symptoms are made up of cognitions, behaviors, and emotions that are linked, so that a change in any element produces changes in the others. An elegant and comprehensive case formulation based on Beck's theory links together all these elements: early upbringing, schema content, precipitating events, and symptom content. Treatment based on Beck's theory entails interventions designed to modify schemas, automatic thoughts, problem behaviors, and activating events and situations.

OTHER COGNITIVE THEORIES AND THERAPIES

Numerous scientists and clinicians have developed alternative cognitive theories and therapies, in some cases borrowing or adapting from Beck's model and in other cases working independently. I describe several here very briefly. They can be used instead of or in addition to Beck's model to guide conceptualization and intervention.

The Oxford Group

Investigators in the United Kingdom have made significant contributions to developing and elaborating cognitive-behavioral and especially cognitive models, especially of various anxiety and mood disorders, including low self-esteem (Fennell, 2006), panic disorder (Clark, 1986), social phobia (Clark, 2001), posttraumatic stress disorder (PTSD; Duffy, Gillespie, & Clark, 2007; Ehlers & Clark, 2000), hypochondriasis (Salkovskis, 1989), and generalized anxiety disorder (G. Butler, Fennell, & Hackmann, 2008; Wells, 2005). Attention to the details of these models will provide invaluable guides to conceptualization using cognitive models.

For example, Ehlers and Clark (2000) propose that PTSD symptoms result when the traumatized individual processes information in such a way that the trauma appears to constitute an immediate, serious danger rather than something that happened in the past. The perception of immediate danger arises from the individual's distorted appraisals of the trauma event and/or its sequelae, including the PTSD symptoms themselves (e.g., "The fact that I can't concentrate means I am going crazy"), from a disruption of autobiographical memory (that is, the inability to correctly "file" the memory, placing it in the context of the individual's past and future), and from use of maladaptive cognitive and behavioral coping strategies (especially avoidance and attempts to push away reminders of the trauma). Interventions flowing out of this conceptualization help the individual integrate memories of the event into the context of his or her biographical memory, block maladaptive responses, and adopt adaptive coping strategies.

Attributional Theories

The reformulated learned helplessness theory (Abramson, Seligman, & Teasdale, 1978) and hopelessness theory (Abramson, Metalsky, & Alloy, 1989) offer alternative diathesis–stress models of depression. Both theories conceptualize vulnerability to depression in terms of a depressogenic or pessimistic explanatory style (the tendency to view negative events as arising from stable, global, and internal causes). Although these theories did not lead directly to therapies, they provide some of the empirical underpinning to Beck's theory. A fascinating clinical example of the use of attribution theory is the proposal by Kingdon and Turkington (2005) that auditory hallucinations can be conceptualized as cognitions that are falsely attributed as having an external source.

Mindfulness-Based Cognitive Therapy and Other Acceptance-Focused Therapies

Mindfulness-based cognitive therapy (Segal, Williams, & Teasdale, 2002) proposes that individuals who have a history of depression are vulnerable to getting pulled, without their awareness, into negative thinking that can trigger symptoms and fuel a relapse. Therefore, Segal et al. (2002) proposed helping these individuals prevent relapse by helping them identify and disengage from their negative thoughts, that is, giving them "a cognitive set in which negative thoughts/feelings are experienced as mental events, rather than as the self" (p. 275).

Mindfulness-based cognitive therapy strives to accomplish its effects by changing people's *relationships to* their thoughts, whereas Beck's cognitive therapy strives to change the *content of* people's thoughts. Nevertheless, these two notions are at times indistinguishable. For example, a person might use Beck's cognitive therapy to respond to the automatic thought "I am worthless" with a mindfulness-type of coping response, such as "Just because I have that thought doesn't mean it's true." In fact, it is possible that some or all of the change in Beck's cognitive therapy is due to patients' changed relationships to their thoughts.

The notion that cognitive therapy may operate in part by changing patients' relationship to their thoughts suggests the possibility that mindfulness-based cognitive therapy, which was designed to prevent relapse, might also be helpful in treating depressive and other symptoms themselves. This notion opens up for the cognitive therapist a myriad of new interventions, including many of those described in acceptance and commitment therapy (S. C. Hayes et al., 1999), dialectical behavior therapy (Linehan, 1993a), and mindfulness-based treatment for generalized anxiety disorder (Borkovec, 2002; Roemer & Orsillo, 2002). More generally, mindfulness-based therapy offers a new approach to maladaptive and distressing thoughts and feelings, that is, the stance of working to accept them rather than to change them.

The Role of Metacognition

Adrian Wells (2000) proposed that metacognition, that is cognition about cognition, plays an important role in producing emotional disorders. Thus, for example, patients with generalized anxiety disorder have dysfunctional beliefs about worry (e.g., "worry is harmful to my health" and "worry helps me solve problems") that cause and maintain their symptoms. Wells proposes that targeting those beliefs will alleviate the symptoms. Data are beginning to accumulate to support these ideas (Wells & Carter, 2001).

Rational Emotive Behavior Therapy

Albert Ellis (1962) developed rational emotive therapy (RET), later modified to rational emotive behavior therapy (REBT). Ellis's theory preceded Beck's theory and proposed that faulty or irrational thinking causes emotional problems and disorders and therefore changing thinking ought to lead to emotional relief.

Ellis's therapy places less emphasis on Socratic questioning as a way to guide a person to a new perception. Instead, it is more directive. Linehan (1993a) uses RET techniques in dialectical behavior therapy and Becker and Zayfert (2001) suggest that RET may be particularly well suited to patients, including many with borderline personality disorder, who can experience Socratic questioning as invalidating. Direct instructions to shift thinking or behavior are especially helpful when emotional arousal is high. Imagine that you have fallen off a boat in high waves, fear you are drowning, and don't know how to get back onto the boat. Which would be more helpful to you: Socratic questioning to help you figure out how to solve the problem or emphatic statements telling you what to do in order to get back on the boat?

A Retrieval Competition Account

Chris Brewin (2006) proposes that individuals have multiple cognitive representations that compete for retrieval and that the goal of cognitive therapy is to help individuals construct and strengthen their positive and adaptive representations so that those representations, rather than the negative and dysfunctional ones, guide perceptions and behavior. This notion has multiple theoretical and clinical implications, including that cognitive therapy is essentially a construction enterprise rather than a modification one.

The Role of Imagery

Ann Hackmann (G. Butler et al., 2008; Hackmann, 1998; Wheatley & Hackmann, 2007) and colleagues, and others (Arntz & Wertman, 1999; Holmes & Mathews, 2005), have elaborated on the role of imagery in psychopathology and its treatment. Imagery, of course, can be seen as a type of cognition or mental representation. There is some evidence that images are more tightly linked to emotion than verbal representations (see Holmes & Mathews, 2005) and therefore some suggestions that interventions to manipulate images can be particularly effective in ameliorating psychopathology (Hackmann, 1998). This work is in its early stages and only case reports and uncontrolled trial data are available as yet (Rusch, Grunert, Mendelsohn, & Smucker, 2000; Smucker & Niederee, 1995; Wheatley & Hackmann, 2007).

Note that for the most part the alternate cognitive theories and interventions described in this section do not contradict Beck's theory but in fact complement and elaborate on it.

ASSESSMENT AND INTERVENTION
GUIDED BY COGNITIVE THEORIES

In this section I describe strategies the clinician can use to guide conceptualization and intervention using cognitive theories. I focus primarily on Beck's theory and therapy, offering some suggestions about using other cognitive models.

Assessment: Collecting Information about the Key Elements of the Formulation Based on Cognitive Theories

Beck's theory proposes that symptoms (which consist of reciprocally causal emotions, automatic thoughts, and maladaptive behaviors) result when schemas learned in childhood are activated by stressful events. An elegant and comprehensive case formulation based on Beck's theory links together all these elements: early upbringing, schema content, precipitating events, and symptom content. Below I describe strategies the therapist can use to assess automatic thoughts, maladaptive behaviors, and schemas. Assessment of the precipitants of the symptoms and the origins of the schemas (these are part of the case-level formulation based on Beck's model) is described in Chapter 6.

Assessing Automatic Thoughts and Maladaptive Behaviors

One of the most useful strategies to get the information needed to conceptualize a case using Beck's model is to use a Thought Record (Figure 2.3). The form is used to help the patient identify the automatic thoughts, problem behaviors, and emotions that arose in a recent upsetting situation. The assumption is that if the person is distressed, then one or more pathological schemas are activated and the person's automatic thoughts, emotions, and behaviors are products of those schemas.

Often patients can report automatic thoughts and describe problem behaviors (or urges) in an upsetting situation in response to the therapist's direct request for this information. If patients have difficulty reporting this, it is often useful to ask them to imagine that the situation is happening again, and then describe the details of who was there, when and where it occurred, and exactly what happened. Evoking the details of the situation usually facilitates the retrieval of information about thoughts, emotions, and behaviors in the situation. Another strategy for helping patients who have difficulty reporting their thoughts and feelings is to offer some options. For example, the therapist can ask, "Were you thinking, 'I can't handle this situation?'" The therapist can also ask patients to "take a wild guess" or "make up" what thoughts they might have been having in the situation. It can also be useful to invite the patient to report visual and other sensory images, not just verbal representations. Wells's metacognitive model alerts us to the fact that cognitions about cognitions can also be clinically important, as can attributions. Brewin's retrieval competition account alerts us to the fact that multiple automatic thoughts are likely present in any particular situation.

The Thought Record is useful in identifying problem behaviors because it links the behaviors to the emotions and automatic thoughts that accompany them. To identify avoidance behaviors, it is often useful to focus on a situation like "having the thought that it is time to do my therapy homework" or "thinking about calling my mother."

Another useful tool for assessing maladaptive behavior is the Activity Schedule (Figure 2.2). In fact, A. T. Beck et al. (1979) assign the Activity Schedule to all patients with depression after the first session, as it provides detailed information about how they are spending their time.

Assessing Schemas

A variety of strategies can be used to assess schemas. As Brewin (2006) points out, it is useful to assess multiple schemas, both maladaptive and adaptive ones.

USE THE DOWNWARD ARROW METHOD

Burns (1980) developed the *downward arrow method* to obtain hypotheses about patients' maladaptive schemas. To use the downward arrow method, the therapist begins by using a Thought Record to identify an episode of emotional upset and the emotions and automatic thoughts triggered during it. It is ideal if the therapist can select a situation that is tied to a high-priority problem on the Problem List, so as to facilitate identifying schemas that are tied to the patient's main problems. When the automatic thoughts have been identified, the therapist asks the patient about each thought: "Imagine that were true. Why would that be upsetting? What would it mean about you if that were true?" The downward arrow method yielded the following string of automatic thoughts for a man who feared asking out a woman he was interested in: "She won't be interested in me" (if that were true why would that be upsetting?), "If I ask her out she'll say no" (if that were true why would that be upsetting?), "I'll be humiliated and devastated" (if that were true why would that be upsetting?), "I won't be able to recover" (if that were true why would that be upsetting?), "I'll be alone forever." The patient's responses indicate that his thinking seems to "bottom out" in automatic thoughts that reflect his view of himself as helpless, fragile, and unlovable.

EXAMINE THEMES OF AUTOMATIC THOUGHTS ACROSS SITUATIONS

A pastor who had recently been diagnosed with cancer was depressed and anxious. Over a series of sessions, he reported Thought Records of a variety of problem situations that included all these thoughts: "I won't be able to cope with side effects of my medication," "The committee I'm chairing at church will split apart in conflict and I won't be able to handle the situation," "My wife, who is depressed, will become suicidal, will call on me for help, and I'll get overwhelmed and incapacitated by her problems," "I'll get overwhelmed and incapacitated by my symptoms," "I'll get overwhelmed and incapacitated by my anxiety and depression." The theme of this man's automatic thoughts across all these situations suggested that he held a self-schema of "I'm helpless and can't cope" and a future-schema of "Bad things will happen." J. S. Beck (1995) uses this strategy to develop schema hypotheses in her method of case conceptualization.

EXAMINE THEMES ACROSS PROBLEMS

This strategy is similar to the one just described but emphasizes seeking themes across the patient's problems, rather than across situations that are tackled in therapy. Sara, a depressed and anxious marketing executive, had problems at work (she procrastinated on projects due to her thought, "I'll do a bad job and my boss will fire me") and social problems (she avoided going to the lunchroom at work because of the thought "No one will sit with me and I'll be alone"). Examination of the behaviors and automatic thoughts that cut across all of Sara's problems revealed a behavioral pattern of passivity and the automatic thought "If I try, I'll mess up, and then I'll get rejected," and this cognitive-behavior pattern suggested that Sara had schemas of herself as inadequate, and schemas of others as critical and rejecting.

ATTEND TO TOPOGRAPHY OF SYMPTOMS

Beck's theory proposes that the topography of symptoms reflects the schemas that are hypothesized to underpin the symptoms. Thus, behavioral passivity suggests a self-schema of helplessness, anger suggests a view of others or the world as unfair, depressed mood suggests a view of the self as worthless or unlovable, hopelessness and suicidal behavior suggest a view of the future as hopeless, self-harm suggests a view of the self as loathsome and deserving of punishment, and automatic thoughts of "I'm worthless" reflect a self-schema of worthlessness.

USE DIAGNOSIS AS A STARTING POINT

Diagnosis can suggest schema hypotheses. For example, Clark (2001) reviews data showing that people with social phobia focus their attention on a negatively distorted mental image of themselves as inept, unattractive, or defective. Foa and Rothbaum (1998) suggest that the typical pathological memory structure of a person with PTSD includes views of the self as incompetent and of the world as dangerous. Numerous investigators have shown that depressed patients hold views of themselves as inadequate/incompetent/a failure and/or unlovable/unacceptable to others (see review by Ingram, Miranda, & Segal, 1998).

USE A PAPER-AND-PENCIL MEASURE

Paper-and-pencil measures for assessing schemas include the Dysfunctional Attitude Scale (DAS; Weissman & Beck, 1978; see also Burns, 1980) and the Young Schema Questionnaire (Young & Brown, 2001). Versions of these scales have been published in Burns (1999), which includes a 35-item adaptation of the DAS, and Young & Klosko (1993), which publishes the 22-item Lifetrap Questionnaire, an early adaptation of Young's Schema Questionnaire. These versions have not been formally psychometrically validated but can be useful in a collaborative search with the patient to identify potential schema vulnerabilities.

OBSERVE THE PATIENT'S BEHAVIOR TOWARD THE THERAPIST

A patient who has the self-schema that she is worthless and the schema of others as abandoning flies into a panic and becomes suicidal when the therapist is delayed in returning her phone call. A patient who views others as likely to hurt and betray her leaves angry telephone messages for the therapist after she feels slighted or poorly treated during the therapy session. A patient who has the schema that he is inadequate and unacceptable to others and that others are rejecting becomes quite anxious when the therapist makes a homework assignment because he fears that if he does the homework incorrectly, the therapist will refuse to treat him. Thus, a detailed examination of the behaviors, emotional responses, and automatic thoughts of the patient during interactions with the therapist can yield schema hypotheses.

USE ALL AVAILABLE INFORMATION

It is important to take advantage of all sources of information, including the patient's appearance and what the patient does not say. For example, a teacher was suffering a financial crisis and was working in therapy on his catastrophic cognitions that he would run out of money and be unable to pay his mortgage. The observation that he was driving a brand-new mega-sized Mercedes lent support to my formulation hypothesis that this man was less afraid of running out of money than he was of feeling inadequate and losing the respect of others.

Whatever strategy the therapist uses to develop schema hypotheses, it is always a good idea to work collaboratively with the patient. When I proposed to a young woman who sought treatment for panic symptoms that she held the belief "I can't handle these symptoms, I'm out of control," she responded: "Maybe. But my main belief is "*I shouldn't have to handle* these symptoms. *It's not fair!!!*" Her view was superior to mine—

it accounted, as mine did not, for her resentment about having the symptoms and her unwillingness to learn coping tools to manage them.

Intervention Guided by Cognitive Theories

Beck's theory proposes that symptoms (made up of automatic thoughts, behaviors, and emotions) arise when life events trigger schemas in a vulnerable individual. Flowing out of this theory, Beck's cognitive therapy strives to produce changes in the mechanisms that cause symptoms, so that when the individual encounters events that previously activated pathological schemas, the schemas do not get activated to cause negative automatic thoughts, maladaptive behaviors, and painful emotions. This is the *mechanism change goal* of Beck's cognitive therapy.

Intervention guided by Beck's cognitive theory also strives to teach the patient skills to prevent and manage symptoms that arise when mechanisms are activated. These can be skills to avoid or manage precipitating situations or skills to manage upsetting emotions that are caused by schema activation. These interventions teach *compensatory skills.* They do not change the mechanisms that the theory describes as causing the symptoms. Barber and DeRubeis (1989) proposed that the mechanism of action of cognitive therapy does not entail changing a patient's schema, automatic thoughts, or maladaptive behaviors but instead entails teaching patients compensatory skills they can use to manage symptoms when they arise.

When both mechanism change goals and compensatory strategies goals are considered, the *treatment targets* of Beck's cognitive therapy are the problematic schemas, negative automatic thoughts, maladaptive behaviors, and precipitating situations that typically trigger symptoms for the individual.

As described above, cognitive theories developed by other investigators and researchers have identified other useful mechanism change goals and treatment targets, including teaching the patient to identify and disengage from maladaptive thoughts that are tied to depressed emotions; increasing the relative strength of adaptive schemas, automatic thoughts, and behaviors; and modifying attributions, metacognitions, and images. Because these alternative cognitive models do not conflict with Beck's model, the clinician can consider using more than one of these intervention tactics simultaneously.

* * *

Beck's model and other cognitive theories and therapies offer powerful tools for conceptualizing and treating a wide range of psychopathology. However, they are not enough. Not all patients respond to them. The learning theories, described in the next chapter, offer another set of useful models and tools.

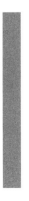

THREE

Learning Theories
and Their Clinical Implications

When I returned a telephone call from my patient Paul, he answered the phone in a bright and cheery tone. As soon as he heard my voice, his tone shifted to one of despair and despondency and he began telling me how hopeless and suicidal he felt.

The above exchange definitely got my attention. Of course, it is normal to answer the phone in a bright cheery manner, and interacting with a caring person who is responsive to one's emotional needs is the appropriate time to let one's emotional expression reflect private experience. Nevertheless, I felt confused and surprised by how abruptly Paul's behavior shifted when he identified me as the caller. I asked myself: What is going on? What am I going to do about it?

The theory of operant conditioning gave me a framework for thinking about the answers to those questions. It suggested the hypothesis that I had inadvertently slipped into reinforcing Paul's hopeless and suicidal verbalizations. The theory also offered some ideas (that I'll describe later) for intervening to address the problem. Learning theories are a useful guide to moment-to-moment clinical hypothesis generation and decision making, such as in the situation illustrated above. The theories also help the clinician develop case conceptualizations and treatment plans, develop and sustain a positive and productive therapeutic relationship, and handle noncompliance and treatment failure.

This chapter describes the fundamental principles of three major learning theories (operant conditioning, respondent conditioning, and observational learning) and offers examples of clinical applications of these principles. I also compare the learning theories with each other and with the cognitive theories described in the previous chapter and I describe combined conditioning-cognitive models. I conclude the chapter with a brief overview of methods for using learning theories to guide formulation and intervention. For more detailed information about the three learning theories, including reviews of the extensive empirical support underpinning them, see Kazdin (2001); Lieberman (2000); Masters, Burish, Hollon, and Rimm (1987); Martin and Pear (2003).

All of the learning theories propose that behaviors (B) are controlled by their context—that is, by their antecedents (A) and/or their consequences (C). Behaviors include those that are voluntary (e.g., leaving the room), or autonomic and involuntary (e.g., heart rate), as well as thoughts and emotional reactions. Antecedents are events that occur *before* a behavior or set of behaviors (B) and that cue or elicit the behaviors. Consequences are events that *follow* the behavior or behaviors. As, Bs, and Cs can be internal (e.g., thoughts, emotional experiences) or external (e.g., physical assault).

OPERANT CONDITIONING: WHEN CONSEQUENCES CONTROL BEHAVIORS

An *operant* is a behavior that is controlled by its consequences. In the operant model a behavior is controlled by something that happens *after* the behavior. Thus, as D. L. Watson and Tharp (2002) elegantly state, "Through operant behaviors, we act, function, and produce effects on ourselves and on our environment. Through the effects—the consequences—the environment acts once again on us" (p. 112). As Kazdin (2001) points out, "Most of the behaviors performed in everyday life are operants" (p. 17). For this reason, a solid understanding of the principles of operant conditioning is essential to the therapist, whose job is to help patients make changes in their behavior.

Operants *serve functions.* Common functions include getting attention, assistance, or approval from others; escaping painful or aversive emotional or physical states; and escaping overwhelming or burdensome life situations. Of course, the fact that a behavior may serve a certain function doesn't mean that the person is doing the behavior on purpose to achieve the function. For example, the fact that Paul's verbalizations about suicide were functioning to gain my attention and assistance doesn't mean that Paul was purposely talking about suicide in order to get my attention. In fact, most likely he was not. Individuals are typically unaware of the consequences that are controlling their behavior.

Reinforcers (positive and negative reinforcement) are consequences that *increase* the probability of a behavior. *Punishment and extinction* are consequences that *decrease* the probability of a behavior. Here (and summarized in Figure 3.1) I give details of these and other principles of operant conditioning. I also illustrate the principles with numerous clinical examples.

Reinforcement Is a Consequence That Increases the Probability of a Behavior Recurring

There are two types of reinforcement: positive and negative. *Positive reinforcement* is the *occurrence* of an event (e.g., receiving a paycheck) that leads to an increase in the probability of behavior (work) that preceded it. *Negative reinforcement* is the *removal* of an event (e.g., reduction in anxiety) that leads to an increase in the behavior that preceded it (e.g., leaving a social event, for the person who has social anxiety). Both positive and negative reinforcement lead to increases in behaviors. However, negative reinforcement involves the presence of aversive stimuli or events that often elicit painful emotions (Pryor, 1999). For that reason, when a choice is available, positive reinforcement is preferable to negative reinforcement as a strategy for increasing the probability of desired behaviors.

- Reinforcement is a consequence that increases the probability of a behavior recurring.

- To effectively control behavior, the consequence must be contingent on the behavior.

- Behavior that is controlled by an intermittent consequence is more resistant to extinction than behavior that is always followed by a consequence.

- Consequences exert more control over behavior when they occur immediately.

- Natural consequences are better than artificial ones.

- Reinforcement of a response increases the probability that it will occur.

- Shaping is developing a new behavior by rewarding successive approximations to that behavior.

- Individuals are typically unaware of the contingencies controlling their behavior.

- Negative reinforcement occurs when the removal of an event leads to an increase in a behavior.

- Extinction occurs when a response that was previously reinforced is no longer followed by the reinforcement.

- Punishment is the presentation or removal of an event after a response that decreases the probability of the response occurring again.

- Extinction and punishment are most effective when combined with reinforcement of behaviors that are incompatible with and serve the same function as the behavior that is being extinguished.

- Even operants are also controlled to some degree by antecedents.

- For maximum leverage, change as many As, Bs, and Cs as possible.

FIGURE 3.1. Principles of operant conditioning. From Jacqueline B. Persons (2008). Copyright by The Guilford Press. Permission to photocopy this figure is granted to purchasers of this book for personal use only (see copyright page for details).

Reinforcers are *defined functionally.* The therapist cannot assume that behaviors or events are reinforcing to the patient because they are appealing to the therapist or they logically *ought* to be reinforcing. Thus, some individuals find self-harming behaviors such as cutting or burning to be (negatively) reinforcing because they reduce painful arousal (M. Z. Brown, Comtois, & Linehan, 2002). Surgical procedures appear to be reinforcing to some individuals (who are thereby diagnosed with Munchausen's syndrome). The *New York Times* (Hoge, 2002) described a British physician who was found to have murdered more than 200 of his patients, perhaps because the death of a patient gave him "a buzz" (Hoge, 2002). The therapist who does not understand the function of a problem behavior is not likely to be able to effectively treat it.

Observation is often the best way to determine what behaviors are reinforcing to a person. Premack (1965) argued that when behaviors are freely chosen, the ones a person chooses more often are more reinforcing than those chosen less often. Boice (1983) used the *Premack principle* to help assistant professors increase their writing behavior by setting up contingency management schemes in which (frequently chosen) activities like reading the newspaper or taking a shower were contingent on meeting a small daily writing quota.

To Effectively Control Behavior, the Consequence Must Be Contingent on the Behavior

The consequence must be *contingent* (i.e., likely to happen given the behavior and not likely to happen in the absence of the behavior) in order to have an effect on the behavior. If the consequence occurs whether or not the behavior occurs, then the behavior will not be under the control of the consequence. If the mother reads her child a story whether or not he puts on his pajamas and gets ready for bed, the story-reading consequence does not control the behavior of getting ready for bed. To control the (getting-ready-for-bed) behavior, every single instance of the behavior need not be followed by the (story-reading) consequence; the consequence can be intermittent.

Behavior That Is Controlled by an Intermittent Consequence Is More Resistant to Extinction Than Behavior That Is Always Followed by a Consequence

If individuals are accustomed to receiving reinforcement only some of the times they emit a behavior, they will continue to emit the behavior longer when the reinforcer disappears than if they are accustomed to receiving reinforcement every single time they emit the behavior. The notion that intermittent reinforcement makes a response more persistent across situations has a variety of clinical implications. For example, once the patient has begun doing therapy homework, if I review his or her completed assignments at only some sessions, not all sessions, it will take longer for the patient's homework behavior to extinguish when I stop reviewing the homework than if I review it at every single session before I stop reviewing it. This principle can explain why a client (or therapist) works like a slave for a boss who only intermittently acknowledges the employee's effort or stays in a relationship with a person who is only intermittently pleasant to be around. It also implies that the therapist ought to take care when teaching new client behaviors, such as assertiveness. At first, to get the new behavior going, the therapist must reinforce every instance of the new behavior. But later, the therapist would do well to shift to an intermittent schedule that better resembles the client's out-of-session environment in order to ensure that the behavior generalizes and is robust to extinction. This principle also affects the therapist, too, as in the case of a client who has several sessions that the therapist views as quite successful but who then misses several sessions, thus shaping the therapist into persistence.

Consequences Exert More Control over Behavior When They Occur Immediately

This principle can be particularly helpful in thinking about the therapy session itself, where patient and therapist mutually affect each other in a sequence that plays out over time (Kohlenberg & Tsai, 1991). For example, suppose the therapist asks a question that evokes the client's shame and the associated action urge, which is to escape. As the therapist asks the question, the client flushes, looks uncomfortable, and shifts the topic. If the therapist accedes to the change in topic (i.e., removes the aversive contingency), the client becomes more likely to try to escape in the future when this topic is raised. The therapist, too, is getting shaped. The therapist asks a question and receives the aversive contingency of the client looking uncomfortable. Then when the therapist changes the topic, the client looks more comfortable. In this sequence, the therapist is negatively reinforced for shifting the topic when the client appears uncomfortable.

Natural Consequences Are Better Than Artificial Ones

Approval and attention are natural consequences (consequences that occur naturally in the world), and when given by therapists they are typically (but not always!) reinforcing to patients. This point can be used repeatedly and in multiple ways. For example, the therapist can respond promptly and warmly to patient behaviors that the therapist wishes to strengthen, for example, an assertive appropriate request. The therapist can be less responsive to patient behaviors that the therapist wishes to extinguish, such as hostile remarks, passivity, or blaming others. Natural consequences are better than artificial ones because they promote generalization of learned behaviors to other situations.

Shaping Develops a New Behavior
by Rewarding Successive Small Increments of That Behavior

Many of us fail to manage our behavior effectively because we do not understand shaping. We set the bar too high, fail, and give up (the behavior is extinguished). One of my patients, who had a long history of making this error, had stopped scheduling any tasks at all and did not even own a calendar. Another, who wished to resume regular jogging, proposed a plan of daily jogging for the following week in spite of the fact that he had not jogged for months and did not even remember where his running shoes were. The concept of shaping suggests that this man would be more likely to achieve his goal if he set a goal of finding his shoes and jogging once than if he insisted on a plan of jogging daily.

Kazdin (2001) provides a delightful example that illustrates shaping. He and his fellow students used contingencies to shape their professor's behavior so that he would stand in the right back corner of the room while lecturing. Shaping was needed because it was not possible to reward the professor for lecturing in the corner because this behavior never occurred—he routinely lectured from a lectern in the middle of the room. The students used natural consequences to shape their professor's behavior. They rewarded, with head nods and other signs of interest, any step he took to the right and they leaned back and turned their eyes away when he moved to the left. After the professor routinely took small steps to the right, the students rewarded only more extreme steps to the right. That is, they required a bigger change in behavior in order to give the reinforcer. After six classes, the professor was leaning against the right corner of the room while giving his lecture. All of these behavior changes appeared to take place completely outside the professor's awareness.

Individuals Are Typically Unaware of the Contingencies
Controlling Their Behavior

The example just given and the one of Paul at the beginning of the chapter illustrate that we are not usually aware of the contingencies controlling our behavior. Although I hypothesized that Paul's hopeless verbalizations served the function of attracting my attention, I did not perceive him as manipulative because I did not believe that he was aware of the contingencies driving his behavior. In fact, I suspected that I had been reinforcing his behavior without being aware that I was doing so.

This example, as well as many of the others already presented, highlights the fact that it is easy for therapists to inadvertently reinforce their patients' maladaptive and even harmful behaviors. Therapists can also inadvertently extinguish or punish adaptive behaviors. Thus, awareness in the moment of the dyadic interplay between patient and therapist and a solid understanding of the principles of operant conditioning are essential tools of the effective psychotherapist.

Negative Reinforcement Occurs When the Removal of an Event or Stimulus Leads to an Increase in a Behavior

As one of my students (thanks to Megan McCarthy) noted, a classic example of negative reinforcement is seat belt fastening, which is reinforced by the cessation of that awful bleeping noise. Many problem behaviors for which patients seek help are negatively reinforced. For example, behaviors like excessive drinking, binge eating, and social isolation often lead to the cessation of unpleasant emotional or physical states. Until I recognized what was happening, I negatively reinforced one of my patients, Juana, for verbally attacking me during therapy sessions by attending to her attacks, which allowed her to avoid the topic we were discussing before she attacked me.

Extinction Occurs When a Behavior That Was Previously Reinforced Is No Longer Followed by the Reinforcement

Therapists can use extinction (also called extinguishing) strategically to abolish maladaptive behavior behaviors, as I did when I stopped responding to Juana's verbal attacks. Carelessness can lead to inadvertent extinction of adaptive behavior. For example, a therapist can inadvertently extinguish a patient's therapy homework by forgetting to review it.

When using extinction, it is important to be aware of the phenomena of *extinction burst* and *spontaneous recovery*. The *extinction burst* is a recurrence of the problem behavior, often in a more intense form, which can occur soon after extinction is imposed, usually after the behavior has started to decrease but before it has completely stopped. *Spontaneous recovery* refers to the fact that after extinction, an extinguished behavior can reappear at a later time, usually in a weaker form. When extinction bursts and spontaneous recoveries occur, it is essential not to reward the behaviors. Doing this places the behaviors on an intermittent reinforcement schedule that makes them more resistant to extinction than they were before. Thus, when I put Juana's verbal attacking behavior on extinction, I had to be aware that her attacking behavior might increase soon after I began the extinction process, that the behavior might reemerge later, and that it was *essential* that I not reinforce it on any of these occasions.

Extinction typically has unpleasant emotional side effects like frustration and anger. Notice how you would feel if you went to your doctor's office for an appointment and found the office closed or to the ATM you regularly use and found it out of order. Patients may need extra support to get through an extinction process successfully.

Punishment Is the Presentation or Removal of an Event after a Behavior That Decreases the Probability of the Behavior Recurring

Punishing consequences can be instituted to stop undesirable behaviors. Thus, when Annette tells me, "I want to die" and then hangs up the phone, I immediately call her back and when she does not respond, I leave her the message that unless she calls me within 5 minutes, I will send the police to her home. This intervention is effective both because it addresses the danger of the situation and because I know Annette will experience a visit from the police as punishing.

An advantage of punishment is that it can produce immediate results, whereas extinction typically takes more time. One valid use of punishment is when dangerous behaviors must be stopped immediately. However, punishment often breeds anxiety, disorganization, and resentment, and therefore is best used sparingly. Thus, I would use the intervention just described only if I assessed the situation as one involving imminent danger.

Extinction and Punishment Are Most Effective When Combined with Reinforcement of Behaviors Incompatible with the Behavior That Is Being Extinguished

This principle points out that the therapist would only want to institute a punisher (e.g., call the police, as in the example above) if the patient's life was truly in danger and in the context of other interventions designed to teach and reinforce alternate, more adaptive behaviors designed to accomplish the same function. For this reason, cognitive-behavior therapists often teach their patients new skills (Bs). However, before teaching a new B, it is important to conduct a careful assessment to determine whether the patient lacks the skill, or has the skill but is not exhibiting it. If the patient doesn't have the skill, the therapist may need to teach it. If the patient has the skill but is not displaying it, the therapist will want to work to identify and overcome the obstacles to displaying it.

In the case of Annette, I would want to offer and teach her methods of communicating distress other than the one that I am punishing and I would also take care to be immediately responsive to any communications of distress and misery she emitted, even low-level ones, so that suicide threats are not needed to get my attention.

To extinguish the hopeless and suicidal verbalizations of Paul, the patient described at the beginning of the chapter, I first stopped reinforcing them with sympathy and extra attention. Instead, I responded to them with tedious suicide assessments that I carried out in a matter-of-fact way. To speed and ease the extinction process, I also worked to identify and reinforce healthier behaviors that could serve the same purpose as Paul's hopelessness and suicidal verbalizations, which I hypothesized served the function of eliciting concern and caring from me. I began purposefully giving extra attention to Paul's reports of adaptive problem-solving efforts.

In the case of Juana, the patient who verbally attacked me, I needed to stop changing the subject when difficult topics arose—this was negatively reinforcing the attacks. But this tactic alone might not eliminate the attacks because they were the only way Juana knew to cope with my requests to discuss anxiety-producing topics. The attacks stopped when I taught her to be mindful of how her anxiety arose when I raised certain topics and to break scary topics down into manageable bits, and showed her skills for assertively asking for help managing the anxiety.

Even Operants Are Also Controlled to Some Degree by Antecedents

Operants, by definition, are controlled by consequences. But most operant behavior is eventually also guided or constrained by antecedents. Organisms learn not only what behaviors bring rewarding consequences but they also learn something about the conditions, or stimuli, that indicate a reward is available. A *discriminative stimulus* is an antecedent event or stimulus that indicates that a certain response will be reinforced. For example, the patient learns to come to the therapist's office at the time of his or her appointment; the reinforcement of meeting with the therapist is *available only at that time and place.*

A behavior is said to be under *stimulus control* if the probability of its occurrence depends on what stimuli are present. For example, a dissertation writer found himself eating, watching TV, and reading the newspaper instead of writing his dissertation. Using stimulus control, he increased his writing behavior significantly by spending the hours of 9 A.M. to 3 P.M. every day at the library. The library was less conducive to distracting activities than his apartment. Behavioral treatments of many problem behaviors, including self-harming and substance use behaviors, typically include interventions to increase control of these behaviors by modifying their antecedents (Linehan, 1993a; McCrady & Epstein, 2003; Opdyke & Rothbaum, 1998).

Here is another example.

> An air force cargo plane was preparing for departure from Thule Air Base in Greenland. They were waiting for the truck to arrive to pump out the aircraft's sewage holding tank. The aircraft commander was in a hurry, the truck was late in arriving, and the airman performing the job was extremely slow in getting the tank pumped out. When the commander berated the airman for his slowness and promised punishment, the airman responded: "Sir, I have no stripes, it is 20 below zero, I'm stationed in Greenland, and I am pumping sewage out of airplanes. Just what are you going to do to punish me?"

In this case, the context, or *setting events* (also called *establishing operations*), influence the effectiveness and nature of the consequences that can be imposed. Linehan (1993a) points to a clinical implication of this notion in the treatment of patients with borderline personality disorder whose personal lives are often so torturous and painful and their interpersonal lives so devoid of positive support and encouragement that the therapist's warmth and support become a powerful positive reinforcer.

For Maximum Leverage, Change As Many As, Bs, and Cs As Possible

D. L. Watson and Tharp (2002) recommend that the therapist manipulate as many As, Bs, and Cs as possible in order to have the best possible chance of affecting the B in question. Thus, to increase the B of writing this book, I manipulated As by writing at the same time and place whenever I could and by discussing the book with my colleagues so they would ask me about it and prompt me to think about it and so work on it. I manipulated Bs by starting each writing period with an easy task (e.g., reworking some of what I had done the day before) and by setting myself small and manageable writing targets each time I sat down to write. I manipulated Cs by using the Premack principle (permitting myself to do other work only after I had fulfilled my book-writing quota) and by eliciting congratulations from my colleagues and husband when I finished a draft of a chapter.

RESPONDENT (PAVLOVIAN) CONDITIONING: WHEN ANTECEDENTS CONTROL BEHAVIORS

Respondent behavior is controlled by antecedents, in contrast to *operant* behavior, which is controlled by consequences. The clearest example of respondents is a reflex. The doctor taps your knee with an instrument and in response your lower leg jerks out. Of course, reflexes are not learned behaviors. They are hardwired responses to certain stimulus situations and so they are called *unconditioned* (i.e., unlearned) respondents (responses).

Respondent conditioning (also called *classical conditioning* or *Pavlovian conditioning*), has its origins in the work of Pavlov (1927). In his famous experiment with a dog, Pavlov repeatedly paired food (which automatically elicits salivation) with a bell until the bell alone without food made the dog salivate. In behaviorist terminology, the food is the *unconditioned stimulus (UCS)* and the dog's salivation is an *unconditioned response (UCR)*. The bell is at first a neutral stimulus that elicits no response but, after repeated pairings with food, it becomes a *conditioned stimulus (CS)* that elicits salivation. The salivation response to the bell is the *conditioned response (CR)*.

Modern views of respondent conditioning propose that it is not simply "a stupid process by which the organism willy-nilly forms associations between any two stimuli that happen to co-occur" (Rescorla, 1988, p. 154). Rather, it involves "the learning of relations among events so as to allow the organism to represent its environment" (p. 151). One of the key experiments underpinning this view is the demonstration by Garcia and Koelling (1966) that when rats were presented with a compound stimulus consisting of a taste, a light, and a noise that was followed by illness, the rats learned to avoid the taste but not the light or noise. In contrast, when the taste–light–noise stimulus was followed by electric shock, the rats learned to avoid the noise and light but not the taste. Thus, conditioning is not simply a function of contiguity but is also a function of information value. That is, taste typically provides more information about illness than does light or noise and therefore rats learned the relationship between taste and illness but not the relationships between light or noise and illness.

The hypothesis that respondent conditioning could explain the acquisition of phobias was tested in the "Little Albert" experiment. J. P. Watson and Rayner (1920) presented a sudden loud noise (the UCS) when 2-year-old Little Albert was playing with a white rat (the CS). Little Albert had a fear reaction (UCR) to the noise and later exhibited anxiety symptoms (CR) to white rats. Respondent conditioning can also account for the fact that cancer patients who experience nausea (UCR) following chemotherapy (UCS) can come to experience nausea (CR) in the presence of stimuli (CSs) that were present before chemotherapy, including the sight of the waiting room of the chemotherapy clinic.

The clinician can make good use of a detailed understanding of the principles of respondent conditioning, which are presented here and summarized in Figure 3.2.

- Respondent, also called Pavlovian or classical conditioning, is a type of learning that results from the pairing of a neutral stimulus with an unconditioned stimulus that elicits a reflexive response. After repeated pairings, the neutral stimulus comes to elicit a response similar to the reflexive one.

- The greater the number of pairings, the more likely the conditioned stimulus (CS) is to elicit the conditioned response (CR).

- If the CS is always paired with the unconditioned stimulus (UCS), it is more likely to elicit the CR than if the pairings occur less consistently.

- Conditioning occurs more strongly and quickly if the UCS or CS or both are intense.

- Conditioning is most likely to occur if the CS precedes the UCS by a half-second.

- Conditioning is often unconscious.

- Some stimuli are more readily paired than others.

- Counterconditioning is a method of eliminating a conditioned response by pairing a CS to a US that elicits a new response that is incompatible with the old one.

- Extinction occurs when the CS is repeatedly presented without the UCS.

- Higher-order conditioning occurs when a CS1 that has been conditioned to a UCS is now paired with a CS2, so that CS2 now comes to elicit a conditioned response similar to the one elicited by CS1.

FIGURE 3.2. Principles of respondent conditioning. From Jacqueline B. Persons (2008). Copyright by The Guilford Press. Permission to photocopy this figure is granted to purchasers of this book for personal use only (see copyright page for details).

The Greater the Number of Pairings of the CS and the UCS, the More Likely the CS Is to Elicit the CR

Until a ceiling is reached, the more often a person experiences a pairing of a spontaneous panic attack (a UCS that elicits a UCR of fear) and a CS (e.g., the approach to the Bay Bridge), the more likely it is that the CS will elicit a CR in that person.

If the CS Is Always Paired with the UCS, the CS Is More Likely to Elicit the CR Than if Pairings Occur Inconsistently

If every time a person approaches a large dog (the CS), he experiences a severe bite (the UCS that elicits a UCR of fear), large dogs are more likely to elicit fear than if the person approaches large dogs often but experiences the UCS only occasionally.

Conditioning Occurs More Strongly and Quickly if the UCS or CS or Both Are Intense

Foa, Steketee, and Rothbaum (1989) invoke this principle to account for the fact that in PTSD (when the UCS is a traumatic event), individuals have stronger fear responses than in other phobias.

Conditioning Is Most Likely to Occur if the CS Precedes the UCS by a Half-Second

If the delay between the CS and UCS is longer than a half-second or the order reversed, conditioning is less likely (Kazdin, 2001). For example, fear conditioning to the sight of a large man is more likely to occur if the sight of the large man (CS) occurs before the gunshot noise (UCS) than if the sight of the large man follows the gunshot noise.

Respondent Conditioning Is Often Unconscious

Humans can learn to associate fear with a stimulus they do not consciously perceive (Ohman & Mineka, 2001). This fact may explain why phobic patients are frequently unable to report conditioning events. It can also explain emotional reactions that appear to come "out of the blue." They may be conditioned emotional reactions to subtle stimuli that are outside awareness.

Some Stimuli Are More Readily Paired Than Others

Conditioning is not simply a matter of contiguity, as noted earlier. Seligman (1971) used the term *preparedness* and proposed an evolutionary account of the fact that some stimuli are more readily conditioned than others. The evolutionary hypothesis explains why humans are more likely to develop phobias (which are conceptualized as learned fear responses) to small animals, snakes, spiders, and heights, which posed dangers to our early ancestors, than of flowers and even items like electrical outlets and dentist chairs that, although dangerous to us now, were not dangerous to our forebears (Ohman & Mineka, 2001).

Counterconditioning Eliminates a CR by Pairing a CS to a UCS That Elicits a New Response Incompatible with the Old One

Counterconditioning is analogous to the phenomenon in operant conditioning that a response can be extinguished more quickly if an alternate, competing response is reinforced. Mary Cover Jones (1924) first demonstrated the clinical utility of counterconditioning when she treated a boy who was terrified of rabbits by gradually introducing rabbits while he was eating something he enjoyed. Wolpe (1958) relied on the notion of counterconditioning when he developed systematic desensitization to treat phobias, using relaxation as the competing response. However, although Wolpe relied on the principle of counterconditioning to develop systematic desensitization, which has proved to be quite effective in reducing pathological anxiety, it is not at all clear that counterconditioning is in fact the mechanism of action of the therapy (Goldfried & Davison, 1994). Numerous accounts of the mechanism have been proposed, including extinction (due to repeated presentations of the CS without the UCS) and cognitive explanations.

Counterconditioning is also used in aversion therapy, which pairs a problem behavior (e.g., ingestion of alcohol or inappropriate sexual behavior, the CS), to a UCS (e.g., a drug) that produces an unpleasant UCR (e.g., vomiting). Cautela (1967) developed covert sensitization, a type of aversive conditioning in which the UCS is an unpleasant image (e.g., of eating vomit). Kearney (2006) provides a useful primer with details on conducting covert sensitization.

Extinction Occurs When the CS Is Repeatedly Presented without the UCS

Extinction (see Figure 3.3) occurs when a response that was previously reinforced is no longer reinforced. Thus, for example, if a woman who was raped in her college auditorium and, as a result, is fearful of the auditorium, forces herself to go to the auditorium repeatedly and is not raped, the auditorium will lose the ability to produce a fear reaction. This principle led to the development of exposure-based treatments for anxiety disorders.

More recently, Bouton (2002) and others proposed that extinction does not so much involve unlearning of associations as it involves learning of new associations, so that new information about the fear cue is stored alongside the old learning. (In fact, Pavlov pointed to this idea.) Similar principles apply to the extinction of operants (Bouton, 2002). Bouton proposed that after extinction the new learning makes the meaning of the CS ambiguous, because both "meanings" (the fear meaning and the new nonfear meaning) are retained and the organism relies on context to resolve the ambiguity. Thus, after extinction, the process of figuring out the meaning of the CS (that is, determining whether the auditorium is safe or dangerous) is similar to the process required to figure out the meaning of an ambiguous word like *bank*. To determine the meaning, the listener relies on context (Is the discussion about finances or about a river?). Stated differently, this view of extinction proposes that exposure treatment teaches the patient accurate safety cues, for example that a big dog is safe in the context of an owner, a leash, and a wagging tail (Zayfert & Becker, 2007).

The idea that extinction is context dependent has several implications for exposure-based therapy for anxiety disorders (Bouton, 1988). The main one is that extinction does not erase the CS–UCS connections; therefore, a return of fear is always possible. Another is that return of fear appears to be controlled in part by context. Exposure treatment carried out in the context of pharmacotherapy may be to some degree dependent on the pharmacotherapy (Otto, 2002). This proposal offers one explanation of the finding that people with panic disorder who received CBT alone had better long-term outcomes than those who were treated with CBT plus imipramine (Barlow, Gorman, Shear, & Woods, 2000).

Another implication of the idea that extinction is context dependent is that *safety behaviors* can undermine the effects of exposure (Sloan & Telch, 2002; Smits, Powers, Cho, & Telch, 2004). *Safety behaviors* are anything that the person uses to feel safe in a feared situation, such as carrying a bottle of anti-anxiety medication or holding on to a companion. Bouton (2002) proposed that the presence of safety signals prevents the effects of exposure from generalizing to situations in which the safety signals are not present.

The idea that safety behaviors can undermine the effects of exposure leads to dilemmas for the therapist because often patients are unwilling to approach feared situations without using safety behaviors (Rachman, 1983). A pragmatic solution to this dilemma may be to allow the use of safety behaviors in early exposure trials if they permit patients to approach situations they would otherwise avoid but to strive to drop out all of the safety behaviors over the course of the therapy.

A: Antecedent of a target behavior.

B: A target behavior.

C: Consequences of a target behavior.

Conditioned stimulus (CS): In respondent conditioning, a previously neutral stimulus that is able to elicit the same response as another (unconditioned) stimulus that has been repeatedly paired with it.

Conditioned response (CR): In respondent conditioning, the learned response to the conditioned stimulus.

Contingent: When a consequence follows only from a specific behavior.

Discriminative stimulus: An antecedent event or stimulus that indicates that a certain response will be reinforced.

Extinction: A procedure in which a reinforcer is no longer delivered for a previously reinforced response, resulting in a decrease in the probability of the response.

Extinction burst: Recurrence of a learned behavior soon after reinforcement is withdrawn.

Higher-order conditioning: The pairing of a conditioned stimulus (CS1) with a second conditioned stimulus (CS2) so that the CS2 comes to elicit a conditioned response similar to the one elicited by CS1.

Negative reinforcement: The removal of an event that increases the probability of the behavior that preceded it.

Observational learning: A type of learning in which behaviors are learned by watching another individual engage in them. Also called Modeling.

Operant: A behavior controlled by its consequences.

Operant conditioning: A type of learning in which behaviors are controlled primarily by their consequences.

Positive reinforcement: An event that increases the probability of the behavior that preceded it.

Punishment: An aversive event, or the lack of a positive event, that decreases the probability of occurrence of the behavior that preceded it.

Reinforcement: A consequence that increases the probability that a behavior will occur again.

Respondent: A behavior controlled by its antecedents.

Respondent conditioning: A type of learning in which behaviors are controlled by their antecedents. Also called classical conditioning or Pavlovian conditioning.

Safety behavior: Any behavior that a person uses to feel safe in a feared situation, such as carrying a bottle of antianxiety medication or holding on to a companion.

Spontaneous recovery: Temporary reappearance of an extinguished behavior.

Unconditioned stimulus (UCS): A stimulus that automatically elicits an unlearned response.

Unconditioned response (UCR): An automatic, unlearned response elicited by an unconditioned stimulus.

FIGURE 3.3. A glossary of selected learning theory terms. From Jacqueline B. Persons (2008). Copyright by The Guilford Press. Permission to photocopy this figure is granted to purchasers of this book for personal use only (see copyright page for details).

Another implication of Bouton's ideas is that the effects of exposure-based treatment can be made more resilient if multiple contexts are used, that is, if people who are afraid of humiliating themselves in public are exposed to a variety of types of public settings (e.g., on the bus, in a restaurant, giving a public talk) at various times of day, in various emotional states, and so on. Yet another implication is that separate exposures to panic symptoms and Bay Bridge driving may not be sufficient to treat a patient who fears *having panic symptoms while on the Bay Bridge.* Exposure to *panic symptoms while driv-*

ing on the Bay Bridge may be needed. Other efforts to strengthen extinction learning are drawn from recent basic science findings about the biological mechanisms of extinction learning and suggest that D-cycloserine may potentiate the effects of extinction learning during exposure-based treatments for anxiety disorders (Hofmann et al., 2006; Ressler et al., 2004).

Higher-Order Conditioning Occurs When a CS (CS1) Is Paired with a Second Stimulus (CS2), So That CS2 Now Elicits a CR Similar to That Elicited by CS1

A hot swirling wind on a fall day is a CS1 that triggers a fear reaction for me because that kind of wind was present on the day of the Oakland fire (UCS) in 1991 that came very close to destroying my home. Recently I met a new person (CS2) on a day I was experiencing the CS1 of the hot swirling wind. Now whenever I see that person (CS2) I experience a fear reaction, although it is milder than the one cued by the hot swirling winds (CS1). Higher-order conditioning might also account for anniversary reactions that are often reported by people who have experienced bereavement or trauma.

Stimulus Generalization Is the Transfer of a Learned Response to Situations Other Than Those in Which the Response Was Learned

Stimulus generalization is the phenomenon that stimuli similar to the ones that have been associated with the UCS also come to elicit the conditioned response. Thus, I experience a fear reaction in response to swirling winds even when they are cold, and the rape victim finds that a large room similar to the auditorium in which she was raped can evoke a fear reaction.

The fact that conditioning is often unconscious and can involve higher-order conditioning and stimulus generalization can result in complex and unexpected emotional reactions that are difficult to predict and explain. Thus, patients who have PTSD symptoms can experience fear reactions "out of the blue" that may reflect the presence of higher-order CSs of which they are unaware, such as a particular flash of light on a silver car bumper that is similar to one they saw at the time they were mugged.

OBSERVATIONAL LEARNING

Observational learning, also called *vicarious learning,* was defined by Bandura (1977) as behavior that results from watching a model's behavior be rewarded or punished. People learn both undesirable and desirable behaviors via observational learning. An example: I don't cross the street against the light in Los Angeles because I saw my husband get a ticket for doing this. However, in New York City, where it is vicariously reinforced (I see others being rewarded for this behavior), I do it all the time. Thus, therapists, who model behavior constantly for their patients, must take care to model adaptive, not maladaptive, behavior. However, they need not model perfect behavior at every moment. In addition to modeling skillful behavior, which is called *mastery modeling,* it can also be helpful to provide *coping modeling.* In coping modeling, the model makes some mistakes or shows weaknesses and then recovers and masters the behavior.

Some theorists argue that observational learning can be explained via the principles of operant and respondent conditioning. For example, as in the case of the traffic light example above, behaviors that are observed to be followed by desired consequences are more likely to be repeated than those that are observed to be followed by punishment. Similarly, consequences experienced by the model must be contingent in order to control behavior; the conditioning will be more effective if the consequences are immediate and if they are natural rather than artificial. And because conditioning often takes place outside awareness, the relationships between antecedents and consequences or between CSs and UCSs are not always reportable by the individual who is learning them.

Additional principles have been shown to apply to the acquisition of behavior via modeling, namely that a person is more likely to imitate a model when the model is similar to the observer, when the model is friendly, and when the model is higher in status, expertise, and prestige than the observer (Rosenthal & Bandura, 1978). The implication of these findings is that the therapist can be a powerful model for the patient. Thus, people with phobias can learn to become less fearful of an object or situation by observing their therapists interact with the fear stimuli in a nonfearful way. Remembering that I am a model can be helpful when I need to do something difficult, such as assert myself to a patient who is annoying me by constantly rescheduling her appointment. I remind myself (when it is true) that the skills I am displaying (making a reasonable assertive request) are skills the patient needs to learn and that I can help her do this by modeling them.

COMPARING THE LEARNING THEORIES WITH EACH OTHER AND WITH COGNITIVE THEORIES

Although I discuss them separately and they have distinct historical traditions, the distinction between classical and operant conditioning is relatively arbitrary. An operant can be described in respondent terms (i.e., the discriminative stimulus is classically conditioned to the response, which in turn is classically conditioned to the consequence). Often the main reason to distinguish the two processes is practical utility. That is, the question the therapist asks is: Do I gain more control over the target behavior by viewing it as a respondent (primarily controlled by antecedent stimuli) or as an operant (primarily controlled by consequences)?

Conceptualizing whether a problem behavior is primarily respondent or operant has important treatment implications. For example, suicidal behavior can appear to be primarily a respondent behavior (e.g., a response to perceptions of hopelessness or auditory hallucinations) or primarily an operant (to achieve the function of getting relief from burdens) (Linehan, 1993a). If the behavior is conceptualized as primarily respondent, the therapist intervenes to change the antecedents that trigger the behavior and doesn't have to worry about strengthening the behavior by attending to it. If the behavior is conceptualized as an operant, consequences are important and the therapist has to be careful not to inadvertently reinforce it.

Learning theories explain behavior differently than cognitive theories. Learning theories are *functional*—that is, they explain behavior by examining its functions (Nelson & Hayes, 1986). Thus, for example, a behaviorist might propose that the function of Paul's behavior (in the opening vignette) was to elicit my caring and concern. In contrast, Beck's cognitive model is a *structural* one. Structural theories explain psychopathology by examining its topography, viewing topographical details as reflections of underlying structures (e.g., schemas). Thus, the cognitive therapist might conceptualize Paul's behavior as caused by schemas of himself as helpless and the future as hopeless. The *structural/functional* distinction comes from biology: one branch of biology studies the *functions* of organs and tissues, and the other branch studies their *structure.*

COMBINED MODELS

Several theorists have pointed to limitations of the operant, respondent, and observational learning models, and have made various proposals, including combined models, to address these limitations. Three are described here: Rachman's proposals about fear acquisition, Mowrer's two-factor theory, and Seligman and Johnston's theory of avoidance learning.

Rachman's Proposals about Fear Acquisition

Rachman (1977) pointed out inadequacies in the conditioning account of fear acquisition, including the following: that people often fail to acquire fears when the conditioning theory suggests they should (e.g., during air raids or traumas); that the distribution of human fears is not consistent with the conditioning theory (otherwise people would be more afraid of dentists and less afraid of snakes); and that people are afraid of many situations and stimuli they have never encountered. A fascinating example of fear acquisition that is not easily accounted for by conditioning theory is the report by Foa et al. (1989) of a rape victim who developed PTSD only after she learned that her assailant had murdered the next woman he raped. Some of these problems are addressed by preparedness and observational learning. Rachman further suggested that fear could also be acquired by the transmission of information and instruction (e.g., the child being told by a parent that going out alone at night is dangerous). This proposal is particularly helpful in accounting for fears of situations that the person has never encountered.

Mowrer's Two-Factor Theory

Avoidance behavior is a prominent feature of anxiety disorders and in fact it often causes the greatest functional impairment. It is not uncommon to meet a person with agoraphobia whose life course has been completely altered because she has avoided driving on bridges or freeways for 10 to 20 or more years. Operant and respondent models alone have difficulty accounting for avoidance. One partial solution is offered by Mowrer's (1960) two-factor theory. It is called a two-factor theory because it involves both respondent (stage 1) and operant (stage 2) conditioning processes. The theory proposes that in stage 1, neutral stimuli (e.g., driving on a bridge) are paired with innately fear-evoking stimuli (e.g., a spontaneous panic attack) and, via *respondent conditioning,* come to elicit conditioned fear responses. In stage 2, escape and avoidance behaviors are negatively reinforced *operants* that allow the individual to escape and avoid the conditioned fear responses. Thus, for example, Bouton, Mineka, and Barlow (2001) propose that panic disorder arises when internal and external stimuli (CSs) that were present during a spontaneous panic attack (the UCS) become associated with the attack. The CSs then trigger anxiety and panic reactions similar to those elicited by the original panic attack and the behaviors of escaping and avoiding the CSs are negatively reinforced.

Seligman and Johnston's Theory of Avoidance Behavior

Seligman and Johnston (1973) argued that although Mowrer's theory accounts for the acquisition of avoidance behavior, it does not account for its maintenance. To address this weakness of Mowrer's theory, Seligman and Johnston (1973) developed a cognitive theory of the maintenance of avoidance behavior. Dogs learned to jump over a barrier to escape an electrical shock. Next, a bell (the CS) was paired with the shock (UCS) and the dogs learned to jump after the bell and thus to avoid the shock. Mower's two-factor theory explains the acquisition of this avoidance behavior.

What Mowrer's theory does not explain is the persistence of the avoidance behavior after the shock (the UCS) was turned off. Despite the fact that the UCS was no longer present, the dogs' jumping behavior (the avoidance behavior) persisted for hundreds of trials. Conditioning principles state that if the UCS is removed, the behavior should have extinguished. But it did not.

To account for the persistence of avoidance behavior, Seligman and Johnston's cognitive theory states that the dog, as a result of his initial conditioning trials, comes to hold two beliefs: "If I jump I will not get shocked" and "If I do not jump, I will get shocked." Each instance of avoidance behavior generates a piece of evidence consistent with the belief "If I jump I will not get shocked" and thus strengthens the belief and the jumping behavior. This cognitive model accounts for the resistance to extinction of avoidance behavior in the absence of the UCS. In fact, the model even suggests that the avoidance behavior should become more entrenched over time, as appears to happen.

The Seligman–Johnston theory has two fascinating clinical implications. First, to stop the avoidance behavior, the organism must obtain information that disconfirms his beliefs, which are inaccurate (the shock is no longer present). In the lab, Seligman taught the dog that the shock was gone by using a harness to prevent the dog from jumping after he heard the bell. Similarly, effective exposure treatment for anxiety disorders requires blocking the patient's avoidance behaviors, including obsessive–compulsive rituals and other more subtle avoidance and safety behaviors.

The second clinical implication is that avoidance behavior is not benign. Behavior that is driven by inaccurate beliefs often produces evidence that strengthens those beliefs. Every time the person with social phobia does not raise his hand in class to ask a question for fear of looking stupid and humiliating himself and has the experience of not looking stupid and humiliating himself, his belief that if he asks a question he will look stupid and humiliate himself gets stronger. This account is similar to the explanation offered by Sloan and Telch (2002) for why the presence of safety signals undermined the effectiveness of exposure to feared situations. They proposed that the use of or focus on availability of safety cues reduces the processing of threat-related information, which prevents the individual from perceiving that the situation is not in fact dangerous. Similarly, Wells, Clark, and Salkovskis (1995) propose that safety behaviors undermine exposure by leading to faulty attributions for safety (e.g., it is because I knew I had the pill bottle that I was able to cope with driving on the Bay Bridge). Consistent with this thinking, conceptualizations of anxiety disorders that attend to the role of safety behaviors and treatments that involve interventions to identify and block safety behaviors are increasingly important in understanding and treating anxiety disorders, including panic and agoraphobia (White & Barlow, 2002), social phobia (Clark, 2001), and generalized anxiety disorder (Schut, Castonguay, & Borkovec, 2001).

ESTs BASED ON LEARNING THEORIES

Interventions based on operant conditioning theory have traditionally been used with children and in institutional settings, where parents and therapists can easily control As, Bs, and Cs. However, operant conditioning is increasingly used to conceptualize and treat problems in outpatient therapy (Dougher, 2000; Kohlenberg & Tsai, 1991). A comprehensive discussion of empirically supported treatments (ESTs) based on learning theory would require another book. Therefore, the discussion here focuses on depression and anxiety, with some highlights and examples of other problem areas.

Depression

Lewinsohn's Behavior Therapy

Lewinsohn (1974) conceptualized depressive symptoms as resulting when individuals have experienced life events or stressors that caused them to lose the ability to obtain positive reinforcers (Lewinsohn & Gotlib, 1995). This can result from being in an environment that does not offer many opportunities to obtain reinforcers, from the failure to carry out the instrumental behaviors that will get the reward (sometimes due to skills deficits), or from an increased frequency of punishment (sometimes due to skills deficits). Based on this conceptualization, Lewinsohn developed a therapy based on his theory that helps individuals with depression increase the positive reinforcement they experience by teaching them to identify and carry out activities they find rewarding, including relaxation, and to improve their social skills in order to increase the amount of response-contingent positive reinforcement and decrease the amount of response-contingent punishment they receive.

Behavioral Activation

Ferster (1973) proposed that depression arises and is maintained because individuals have oriented their lives in service of escape or avoidance instead of the pursuit of positive reinforcement. Ferster's model leads to the proposal that depression can be treated by helping the person with depression reduce his reliance on escape and avoidance behaviors and expand his behavioral repertoire so as to increase the availability of positive reinforcements. Although Ferster did not develop a therapy based on his approach, his model is well represented in the work of Neil Jacobson and colleagues (Jacobson, Martell, & Dimidjian, 2001; Martell et al., 2001), who developed behavioral activation (BA), a treatment for depression that strives to help depressed patients expand their behavioral repertoire so as to regain old and obtain new sources of reinforcement and to reduce escape and avoidance behaviors, including rumination. Initial efficacy trials have shown that BA is effective in treating depression (Dimidjian et al., 2006; Jacobson et al., 1996).

Cognitive Behavioral Analysis System of Psychotherapy

McCullough (2000) developed an EST for chronic depression—the cognitive behavioral analysis system of psychotherapy (CBASP)—that is based on a combined learning-cognitive conceptualization. He proposes, as do the learned helplessness and learned hopelessness theories (cf. Abramson et al., 1989), that the chronically depressed person does not have "perceived functionality." Perceived functionality is "one's perception of a contingency relationship between one's behavior and consequences" (p. 71). Without perceived functionality, the patient loses the motivation to take action and suffers a dearth of positive reinforcers and an excess of punishers. Stated differently, these individuals are not capable of "if this-then that" thinking. To address this deficit, McCullough developed CBASP. CBASP makes elegant use of negative reinforcement, carefully producing unpleasant emotional states in the therapy session and then working to teach patients experientially that they can, in fact, take action to escape the misery they are feeling. CBASP also often involves modeling and skills training, as many chronically depressed individuals have deficits (for example, of assertion skills) that prevent them from obtaining desired outcomes. CBASP has been shown in a large controlled trial (Keller et al., 2000) to provide effective treatment for chronically depressed outpatients when combined with nefazodone. Patients who received CBASP plus nefazodone had outcomes that were superior to either monotherapy (CBASP alone or nefazodone alone).

Anxiety, Fears, and Phobias

Many ESTs for fears and phobias are based directly on Mowrer's (1960) two-factor theory, described above, which proposes that pathological anxiety arises as a result of a respondent conditioning process. Thus, Janet, who was held up at gunpoint by a tall man in a blue shirt, now experiences conditioned fear responses (CRs) that are elicited by the many CSs (cash register, tall man with blue shirt, increased heart rate) that were paired with the UCS (the holdup). In addition, in stage 2 of the model, escape and avoidance responses are operants that are negatively reinforced by the anxiety reduction that follows them. The model proposes that if Janet exposes herself to the anxiety-evoking CSs without the UCSs being present while blocking escape and avoidance behavior, the CR fear responses will extinguish. Large numbers of therapies based on this model rely on a variety of exposure strategies, including *in vivo* exposure, imaginal exposure, gradual exposure, flooding, and others, and also work to block the patient's escape and avoidance responses, including both flagrant rituals, as in obsessive–compulsive disorder (OCD), and more subtle avoidance and safety behaviors. Numerous ESTs have shown these therapies to provide effective treatment for anxiety disorders and related problems (e.g., hypochondriasis) (Nathan & Gorman, 2002).

Other Problems

Linehan's (1993a, 1993b) dialectical behavior therapy (DBT, which is described in more detail in the next chapter) relies extensively on operant principles to treat suicidality, self-harm, and other problem behaviors of borderline personality disorder. In DBT, the therapist conducts behavioral analyses to identify antecedents and consequences of these problem behaviors and to treat them by modifying antecedents and consequences and by teaching the patient new behaviors that can serve the same function as the maladaptive ones.

Another EST based on learning theory is the community reinforcement approach (CRA) for treating substance abuse problems (Smith & Meyers, 2000). CRA is based on the formulation that environmental contingencies play a powerful role in controlling drinking and drug-using behavior, and changes in those contingencies in multiple environments (social, familial, recreational, vocational) can help clients change their substance use.

Evidence-based therapies based on operant conditioning have also been developed for many other problems, including anorexia nervosa, pain, psychotic symptoms, and trichotillomania (Mansueto, Golomb, Thomas, & Stemberger, 1999).

ASSESSMENT AND INTERVENTION GUIDED BY LEARNING THEORIES

Here I describe some assessment procedures to obtain information for a formulation based on learning theories, and a brief account of intervention based on learning theory.

Collecting Information for Key Elements of the Formulation

A formulation of a behavior (B) based on learning theory describes the antecedents (As) and consequences (Cs) that are controlling the B. The clinician who is relying on learning theory to understand his or her client's behavior conducts a careful assessment (a functional analysis) in order to identify the As and Cs that are controlling the Bs of interest. I provide brief guidelines for conducting a functional analysis. This is a huge topic that I cannot do justice here. Additional details are provided in Haynes and O'Brien (2000), Kazdin (2001), D. L. Watson and Tharp (2002), and the outstanding chapter by Hawkins (1986) on the topic of selection of target behaviors.

A key first step is to identify the target behavior or behaviors of interest. These are problem behaviors (e.g., binge eating) that the person wants to decrease or adaptive behaviors (e.g., exercise) that the person wants to increase. More information on this topic is provided in discussions in Chapters 5 and 6 on identifying problems and setting treatment goals. Good brief guidelines are:

- Select a behavior that is a high-priority problem behavior (e.g., life threatening and/or therapy threatening).
- Select an adaptive behavior and work to increase it (e.g., work to increase dissertation-writing behavior instead of to decrease TV-watching behavior).
- Identify behaviors that are concrete, specific, and can be easily identified and measured.

After identifying a target behavior, the clinician collects data to identify the As and Cs that are controlling the behavior. Interviewing the patient, family members, and other

Antecedents (A)	Behaviors—actions, thoughts, or emotions (B)	Consequences (C)
• When did it happen? • Whom were you with? • What were you doing? • Where were you? • What were you saying to yourself? • What thoughts were you having? • What feelings were you having?	• What were you saying to yourself? • What thoughts were you having? • What feelings were you having? • What actions were you performing?	• What happened as a result? Was it pleasant or unpleasant?

FIGURE 3.4. Assessing the As, Bs, and Cs. Adapted from Watson and Tharp (2002, p. 68). Reprinted with permission of Wadsworth, a division of Thomson Learning: *www.thomsonrights. com.* Fax 800-730-2215.

professionals who are working with the patient can yield useful information. However, monitoring data, usually collected by patients themselves, are essential to flesh out a functional analysis because, as noted above, people typically don't know the contingencies controlling their behaviors. Questions that are useful in assessing As, Bs, and Cs are provided in Figure 3.4, and an Event Log that the patient can use to track As, Bs, and Cs is provided in Figure 3.5. The therapist can also conduct a behavioral chain analysis during the session and can teach the patient to use these strategies outside the session. A behavioral chain analysis identifies the antecedents (As) and consequences (Cs) of a problem behavior (B). A detailed chain of As leading up to the behavior is particularly useful to aid the work of generating strategies the patient could have used (and can use next time in a similar situation) to interrupt the chain and prevent the behavior. The steps of conducting the chain analysis are described in Figure 3.6 and borrow heavily from Linehan (1993a).

Intervention Guided by Learning Theory

Information about the As and Cs that control a target behavior, B, is used to devise an intervention plan. The treatment targets of an intervention plan based on a functional analysis are the As, Bs, and Cs that were identified in the functional analysis. Tips on strategies for changing the As, Bs, and Cs are shown in Figure 3.7. It's a good idea to consider an intervention plan that involves changing as many of the relevant As, Bs, and Cs as possible (D. L. Watson & Tharp, 2002). Therapeutic work to change As, Bs, and Cs can involve a multiplicity of interventions, ranging from things as simple as changing the A by inducing the patient to set an alarm clock to changing a B by teaching a complex set of social skills.

The following clinical examples of the use of operant principles to change behavior include a case of psychogenic vomiting and one of sexual acting-out behavior. Sutherland (2008) provides entertaining examples of a wife's use of operant principles to change her husband's behavior.

(text continues on page 64)

Time	Date	A	B	C

FIGURE 3.5. Event Log. Copyright 2001 by the San Francisco Bay Area Center for Cognitive Therapy. Reprinted by permission in Jacqueline B. Persons (2008). Permission to photocopy this figure is granted to purchasers of this book for personal use only (see copyright page for details).

A behavioral chain analysis identifies the chain of events (cognitions, emotions, behaviors, physiological sensations, external events, etc.) preceding and following a particular behavior. That is, it identifies the antecedents (As) and consequences (Cs) of a problem behavior (B). A detailed chain of As leading up to the behavior is particularly useful when generating strategies the patient could have used (and can use next time in a similar situation) to interrupt the chain and prevent the behavior.

This description of a behavioral chain analysis borrows heavily from Linehan (1993a); behavioral chain analysis is a key component of DBT. The first step is to identify the target behavior (B) of interest. It could be an adaptive behavior that the person wants to increase but is typically a maladaptive or problem behavior that the person wants to decrease or stop. Adaptive behaviors include going to work, taking needed medication, or getting out of bed at a particular time. Maladaptive behaviors include self-harming behaviors, suicidal behavior (e.g., Internet research on effective means of suicide, substance use, binge eating, having unprotected sex, or calling the therapist to leave an abusive telephone message).

The next step is to select a specific instance of the target behavior (B) to analyze. Select one that is tied to a life-threatening or other high-priority problem, one the patient can remember well, one the patient wants to investigate, one that seems particularly typical, one that led to a lot of problems (including problems in therapy), or the most recent one.

The next step is to identify the As that preceded and the Cs that followed the behavior. The goal is to identify all the small links of the chain that led up to and followed the B, especially the long link leading up to the B. It is important to get a long link because it is typically easier to interrupt a chain of behaviors leading to a problem behavior earlier in the chain than later, often because emotional arousal is lower earlier in the chain than later.

In identifying the links, I usually start with the B and go backward. Another option is to ask the patient when the problem (i.e., the problem that the patient solved with the behavior) started and to go forward from there. The advantage of this strategy is that it helps the patient tie the behavior to maladaptive efforts to solve particular problems he or she is experiencing. Nevertheless, I usually start with the B and go backward because it is easy to identify the B and it is frequently difficult to identify when the problem started. In addition, sometimes the problem started days or weeks ago, and a good behavioral chain analysis should not cover more than 1 or 2 or at most 24 hours.

I start the process of going backward from the B by asking, for example, "What happened just before you cut your arm?" Here I am asking for thoughts, emotions, physiological sensations, or external events that immediately preceded the B. Often the patient's response is something that happened quite a bit earlier (that is, the patient skips a lot of links). When this happens, I note down the information the patient gives me but then repeat my question about what happened *immediately before* the behavior in question. As you get information about the links, it is essential, as Linehan (1993a) notes in her beautiful description of behavioral chain analysis (pp. 258–264), not to give in to the temptation to assume you understand the connections between the links. Thus, when the patient indicates that one behavior (he told me he hated me and would not talk to me anymore) preceded another (I got on my knees and begged him to talk to me), it is important not to assume that you know the connection between these two events. Ask. In this case, when asked, the patient reported the important link: I felt panicky, as if I was about to die. As I collect information about the links, I write them down (in pencil, to allow for easy revision) on a blank piece of white paper so the patient and I can look at it together.

Patients typically have difficulty reporting information about antecedents. Often they weren't paying attention or were actively avoiding paying attention (this behavior is itself a maladaptive coping strategy). To aid in getting information about the As, the therapist can work with the patient to re-create the situation. Ask questions like: Where were you? What time was it? Who was there? What emotions were you experiencing? These often serve to re-evoke the situation to some degree and jog the patient's memory.

After going backward to identify the As that happened before the B, go forward to identify the Cs that happened after the B. Here the goal is to identify events that may be reinforcing or maintaining the problem behavior (such as relief from emotional distress, escape from aversive situations, or caring or other rewarding responses from others). Another goal is to identify consequences that may be punishing or weakening the problem behavior (such as physical pain, guilt, shame, or negative interactions with others).

FIGURE 3.6. Conducting a behavioral chain analysis. From Jacqueline B. Persons (2008). Copyright by The Guilford Press. Permission to photocopy this figure is granted to purchasers of this book for personal use only (see copyright page for details).

Antecedents (A)	Behaviors (B)	Consequences (C)
You can change the triggering events for a behavior by building in antecedents that lead to wanted behavior, and removing antecedents that lead to unwanted behavior.	You can change actions, thoughts, feelings, or behaviors by practicing desired acts or substituting desired alternatives for undesired actions.	You can change the events that follow your behavior to reinforce desired acts, and not reinforce undesired actions.

FIGURE 3.7. Changing As, Bs, and Cs. From Watson and Tharp (2002). Reprinted with permission of Wadsworth, a division of Thomson Learning: *www.thomsonrights.com.* Fax 800-730-2215.

A Case of Psychogenic Vomiting

Thomas was a 25-year-old young man who was brought by his family to the outpatient clinic where I was an intern for treatment of unexplained episodes of vomiting. Multiple workups had found no medical explanation for the vomiting. The problem had persisted for years. In fact, Thomas was one of those patients who was passed from one trainee to another in the hospital outpatient clinic. Each year a new trainee arrived on the scene and was assigned to his case. Now he was my patient. And the problem was getting worse. As a result of repeated episodes of vomiting, Thomas had an esophageal tear, meaning that each new episode of vomiting exposed him to a risk of bleeding to death. I conducted a behavioral analysis and learned that Thomas had a boring life. He had a low-normal IQ, and he was not working or going to school; he hung around the house, ignored by his family—until he had an episode of vomiting, when his mother mobilized to clean up the vomit, take him to the emergency room and spend hours with him there, bring him home and prop him up in front of the TV, and bring him soothing drinks and foods. Based on this information, I conceptualized the vomiting behavior as an operant that allowed Thomas to escape his boring and isolated life and gain the stimulation of the emergency room and the attention of medical professionals and his family, especially his mother. The functional analysis of Thomas's vomiting behavior is summarized in Figure 3.8.

This formulation led to a treatment plan that involved changing the antecedents by finding a day treatment program for Thomas and changing the consequences by dropping out the rewards for vomiting (his mother did not go with him to ER) and adding some punishments (Thomas cleaned up his own vomit). About four months were required to make all of these changes. However, within weeks of instituting them, Thomas's vomiting had ceased.

Antecedents (A)	Behaviors—actions, thoughts, or emotions (B)	Consequences (C)
Boredom Nothing to do No meaningful relationships	Vomiting	Attention from mother Special treatment at home (TV, food) Stimulation, activity

FIGURE 3.8. Functional analysis of Thomas's vomiting behavior.

A Case of Sexual Acting-Out Behavior

In the case of Helene, a careful analysis of antecedents and consequences, especially antecedents, helped her gain control of sexual acting-out behavior. Helene came to her session reporting, with shame, that she had had unprotected sex on the first date with a man she hardly knew and in fact was not much attracted to. She was upset with herself about this and felt a lack of control over her behavior. She noted that at the time of the behavior she had some dim awareness that she should not go forward, but did it anyway. Antecedents were a really long date on Saturday night and the awareness that she had no commitments the following morning.

We began by working to change some of those things, scheduling shorter dates and making Sunday-morning plans, including to call me and leave me a telephone message about how the date went. Helene viewed this last step as helpful because she knew she would find it very punishing to call me and tell me she had had sex again on a date. Helene reported that these interventions felt helpful but that she still did not feel in complete control of her behavior.

In a later session we worked on another dating issue. Helene was using an Internet dating service, and after beginning an e-mail correspondence with one man, she had lost interest and didn't want to continue to get to know him. A friend pointed out to her that she could just stop contacting him. She had not thought of doing this. She had felt that she needed to compose an elaborate e-mail message to explain why she was withdrawing. As we discussed why she did not just stop contact, it occurred to me that Helene had difficulty doing this because she was intimately involved emotionally with the man at some level, more than would be expected based on the level of their contact. This reminded me of the sexual acting out, where she plunged into a deeper level of intimacy with her date than was warranted by her relationship with him. What was this about?

In response to this question, Helene reported that she had spent hours fantasizing about these men. Even before meeting them she had already projected her relationship with them far into the future, including marriage, buying a home, introducing them to her extended family, and so forth. This fantasizing was a key antecedent to her behaviors of having unprotected sex on the first date and failing to realize she could withdraw as soon as she wanted to stop an introductory e-mail contact. As soon as we identified this antecedent, Helene immediately took action to stop it and was relieved to feel more in control of her behavior in the dating arena.

* * *

This chapter describes basic principles of *learning* theories and some information about how to use them in clinical work. These models provide an invaluable addition to the contributions of the *cognitive* models described in Chapter 2. The next chapter describes one more group of basic psychological models of psychopathology and their clinical applications: models of *emotion*.

FOUR

Emotion Theories
and Their Clinical Implications

Emotion theories offer mechanism hypotheses that can guide case formulation, treatment planning, and clinical decision making. In this chapter, I define emotion, describe its basic features, discuss the functions of emotions, and describe several basic emotion models. I describe cognitive-behavior therapies based on emotion models and flesh out some more general clinical applications of the models. I compare the emotion models presented in this chapter with the cognitive and learning models presented in Chapters 2 and 3. I conclude with a brief discussion of how to collect information to develop a formulation and to intervene based on the emotion models described in this chapter.

DEFINITION OF EMOTION

Emotion researchers typically rely on a definition of emotion that originated with William James (1884), namely that an emotion is *a response of a complex system that is designed to prepare an organism to respond to environmental stimuli that have evolutionary significance.* The most obvious example is the fight–flight–freeze response to a predator.

The notion that emotion has evolutionary significance has many useful clinical implications. As mentioned earlier, it can explain why we are more likely to develop phobias of things that were dangerous to our predecessors (e.g., snakes and humans with angry facial expressions) than of recently invented dangerous objects (e.g., guns and dentists' chairs) (Ohman & Mineka, 2001; Seligman, 1971). Psychoeducation about the survival value of emotions can be useful in helping patients shift from unproductive efforts to suppress or avoid emotional experience (e.g., "I shouldn't feel anxious in this situation") to acknowledgment, validation, and acceptance (e.g., "These reactions are here for a reason") (Barlow, Allen, & Choate, 2002; Borkovec, 1994; S. C. Hayes et al., 1999). For example, teaching patients that anger can be a type of fear response (the "fight" of the fight–flight–freeze response to a frightening situation) can help them understand and manage their anger better.

FEATURES OF EMOTION

Emotions are *brief*, lasting seconds to minutes (Ekman, 1992). Other terms, including *mood, affect,* or even *personality* (Barlow, 2002) are used to refer to longer-lasting states. The fact that emotion is brief suggests that one way to cope with painful emotions is simply to wait for the natural decay process to take place. Thus, in DBT, Linehan (2003a) teaches explicit strategies for tolerating unpleasant emotions and letting them pass without doing anything to worsen them or trigger them again.

Emotions, as Gross and Muñoz (1995) point out, have "an imperative quality." They grab our attention. Thus, fear serves as a signal that a life-threatening predator is on the scene and brings an immediate halt to all other activity. Helping patients understand this aspect of emotional functioning can increase their acceptance of painful emotions and even encourage them to adopt a stance of curiosity, asking "What can I learn from the presence of this emotion?"

Emotions are always a *response to some stimulus,* although, as Izard (1993) points out, the triggering stimulus can be an internal one (e.g., a memory). Information about the stimuli that trigger them can be useful in the process of developing strategies to manage emotions. Given that emotion is a response to a stimulus, one way not to have an unpleasant emotion is to escape or avoid the stimulus that triggers it. Often this strategy is adaptive, for example, escaping fear by leaving a situation that poses real danger (e.g., a violent altercation on the street). However, some clinical problems are the result of the overuse or underuse of this strategy. For example, people with anxiety disorders tend to avoid situations that are actually safe and the avoidance behavior itself often has significant negative consequences.

To the layperson, *emotion* is the subjective experience of feeling states. To the emotion researcher, subjective experience is simply one of several components of emotion. The others are behavioral (purposeful behavior, facial expression, nonverbal postures), physiological, and cognitive components.

The fact that emotion is a multiple-component phenomenon has several clinical implications. First, because the components are linked, changes in one component have the potential to produce changes in another. Levenson, Ekman, and Friesen (1990) showed that when actors used muscle movements to produce *facial expressions* of certain specific emotions, their *autonomic nervous system activity* and *verbal reports of subjective states* changed to match the emotion reflected by the facial expression (see also earlier studies of the James–Lange theory of emotion reviewed by Barlow, 2002). Similarly, Finzi and Wasserman (2006) reported the results of an uncontrolled study showing that Botox injections that eliminated frowning and muscle furrowing (facial expressions of unhappiness) relieved depression in 9 of 10 depressed women. Many cognitive-behavior therapists have developed interventions that capitalize on this insight, including Beck, who strives to change cognitions and behaviors in order to change the experiential component of emotion and Linehan (2000), who teaches the skill of taking action opposite to the action tendency of the emotion as a strategy for changing experiential emotion. The meditation practice of adopting a half smile is also understandable from this point of view.

Second, the degree of synchrony of the emotion's components is often clinically important. The elements of an emotional response are frequently desynchronous. That is, in Peter Lang's (1987) words, "Fear is not a lump." Desynchrony is often adaptive and often the clinician strives to help the patient achieve it. One example is to experience despair without acting on it. Acceptance-based therapies, especially acceptance and commitment therapy (ACT; S. C. Hayes et al., 1999), teach strategies that patients can use to promote desynchony. An example is purposely having the thought "I can't get out of bed" while simultaneously moving the needed muscles to get out of bed.

Desynchrony can also cause problems. For example, Kring, Kerr, Smith, and Neale (1993) showed that individuals with schizophrenia who have a flat emotional expression often have a normal subjective experience of emotion. It is easy to understand how this desynchrony could produce a host of interpersonal miscommunications (Keltner & Kring, 1998). In this type of situation, the therapist may wish to help the person promote synchrony or compensate for desynchrony of the elements of an emotional response.

Finally, desynchrony implies that subjective experience and other components of emotion can occur without cognitions (Zajonc, 1980, 1984; see also Clore & Ortony, 2000). This observation points to the need for noncognitive interventions to help people reduce painful emotional states.

FUNCTIONS OF EMOTIONS

The evolutionary view proposes that emotions serve functions essential to survival. Many of these involve social interactions (e.g., obtaining sex, rearing offspring, promoting cooperation, and avoiding conflict in the social group). Keltner and Kring (1998) proposed that the main social functions of emotions are to *signal important information to oneself and the communication partner, evoke emotional responses in others,* and *provide incentives for others' actions.*

Emotions Signal Information to Self and Others

Imagine what your life would be like if you had no subjective experience of emotion. As Levenson (1999, p. 497) points out, "subjective feeling helps us to clarify the way we feel, to think and talk about the events that led to the emotion, to make future plans concerning these events (e.g., to avoid or pursue situations that might be productive of these emotions), to share our feelings with others in ways that will elicit additional support from them, and to describe our feelings in ways that will cause others to alter their behaviours." Deficient subjective experience of emotion may in part account for the identity deficits of the patient with borderline personality disorder, the negative symptoms of schizophrenia, and the chaotic lives and interpersonal difficulties of patients with bipolar disorder and borderline personality disorder (see (Linehan, 1993a).

Consistent with the hypothesis that information about one's emotional experience aids in coping, Barrett, Gross, Christensen, and Benvenuto (2001) showed that patients who were better at making fine distinctions among emotional experiences, particularly negative emotions, were more able to regulate their emotions. This finding suggests that individuals who have emotion regulation deficits may benefit from psychoeducation about emotions and in particular from training in making fine discriminations in their emotional experience.

Some individuals appear to have emotion systems that undersignal, oversignal, or bounce back and forth between those two extreme positions. Underperception of danger may explain why some people experience multiple traumas. These individuals may have learned to cope with repeated traumas by ignoring internal emotional cues of danger because those cues did not provide any useful information (for example, the child could not escape repeated beatings, so learned to ignore fear cues). As a result of ignoring fear responses, these individuals place themselves in situations they view as safe but that in fact are dangerous. One of my patients, an attractive young woman who had an extensive history of sexual abuse, reported that she allowed a man who was a complete stranger to drive her home after he stopped to help when her car broke down. She gave me this information in passing in a bland tone of voice and did not perceive her behavior as problematic in any way.

Another example of how emotional experiencing provides information to the self is the emotion of embarrassment, which may serve the function of informing a person that he or she has violated social norms (R. S. Miller & Leary, 1992). In support of this notion, Keltner, Moffitt, and Stouthamer-Loerber (1995) showed that adolescent boys who displayed little embarrassment when they made social mistakes tended to have more antisocial behavior.

Emotions also communicate to others. Facial expression is one of the main ways we communicate emotions to others. When this method fails, significant communication difficulties can result. One of my patients had a strikingly mask-like face; she reported that she had learned as a child to inhibit facial expressions in order to avoid triggering rage in her alcoholic father. Several other patients presented a habitually placid, pleasant, or cheerful facial expression that was completely at odds with their subjective experience of distress. All these individuals used facial expression in a way that had helped them cope in the abusive environments in which they were reared but was not very helpful in other environments—including in the therapy session. I often made errors as I worked with these patients because I failed to correctly read their emotional state. These examples demonstrate that it is a mistake for the therapist to assume that the patient's facial expression is accurately signaling his or her subjective experience (Kring et al., 1993).

Many clinical problems result when individuals have deficits in their ability to receive emotional information. Individuals who have autism, Asperger syndrome, and other pervasive developmental disorders have deficits in their ability to read facial expressions and other emotional and social cues. When patients report interpersonal problems or appear to experience communication deficits in the session, therapists may want to investigate whether expressive or receptive deficits in facial expression and other communications of emotion might be present. Sometimes the cognitive-behavior therapist can do this; in other cases, specialized testing is needed (Gaus, 2007).

Emotions Evoke Emotions in Others

Emotion displays evoke emotional responses in others. For example, the expression of anger tends to elicit fear (Dimburg & Ohman, 1996) and the expression of sadness tends to elicit sympathy (Keltner & Haidt, 2001). Patients may be inadvertently receiving punishment or rewards from others as a result of this system, as in the woman with depression who was able to articulate her fear that if she recovered she would lose her husband's solicitous caretaking (Arkowitz & Westra, 2004). It is essential that the therapist remain aware of the possibility that warmth and sympathy can inadvertently reward passivity, crying, suicidality, or other maladaptive behaviors in their patients.

By monitoring their own emotional responses when they are interacting with their patients, therapists can obtain invaluable information, including about the emotional experiences of others in the patient's life. The fact that the patient's expression of emotions elicits emotions in the therapist likely underpins some of the features of multisystemic therapy (MST) for antisocial adolescents (Henggeler et al., 1998) and DBT for borderline personality disorder (Linehan, 1993a). To help therapists manage the negative emotions their patients elicit, both therapies explicitly call for the therapists to focus on clients' strengths and to work as part of a treatment team. The importance of attending to the emotions the patient elicits in the therapist also appears in CBASP for chronic depression (McCullough, 2000). McCullough emphasizes how important it is for the therapist to resist adopting the dominating stance evoked by the passivity of the patient with chronic depression because that stance can reinforce and worsen the patient's passivity.

Therapists can use the fact that emotions in one individual evoke emotions in another to help their patients regulate their emotions. Thus, when I am working with a patient who is experiencing extremely high fear or shame and who needs to modulate that intense state in order to work effectively in therapy, I work to calm my own emotions and to communicate that calmness in my posture, voice tone, and demeanor. By doing this, I can signal to my patient that the situation is safe and evoke calming emotional responses in the patient. Cesar Millan (Millan & Peltier, 2006) uses similar notions in his methods for teaching dog owners to manage fearful and other problem behaviors in their pets. His accounts are fascinatingly relevant to the psychotherapy process (Gladwell, 2006).

Emotions Provide Incentives to Others

Emotions reward behaviors in others. For example, a parent's positive emotional display rewards a child for performing desired behaviors. Depressed and anxious individuals often have facial expressions and other behaviors that negatively reinforce people for keeping their distance. Patients who express anger or hopelessness are not usually the ones that clinicians look forward to seeing.

Several cognitive-behavioral therapies make explicit use of the notion that emotional responses serve as incentives to others. Behavioral marital therapies (Stuart, 1980) typically begin with positive behavioral exchanges and other interventions to evoke positive emotionality that can serve as an incentive for additional behavioral change. Edwards, Barkley, and Robin's (1999) treatment for defiant teens begins by teaching parents to reinforce the teen's prosocial behaviors, often with emotional responses, in order to establish the parent as a positive reinforcer who can shape later behavioral change. As was discussed in the section on operant conditioning in Chapter 3, Kohlenberg and Tsai's (1994) functional analytic psychotherapy rests on the therapist's skill at using his or her behavior and emotional expressions in the therapy session as natural reinforcers to change patient behavior. When I'm working with a passive patient with depression and ask for some response, I try to lay back and let tension build until I get some sort of adaptive response from the patient, at which I point I lean forward and provide a dose of warmth and support. The therapist can also explicitly describe emotional contingencies in order to change patient behavior. A patient who was quite attached to me failed several times to complete her homework assignments. After simple reminders and some other efforts to solve the problem failed, I made a point of telling her explicitly that her failure to do the assignments was demoralizing me (it was). The next week she completed her assignment and when I asked what had changed her behavior, she stated, "I did my homework because I didn't want you to be demoralized."

MODELS OF EMOTION

Two broad views of emotions are the *discrete* view, which identifies and accounts for discrete emotions (such as fear, disgust, and sadness) and the *dimensional* view, which accounts for more general emotional states or dimensions, such as valence and arousal level.

The Discrete Emotions View

The discrete emotions view proposes that the emotional system recognizes a few specific emotions, with all other emotions being admixtures of these (Ekman, 1992). Although there is some disagreement, the list of discrete emotions generally includes fear, sadness, anger, disgust, happiness, and contentment. The discrete emotions model described by Levenson (1994; see also Gross & Muñoz, 1995) further proposes that emotions are governed by two distinct but partially communicating systems. These two systems are a *core system that is* hardwired and designed to accomplish evolutionarily adaptive functions (e.g., escape from danger) and a *control system* that regulates the activities of the core system.

The Core System

The core system scans incoming information from the environment. When it detects information that matches a prototype situation (e.g., a predator) it automatically activates stereotypical responses across multiple systems. The core system is viewed as having evolved a long time ago, being wired in the amygdala, and receiving little cortical input. Thus, as J. B. Rosen and Schulkin (1998, p. 486) point out using the example of fear, "although the experience of fear can be conscious, the brain mechanisms generating fear and the appraisal of stimuli as fearful are unconscious and automatic, similar to the workings of any other body organ." Ohman and Mineka (2001) further proposed that responses of the core system are *encapsulated*; that is, "once activated, a module tends to run its course with few possibilities for other processes to interfere with or stop it" (p. 485).

The Control System

The control system acts to modify the input to the core system by changing our appraisals of *incoming* information (e.g., appraising a bump from my husband in bed at night as an accident) and the *output* of the system (e.g., inhibiting the impulse to punch him)

(Levenson, 1999). Thus, although the activity of the core system is largely automatic and encapsulated, its input and output can be regulated to some degree by the control system.

The control system is viewed as more sensitive to learning than the core system. Gross (1998) described stages of emotion regulation, proposing that emotion can be regulated *before* it occurs (e.g., by choosing to place oneself in a particular situation or to avoid it), *during* its occurrence, and *after* it has been activated (e.g., by suppressing responses after they arise). Furthermore, multiple components of emotion (e.g., facial expression, experiencing) can be regulated.

Some emotion regulation strategies are more effective than others and some even have negative effects. Barrett et al. (2001) review data indicating that suppression strategies are not very effective at reducing negative emotional experience and impose costs by decreasing positive emotional experience and increasing activation of the sympathetic nervous system. Wegner (1994) proposed that the task of suppression requires the person to establish a two-part mechanism, one that monitors the to-be-suppressed material and one that suppresses. When the person is stressed or under a cognitive load, the suppression system breaks down and the monitoring system remains intact, resulting in intrusions of the material the person wants to suppress. Thus, efforts to suppress can produce intrusions (Wegner, 1994; Wenzlaff & Wegner, 2000). Suppressed thoughts just before sleep can even lead to intrusions in dreams (Wegner, Wenzlaff, & Kozak, 2004).

Implications for Conceptualization of Discrete Emotion Models

Many psychopathological disorders and symptoms can be conceptualized as resulting from excessive, deficient, and/or dysregulated discrete emotions. Some clinical problems can be viewed as an excess of emotional responding, including the panic of the patient with panic disorder, the anger of a person who has borderline personality disorder, or the disgust of the person with obsessive–compulsive disorder who fears contamination. Some problems can be seen as a dearth of emotional responding, such as anhedonia in schizophrenia and mood disorders, numbing and dissociation in PTSD, and feelings of emptiness in borderline personality disorder. Sometimes the problem is one of alternation between various intense emotional states, alternation between intense and flat emotional states (as in borderline personality disorder, bipolar disorder, or PTSD), or experiencing two states simultaneously (as in the mixed state in bipolar disorder). And many problems can be conceptualized as resulting from deficient or maladaptive regulation strategies, such as the use of excessive avoidance to manage fear or drugs and alcohol to manage anger and frustration.

Conceptualization using the discrete emotion view is complicated by the fact that emotional responses are driven by two tightly related systems (the core and control systems). As a result, it can be difficult to determine whether any particular emotional phenomenon is the result of the activation of or defects in the core system, the control system, or both (Kring & Werner, 2004). The numbing symptom of PTSD, for example, could result from insufficient activation of the core system, excessive activation of the control system, or both. This means that the therapist may need to consider more than one hypothesis about how core and control systems may be causing the patient's symptoms.

Implications for Intervention of Discrete Emotion Models

Intervention decisions for a problem that is conceptualized as caused by the responses of the core and control systems are based on what we know about those two systems and how they communicate. Treatment targets include the emotional responses generated by the core system and the faulty or deficient control system activities the patient is using in an attempt to regulate those emotions.

EMOTIONS CAN BE CHANGED BY INDUCING OTHER EMOTIONS

Some individuals have learned to use cutting, burning, and other self-mutilation to change their emotional state. These self-harm behaviors may trigger emotions that are of such vital evolutionary significance that they successfully "hijack" the emotional system and induce another emotional state, allowing the individual to escape a painful state that he is otherwise unable to exit. Linehan's temperature skill can be conceptualized as operating in this way. In the temperature skill, a person who is suffering from a painful state of high sympathetic nervous system arousal attempts to escape this state by activating intense parasympathetic arousal by plunging her head in a tub of ice water while holding her breath (Linehan & Korslund, 2004). Other interventions that operate to change an emotional state by activating another emotional state include Linehan's (1993a) use of irreverence, which can trigger surprise or incredulity, and Foa and Wilson's (1991) strategy of defusing the fears of a person with OCD by having the person sing a humorous song about the fear (see also the humorous poetry Bell, 2007, used to defuse his OCD fears).

Intense interpersonal connections (e.g., between patient and therapist) may also have the ability to reach the patient (and therapist!) at a visceral level and shift emotional states in a way that other methods cannot. This fact may explain in part why the therapeutic relationship assumes a more central role in DBT (which was developed to treat individuals who experience intense emotional states) than in other cognitive-behavior therapies. Similarly, Foa (2001) points to the importance of the therapeutic relationship in exposure therapy, which also evokes painful emotional states.

INTERVENTIONS TO PREVENT ACTIVATION OF INTENSE EMOTIONS ARE HELPFUL

If, as the model suggests, core emotion modules can't be stopped once they start, then therapeutic interventions must be developed to prevent activation of the core system. Therapies for mania and bipolar disorder consistently devote quite a bit of time to helping patients prevent manic episodes (see Basco & Rush, 1996; Frank, 2005; Miklowitz, 2002; Newman et al., 2002). A staple of DBT and therapies for anger and substance abuse (substances are often used to reduce painful emotions) is behavioral chain analysis, which can identify events leading up to painful emotional states in order to develop strategies to interrupt the chain the next time it starts or to prevent it from starting at all.

COGNITIVE INTERVENTIONS DO NOT CHANGE SOME EMOTIONS

The two-part discrete emotion model, consisting of core and control systems, accounts neatly for our common experience that we have two modes of knowing: a visceral/emotional/gut one and a logical/intellectual one (see also Barnard & Teasdale, 1991). In fact, this two-system view is part of the DSM (American Psychiatric Association, 2000) definition of phobia. Patients who meet criteria for a phobia experience fear in the presence of an object or situation that they know is not dangerous. As I write this material, I am having both of those experiences as I contemplate an upcoming dental procedure. I'm having both a visceral fear response and cognitions that the procedure is safe. The two-part discrete emotion model tells me that cognitive interventions can modulate the responses of the core system (e.g., can soften my dental fear response a bit) but will not stop it completely. This is because in the discrete emotion model, my visceral fear response results from the activation of a core system located in the midbrain that has only limited communication with my cerebral cortex (LeDoux, 1989). This information is helpful to me as I work to manage my fear. It tells me that efforts to suppress the fear are not likely to be helpful (and may even be counterproductive) and guides me to shift my energy to promote tolerance and acceptance of the fear. So I am working to distract myself so as to feel a bit better while waiting for the fear to dissipate.

INTERVENTIONS TO PROMOTE TOLERANCE OF INTENSE EMOTIONS ARE HELPFUL

If core emotional responses, once started, cannot be stopped, then interventions of acceptance, mindfulness, distress tolerance, self-soothing, and harm reduction (which are staples of DBT, treatments for substance abuse, treatments for anger, and behavioral exposure treatments for anxiety) are essential. These are skills that allow a person, for example, to experience a panic attack without fleeing, intense self-hate, or self-harm. Another way of viewing these interventions is that they attempt to deactivate the behavioral element of the emotional system or detach it from the other elements.

INTERVENTIONS TO REDUCE SUPPRESSION ARE HELPFUL

As noted above in the description of the control system, quite a bit of evidence indicates that suppression of thoughts and feelings leads to negative results. Several cognitive-behavior therapies capitalize on these ideas, including exposure-based treatments (which promote experiencing and approaching feared thoughts and feelings), acceptance-based therapies like acceptance and commitment therapy (ACT; S. C. Hayes et al., 1999), and mindfulness-based interventions for depression (Segal et al., 2002) and generalized anxiety (Mennin, 2004; Roemer & Orsillo, 2002).

PRETREATMENT CONTRACTING CAN HELP REGULATE INTENSE EMOTIONS

Several therapies emphasize the need to obtain a firm commitment from the patient who begins treatment to comply with it and complete it. These commitments are important because when intense emotions appear on the scene, the patient will have compelling urges to do other than what effective treatment requires. Steketee (1993) asks patients seeking exposure and response prevention for OCD to sign a contract before they begin treatment stating that they will adhere to and complete treatment. DBT requires patients to agree to goals of stopping suicidal and self-harming behavior as a condition of treatment.

INTERVENTIONS TO TEACH EMOTION REGULATIONS SKILLS ARE HELPFUL

Many clinical phenomena can be conceptualized as resulting from patients' failure to acquire or use good emotion regulation strategies. Problem behaviors such as avoidance, compulsive rituals, substance abuse, excessive emotional dependence on others, binge eating, self-harming, suicidality, and even rumination and worry (cf. Borkovec, 1994) can all be conceptualized as maladaptive emotion regulation strategies.

Many individuals appear to have learned emotion regulation strategies that were effective in managing abusive situations they experienced in childhood but that are no longer very adaptive. One of my patients learned as a child to use fantasy as a way to escape from her parents' drunken fights, which she could not escape in any other way. Although adaptive when she was a helpless child, this strategy for coping with distress served her poorly as an adult, when more active strategies (e.g., searching for a new job when she was laid off) were needed.

A FOCUS ON PARTICULAR DISCRETE EMOTIONS CAN BE HELPFUL

Discrete emotion models draw nuanced distinctions between emotional states in a way that dimensional models (described below) do not. These distinctions are important in some clinical situations. DBT does a good job of highlighting states that are particularly problematic for patients with borderline personality disorder and that require focused therapeutic attention, such as shame and contempt; Linehan and Manning (2005) propose that contempt is an aspect of disgust. It is therapeutically helpful to identify the emotion of disgust in the patient who has OCD and to distinguish it from fear because the clinician can't assume that disgust will habituate during exposure-based treatment in the same way fear does (Olatunji, Sawchuk, Lohr, & de Jong, 2004).

TREATMENT IN PHASES IS NEEDED FOR SOME PATIENTS

Successful exposure treatment for pathological fears generally requires that patients be able to tolerate painful emotional states without carrying out impulsive and self-destructive behaviors. However, not all patients can do this. To address this dilemma, Linehan (1993a) carries out DBT in stages, teaching emotion regulation skills before treating the PTSD that many patients with borderline personality disorder suffer.

TELEPHONE COACHING CAN BE HELPFUL

When intense emotions are activated, logical reasoning goes off-line and it is easy to forget new coping tools learned in therapy. As Linehan (1993a) points out, the concept here is similar to that of coaching in basketball. During practice the coach teaches new skills. However, in the heat of the game the players become emotionally aroused and forget the skills. When this happens, the coach calls a time out and offers coaching to help the players recall the skills they learned in practice. Similarly, when our patients become emotionally aroused, their core system is activated, their cerebral cortex is not fully engaged, and they forget the skills they learned in the therapy session. They need coaching in the moment to help them remember the skills when they are emotionally activated. For this reason, telephone coaching is an essential component of DBT and also may be needed to effectively treat other patients who experience surges of intense emotion, such as those with bipolar disorder, impulse control disorder, depression, and anxiety disorders.

TEAM TREATMENT CAN BE HELPFUL

As noted above, individuals who experience intense emotions and have problem behaviors can evoke emotions in the therapist that make treatment difficult. To address this issue, therapies like DBT and MST require that treatment be done by a team that can help the therapist manage his or her negative emotions and stay on track with the treatment plan.

CBTS BASED ON DISCRETE EMOTION MODELS

Linehan's (1993a, 1993b) DBT is based on a conceptualization of the symptoms of borderline personality disorder as resulting from deficits in both the core and control emotional systems. Linehan uses the term *emotional vulnerability* to refer to the core system deficit in borderline personality disorder. *Emotional vulnerability* consists of high emotional sensitivity to environmental stimuli, intense emotions, and a slow return to baseline after emotions are triggered. The DBT formulation also proposes that individuals who have borderline personality disorder have failed to learn and use good strategies to regulate the intense emotions that arise as a result of the emotional vulnerability deficit, and instead often do so by using maladaptive strategies, including avoidance, self-harm, suicide, or substance use. A review of the (mixed) evidence supporting these propositions is provided by Koerner and Dimeff (2007).

Based on this conceptualization, the treatment targets of DBT (Linehan, 1993a) are the emotional vulnerability and the emotion regulation strategies. DBT strives to teach patients tools to reduce emotional vulnerability and to replace maladaptive with adaptive emotion regulation strategies. DBT has been shown to be effective in treating suicidal behavior, borderline personality disorder, substance use, binge eating, and depression with comorbid personality disorder (Dimeff & Koerner, 2007).

Other cognitive-behavior therapies that rely in some way on aspects of discrete emotion theory include the emotion regulation therapy developed by Mennin (2004) for generalized anxiety disorder, which views worry as a maladaptive emotion regulation strategy; ACT, developed by S. C. Hayes et al. (1999), which proposes that psychopathology often arises from efforts to avoid and suppress emotion; mindfulness-based strategies to treat anxiety and depression (Roemer & Orsillo, 2002; Segal et al., 2002); and behavioral activation (BA; Martell et al., 2001). All of these therapies teach patients to replace maladaptive emotion regulation strategies with more adaptive acceptance-based ones. In addition, Beevers et al. (1999) reviewed evidence that individuals with depression use maladaptive emotion regulation strategies (in particular, they overuse suppression) and described more adaptive emotion regulation strategies that they can use. Many of these strategies were drawn from current cognitive-behavior and mindfulness-based therapies.

The Dimensional View of Emotion

Dimensional models do not contradict discrete emotion models. They simply offer an alternative view. Instead of focusing on discrete states, dimensional models focus on broad overarching dimensions. Two dimensional models, the approach and withdrawal model and Peter Lang's bioinformational theory (Lang, Cuthbert, & Bradley, 1998), have implications for the conceptualization and treatment of psychopathology.

The Approach and Withdrawal System Model

The approach and withdrawal system perspective was originally developed by Gray (1973), who described emotions as resulting from three affective–motivational systems: the behavioral inhibition system (BIS), the behavioral activation system (BAS), and the fight–flight system (FFS). The primary element of the model is the BIS. When the BIS detects certain types of stimuli (nonreward, punishment, novelty), it orients the organism's attention toward the stimulus, suppresses ongoing behavior, activates withdrawal behavior, and generates anxiety and other negative affect. Gray views an overactive BIS as the biological basis of anxiety. The BAS system responds to signals of reward and nonpunishment (safety signals) by facilitating approach and appetitive behavior and positive affect like elation, excitement, and interest. An underactive approach system is seen as causing depression and anhedonia, and an overactive approach system is seen as causing mania and impulsivity. The third system, the FFS, responds to unconditioned pain and frustrative nonreward with surges of autonomic arousal and action tendencies of escape, avoidance, and defensive aggression. The FFS system is viewed as underpinning fear and panic reactions.

Watson and Clark developed a tripartite model of mood and anxiety disorders that they tied to the BIS–BAS model. D. Watson, Wiese, Vaidya, and Tellegen (1999) proposed that emotional states have two dimensions, positive affect (PA) and negative affect (NA), where a high degree of PA results in active, elated, enthusiastic, excited states, and a high degree of NA results in fearful, hostile, nervous, distressed, scornful, guilty states. Sometimes a third dimension of physiological arousal (termed anxious arousal, AA), corresponding roughly to the FF system of Gray, is added, thus creating a tripartite model. D. Watson et al. (1999) argued that NA is the subjective component of BIS activation and PA the subjective component of BAS activation. A revision to the model was later proposed to better account for the heterogeneity among the anxiety disorders (Mineka, Watson, & Clark, 1998). The revised model, termed the integrative hierarchical model, proposes that high AA is more characteristic of panic disorder than other anxiety disorders (T. A. Brown, Chorpita, & Barlow, 1998; Zinbarg & Barlow, 1996).

Clinical Implications of the Approach and Withdrawal System Model

Strauman et al. (2001) have developed a therapy and reported some initial efficacy data (Strauman et al., 2006) for patients with depression that is based in part on the approach and withdrawal model's predictions that these patients would benefit from interventions to help them increase their ability to approach important personal goals and decrease inhibition behaviors. In addition, the approach/withdrawal/tripartite dimensional model has numerous useful clinical implications (see also Barlow, 2002; Kring & Bachorowski, 1999).

HIGH RATES OF COMORBIDITY OF ANXIETY AND DEPRESSION

The model accounts for the high rates of comorbidity of anxiety and depression. D. Watson et al. (1999) have theorized that the BAS and BIS operate in a mutually inhibitory way, so that an underactivation of the BAS (resulting in sadness and anhedonia) is typically accompanied by an overactivation in the BIS (resulting in anxiety) (see also Depue & Iacono, 1989; Kasch, Rottenberg, Arnow, & Gotlib, 2002).

EXTENSIVE OVERLAP OF SYMPTOMS OF ANXIETY AND DEPRESSION

The approach and withdrawal model also accounts for the extensive overlap in symptoms of anxiety and depression. It is difficult, for example, to develop a measure of one that does not include symptoms of the other (e.g., fatigue, insomnia, and difficulty concentrating are symptoms that commonly appear on both anxiety and depression scales (Dobson & Cheung, 1990). D. Watson et al. (1999) accounted for this overlap by proposing that BIS activation produces NA, an undifferentiated negative state that is characteristic of both anxiety and depression.

CONCEPTUALIZING A RANGE OF DISPARATE SYMPTOMS AS NEGATIVE AFFECT

The proposal flowing out of the approach and withdrawal system model is that many patients are troubled by undifferentiated states of negative affect. This suggests that it is not always important for the therapist to determine precisely which emotion the patient is experiencing in order to treat it effectively. Is it anxiety? Is it depression? Using the approach and withdrawal model, a state of NA that shares characteristics of both depression and anxiety can be targeted for treatment. This notion makes good clinical sense. Many patients seek treatment for problems (e.g., an unsatisfying job or an unhappy marriage) that are making them miserable and they are not very concerned about the precise details of their misery. This conceptualization is also consistent with the fact that when anxious depressed patients improve, much of the change they experience is due to changes in NA, which is common to both anxiety and depressive symptoms (Kring, Persons, & Thomas, 2007; Mohr et al., 2005; Schmid, Freid, Hollon, & DeRubeis, 2002; Tomarken, Dichter, Freid, Addington, & Shelton, 2004). It is also consistent with the fact that many of the same psychosocial interventions (e.g., cognitive restructuring, behavioral activation/exposure) and pharmacological compounds are used to treat both anxiety and depression.

DECREASING NEGATIVE AFFECT IS NOT THE SAME AS INCREASING POSITIVE AFFECT

Another clinically useful aspect of the approach and withdrawal model (and also, in fact, of the discrete emotion model) is that it highlights the fact that decreasing negative affect is not the same thing as increasing positive affect. Different interventions may be needed to accomplish these two goals and psychologists would benefit from attending more to increasing positive affect.

Although psychologists have spent quite a bit of time thinking about negative affect and how to reduce it, they have spent relatively little time thinking about positive affect and how to increase it. Exceptions include the positive psychology movement (Seligman, Steen, Park, & Peterson, 2005) and Frederickson's (2001) work on positive emotions. Frederickson proposes that positive emotions widen the array of thoughts and actions that come to mind and help the individual build new approaches through the generation of enduring personal resources. Treatment developers who have made contributions in this area include Linehan (DBT; 1993a) and Gilbert and Procter (compassionate mind training [CMT]; 2006). Both emphasize teaching skills for self-soothing and compassion to patients who are prone to shame, self-criticism, and self-hate. Earlier contributions in this area include progressive relaxation (Bernstein & Borkovec, 1973), pleasant activity scheduling (Lewinsohn, Gotlib, & Hautzinger, 1998), and even systematic desensitization (Wolpe, 1958).

The approach and withdrawal model provides an elegant and parsimonious explanation of the phasic nature of disorders like bipolar disorder, cyclothymia, and borderline personality disorder. The model views the bipolar patient's excitable impulsive states as due to overactivation of the same system (the BAS) that, when underactivated, produces depressed mood and passive behavior (Depue & Iacono, 1989; Gray, 1990). For example, my patient Serena alternated between angry agitated states and disengaged shutdown states. In fact, Serena sought treatment for the angry agitated states and I did not identify the disengaged shutdown states until several months into treatment, when Serena reported spending hours every day playing computer games, an activity she liked for many reasons, including that it helped her avoid and escape her angry agitated states. Conceptualizing Serena's two extreme states as dynamically linked helped me focus on teaching her to modulate her extreme emotional experiencing and behavior (find the middle ground) rather than simply teaching her strategies to manage each state in isolation, without reference to the other.

Using the Approach and Withdrawal System Model to Guide Conceptualization and Treatment of a Complex Case: Susan

Susan met criteria for borderline personality disorder, bipolar disorder, and PTSD, and had a recent history of cocaine and amphetamine abuse. She felt chronically unmotivated, anhedonic, and bored. In fact when I first met her she complained of rarely having feelings at all. She was also poor at "follow-through"—she started lots of things and didn't finish them. All of these problems can be conceptualized as resulting from an underactive BAS.

Susan also had occasional angry episodes. One involved a physical fight with her (former) boss. These episodes can be conceptualized as resulting from an overactive BAS. Susan also used cocaine, amphetamines, shoplifting, partying, and, in general, "living on the edge" to alleviate boredom and add sparkle and interest to her life. These behaviors can be seen as maladaptive strategies to boost an underactive BAS and/or as the result of an episodically overactive BAS.

Finally, Susan tended to disengage (by sleeping, drinking alcohol, watching TV, and reading) in response to any discomfort or problem of even the smallest sort. When stressed, Susan took to her bed, staying there for days or weeks, sleeping and watching TV and refusing to answer the telephone, return calls, or keep appointments with friends or doctors. These disengagement behaviors can be accounted for by the hypothesis that her BIS was overactive and/or because her BAS was underactive, she did not have valued goals that promoted behavior in the service of those goals even in the face of discomfort.

Not surprisingly, Susan's life was stalled in many ways. Despite her high intelligence, she had not finished college and at age 42 was working odd jobs and making very little money (she was supported by an inheritance). She had a boyfriend who was unemployed and, in fact, was married to another woman.

The beauty of using the approach and withdrawal system to conceptualize Susan's case is that it accounts for a multitude of diverse problems with one model, namely that Susan had a BAS that was mostly underactive but occasionally overactive, and a BIS that was overactive. Treatment based on this conceptualization involved teaching Susan the conceptualization and carrying out a variety of interventions to address Susan's approach and withdrawal system dysfunctions. To address BAS underactivation, I used motivational interviewing strategies (W. R. Miller & Rollnick, 2002) to help Susan identify valued goals and to increase discrepancy between her current situation and her goals so as to increase motivation to change. Susan stated that she wanted to learn to follow through with things so she could finish her college degree and get a good job to earn enough money to buy a nice car. I also worked with Susan to identify the dysfunctionality of her BAS overactivity. This too required a bit of motivational interviewing, as Susan was reluctant to give up her reputation (with herself and others) as "having a wild life." However, after quite a bit of work, including reviewing pros and cons of her current lifestyle, including her physical fight with her former boss, Susan decided that "I have to make a change." Once she reached that conclusion, Susan began learning skills to modulate her aggressive feelings and impulsive behaviors. She learned to restrain impulsivity (e.g., the urge to quit her job) by waiting 24 hours before implementing any important decision. She also learned strategies to override her (BIS-activated) tendency to withdraw and disengage. Susan learned to anticipate early signs of disengagement (e.g., the urge to call in sick) before she carried them out and to take steps to reengage quickly when she disengaged (e.g., after she overslept one morning she called her employer promptly to apologize and explain that she would arrive late). Medications also helped, especially lithium, which helped Susan control impulsive aggressive behavior.

Susan made nice progress in getting her life on track. When asked what had helped her most in therapy, she responded: "I learned that when a problem comes up, if I approach it and work to solve it instead of avoiding it, I have a much better life. I also learned to focus on my goals and use those—not my mood at that moment—to decide how to handle a situation."

Peter Lang's Bioinformational Theory

Peter Lang's (1979; Lang et al., 1998) theory of emotion proposes that emotions are represented in memory as linked propositions (cognitions) of three types: propositions about the *stimulus* elements (e.g., a big spider and its hairy legs), *response* elements (e.g., running, increased heart rate), and *meaning* elements (e.g., "I'll get bitten and die an agonizing death") of a stimulus. If a person is presented with information that matches enough of the elements in the network of propositions, the emotion is triggered. The cognitive networks are tied to two primary motivational systems in the lower brain: an appetitive system (food, drink, sex) and a defensive system (safety).

Lang's model is a hybrid of discrete and dimensional emotion models, in that he identifies the discrete emotion of fear but links it to dimensional motivational systems in the lower brain. Cognitions play a central role in Lang's theory. However, the theory allows for subjective emotions to occur without cognitive mediation or awareness if enough stimulus and response elements are matched to trigger the emotion program without activating the meaning elements. Lang views most emotional responses as the product of learning and conditioning, although some can be innate.

Clinical Implications of Lang's Theory

Lang's (1979; Lang et al., 1998) theory has useful implications for the conceptualization and treatment of pathological fears (Foa et al., 2006; Foa & Kozak, 1986; Foa, Hembree, & Rothbaum, 2007; Foa & Rothbaum, 1998). Lang proposes that pathological fears can be conceptualized as arising when the individual learns problematic connections in his or her propositional network, such as the links between the response element of tachycardia and the meaning element of heart attack in the fear network of a person who has agoraphobia (see Figure 4.1). To overcome the pathological fear, Lang's theory proposes that the emotion network must be activated and disconfirming information must be presented in a way that allows the individual to create new response and meaning elements for the stimulus elements in the situation. When these two things occur, *emotional processing* occurs. In the case of the agoraphobia example in Figure 4.1, successful emotional processing results in changing the links between the propositions in the fear network, so that the proposition of "tachycardia" is no longer linked to the "heart attack" proposition (see Figure 4.2).

Although no ESTs were developed on the basis of Lang's theory, Foa et al. (2006) and Foa and Kozak (1986) drew on Lang and on Rachman (1980) to propose that *emotional processing* is the mechanism of action of behavioral exposure treatments for fears and phobias. The emotional processing model proposes that cognitive change happens

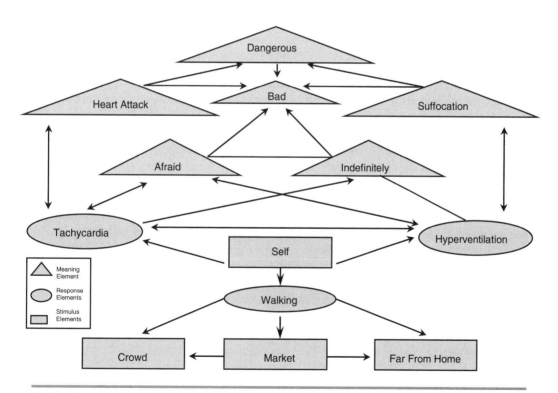

FIGURE 4.1. Schematic agoraphobic fear network. Adapted from Foa and Kozak (1986, p. 29). Copyright 1986 by the American Psychological Association. Adapted by permission.

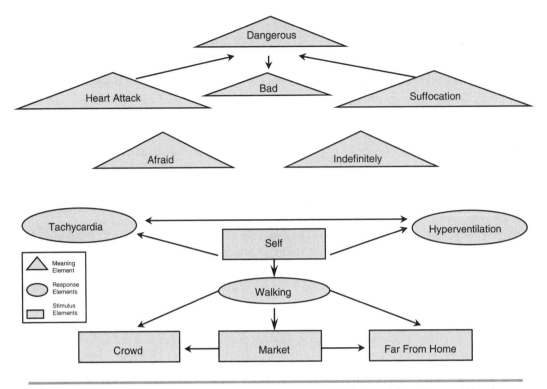

FIGURE 4.2. Schematic network after emotional processing. Adapted from Foa and Kozak (1986, p. 29). Copyright 1986 by the American Psychological Association. Adapted by permission.

in addition to extinction of conditioned responses during exposure-based treatment for pathological fears, and that the cognitive and conditioning processes are related.

The proposal that cognitive change can happen in addition to habituation and extinction during exposure-based treatment has important implications for treatment procedures. One is that the decrease in fear (typically measured by asking the patient to rate subjective units of distress [SUDS] every 5 minutes) may not follow the smooth curve expected by an extinction or habituation model. This is because reorganization of the fear network in response to exposure to corrective information typically produces a more erratic pattern of changes in fear ratings (Foa, 2001). Another is that the therapist must attend to the stimulus, response, and meaning elements of the fear situation in order to promote the needed changes in the fear network. Another is that the therapist can carry out some cognitive interventions to help along the change process, especially the change in the meaning elements of the fear network. In contrast, in an exposure treatment viewed as operating via habituation or extinction, the therapist's role is simply to help the patient confront the fear stimulus and refrain from avoidance behaviors. Thus, the emotional processing model provides an integration of learning and cognitive views of the process of overcoming pathological fears (Foa & McNally, 1996; Foa et al., 1989).

The fact that in the emotional processing model activating the fear network is a precondition of change has many clinical implications. One, as Samoilov and Goldfried (2000) point out, is that cognitive-behavior therapists would benefit from using experiential and other methods to evoke emotion in the therapy session rather than working too quickly to diminish emotional responding. The therapists can also use this idea to remind themselves that it is good news when patients are having problem behaviors or emotional states in the therapy session (e.g., experiencing rage and attacking the therapist): it means that the problematic emotion networks are activated and thus available for change (Kohlenberg & Tsai, 1991; W. R. Miller & Rollnick, 2002).

Lang's model also provides a good account of what is typically called mood-state-dependent thinking and behavior but which, in this discussion, might better be called emotion-dependent thinking and behavior. The model proposes that when a particular memory network is activated, the subjective emotions and behaviors associated with the network are also activated, as are other memory networks that share elements with it. Thus, when the patient's emotional state is sad, he or she is likely to report many negative memories, negative predictions about the future, and negative self-assessments. That is, "emotions act as magnets for like memories" (Levenson, 1999, p. 498). One clinical implication of emotion-state dependence is that accurate assessment of the problematic memory network may require some sort of prime to activate it (Persons & Miranda, 1992; Segal et al., 2006). Barlow's panic control treatment (PCT) uses this idea by evaluating the patient's distress in response to somatic sensations *after* evoking the sensations.

Emotion-state dependence also suggests that if the therapist can in any way shift the patient's emotions, his or her thinking and behavior and other aspects of emotional functioning are likely to shift as well. Bower (1981) illustrated this phenomenon with the example of Sirhan Sirhan, who did not recall shooting Robert F. Kennedy until the intense emotional state he experienced when he carried out the shooting was re-evoked. At that point, he recounted the shooting in vivid detail.

Lang's model also accounts for situations in which individuals who have good coping skills in some situations fail to use them in other situations. The model suggests that the recall and use of skills may be emotion-state dependent (that is, they fail to generalize to other emotion states). The therapist can help by teaching the patient generalization skills or tools that will help him or her recall and implement coping skills when in multiple emotional states. This is one of the rationales for the telephone component of DBT. On the telephone the therapist can help the patient remember and use, in a highly charged emotional situation, skills that were learned in calmer emotional states. This notion also underpins the use of coping cards that patient and therapist develop and write in the therapy session that the patient can read to guide management of emotions, or even a manic episode, outside the session (Frank, 2005). Following this line of thinking, Sheri Johnson is developing an intervention for mania in which she first teaches the patient strategies to calm elated and manic states. Then she uses a musical induction to trigger those states and helps the patient practice using the calming strategies while in the elated state (Johnson, 2007). Similarly, Deffenbacher and McKay (1998) use interventions that involve purposefully activating anger in order to practice anger management skills while angry.

COMPARING COGNITIVE, LEARNING, AND EMOTION-FOCUSED THEORIES AND THERAPIES

The cognitive and learning theories described in Chapters 2 and 3 often view emotions as problems and emotional expression as something to be stopped or decreased. In contrast, emotion theorists view emotions as arising from an evolutionary heritage and serving important functions that facilitate adaptive behavior. In fact, Samoilov & Goldfried (2000) posit that a vital part of psychotherapy is in-session emotional arousal that promotes "reorganization of underlying emotional themes, assimilation of new information, and formation of new implicit meaning structures" (p. 383).

At the same time, there is considerable overlap among theories of emotion (this chapter), cognition (Chapter 2), and learning (Chapter 3). Because it is defined as a multicomponent entity, emotion includes cognitions and behaviors and thus in some sense subsumes the cognitive and learning models described in Chapters 2 and 3. Lang's theory of emotion, for example, explicitly includes cognitive and conditioning elements and Barlow (2002) describes Beck's theory as one of several cognitive theories of emotion. And much of the discussion of learning models in Chapter 3 focuses on conditioned emotional responses—that is, the conditioning of emotional responses to neutral cues.

Although they arise out of different theoretical frameworks, the overlap of the various theories also appears in the way that A. T. Beck's behavioral activity scheduling interventions (Beck et al., 1979), Lewinsohn's behavioral treatment (Lewinsohn & Gotlib, 1995), McCullough's cognitive and behavioral analysis system of psychotherapy (CBASP; 2000), and the behavioral activation treatment developed by Martell et al. (2001) are all consistent with the approach and withdrawal systems view of depression. All of these therapies propose that effective treatment helps individuals with depression become more active and engaged with their environment, especially in ways that increase positive affect.

Despite their overlap, emotion theories and therapies do not make cognitive and learning conceptualizations and interventions superfluous. Emotion theories and therapies cast a different lens on the same phenomena, causing our eye to focus on different aspects of the phenomena and leading to new conceptualizations and interventions that provide useful alternatives to the cognitive and learning ones.

ASSESSMENT AND INTERVENTION GUIDED BY EMOTION THEORIES

Here I describe strategies that can be used to collect the information necessary for a conceptualization based on one of the emotion models described above and I say a bit more about intervention based on the emotion models described in this chapter.

Collecting Information for the Formulation

The assessment information the therapist seeks depends on which emotion model the therapist is using (e.g., a discrete emotion model or a dimensional one like Gray's approach and withdrawal systems model). I discuss details specific to the various models below. However, in all the models, emotions are multifaceted and include behavior and cognitions. Thus, to assess emotions, the therapist can use many of the tools described in Chapters 2 and 3, including the Thought Record (Figure 2.3), the Activity Schedule (Figure 2.2), and the Event Log (Figure 3.5), which is used to assess target behaviors and their antecedents and consequences. In addition, the therapist who is guided by emotion theory attends to facial expression (or lack of it), voice tone, posture, and other aspects of emotion behavior. Paul Ekman's work, including a set of DVDs that teach skills to identify very brief facial expressions of emotion (Ekman, 2003, 2004) can help the therapist with the task of identifying facial expressions. In addition, as described above, emotions in one person can evoke emotions in another. This fact means that therapists can obtain information about the patient's emotions by attending to their own emotional reactions.

Using Discrete Emotion Models

Therapists who are using discrete emotion models to conceptualize a case will want to collect information about the discrete emotions the patient is experiencing (the core system) and the regulation strategies he or she is using (the control system). The therapist can begin by simply asking for a verbal report: "What emotion are you feeling now/ were you feeling then? Fear? Shame? Both?" Sometimes patients can answer this question easily. However, many patients are not very skilled at identifying their emotions and will need help from the therapist. To provide this help, it can be useful to work with the patient to re-evoke memories and images of the problematic situation. Visual and other sensory images may be particularly useful because there is some evidence that they are tied more tightly to emotions than are verbal representations (Arntz & Wertman, 1999; Holmes & Mathews, 2005). This strategy provides information that the therapist can use to help the patient identify his or her emotions. For example, re-evoking the situation may elicit facial expressions in the patient that will give the therapist information about the patient's likely emotional experience in the situation. Sometimes the patient reports secondary emotions that were triggered by primary emotions not immediately apparent to the patient without careful questioning by the therapist.

The patient can also use the Daily Log provided in Chapter 9 (Figure 9.5) or a personal digital assistant or the Event Log (Figure 3.5) to record emotions and regulation strategies. Self-monitoring here serves both as an assessment tool and an intervention, as it will help increase the patient's awareness of emotions and regulation strategies and this is very likely to improve his or her emotion management abilities.

The therapist can also use some of the assessment tools described in Chapter 3 to get detailed information about control system activities the patient is using in an attempt to regulate emotions. The patient can use the Event Log (Figure 3.5) to log maladaptive emotion regulation strategies in the B (Behavior) column and to record the As (antecedents) and Cs (consequences) that precede and follow the B in order to obtain information about the function of the emotion regulation strategy. The therapist can teach the patient to carry out a detailed behavioral chain analysis (Figure 3.6) of the As leading up to particular instances of problem Bs and the Cs that follow. Over the course of repeated chain analyses, patient and therapist gain an increasingly fine-grained picture of the variables controlling a particular problem B.

Using Dimensional Models

To collect information for a conceptualization based on the approach and withdrawal system model, the therapist can use the Mood Chart developed by Michael A. Tompkins (2004) that is presented in Figure 4.3. The patient logs his or her mood at the same time

86

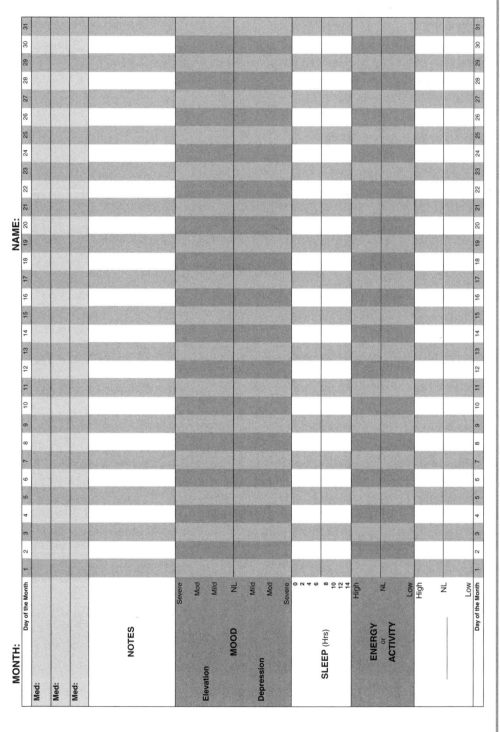

FIGURE 4.3. Mood Chart. Adapted from Tompkins (2004). Copyright 2004 by The Guilford Press. Reprinted by permission in Jacqueline B. Persons (2008). Permission to photocopy this figure is granted to purchasers of this book for personal use only (see copyright page for details).

every day by entering a dot at some point in the Mood section of the chart. The chart can also be used to track activity, energy, medications, sleep, menstrual cycle, or other phenomena that might be tied to mood. A visual inspection of the chart can generate some testable hypotheses about how and whether these phenomena might be related. The chart's monthly format and visual layout allow the patient and therapist to identify dynamic relationships over time that often lend themselves to conceptualization using the approach and withdrawal system model, as in the case of Susan, above. In addition, as with the other self-monitoring tools described here, the Mood Chart increases emotion awareness. Some patients, when I first ask them to complete the chart, report that they have great difficulty identifying the valence of their emotions. With practice, their ability to do this improves.

Another useful assessment tool when using the approach and withdrawal system model is the Positive and Negative Affect Schedule (PANAS) developed by D. Watson, Clark, and Tellegen (1988), which appears in Figure 4.4. The PANAS contains 20 emotion adjectives and was designed to measure PA and NA, where PA assesses the experiential component of BAS activation and NA assesses the experiential component of BIS activation. The scales have been shown to be internally consistent and largely uncorrelated (D. Watson et al., 1988).

This scale consists of a number of words that describe different feelings and emotions. Read each item and then mark the appropriate answer in the space next to that word. Indicate to what extent you have felt this way during the past week. Use the following scale to record your answers.

1	2	3	4	5
very slightly or not at all	a little	moderately	quite a bit	extremely

_____ interested	_____ irritable
_____ distressed	_____ alert
_____ excited	_____ ashamed
_____ upset	_____ inspired
_____ strong	_____ nervous
_____ guilty	_____ determined
_____ scared	_____ attentive
_____ hostile	_____ jittery
_____ enthusiastic	_____ active
_____ proud	_____ afraid

FIGURE 4.4. The Positive and Negative Affect Schedule (PANAS). From D. Watson, Clark, and Tellegen (1988). Copyright 1988 by the American Psychological Association. Reprinted by permission.

To complete the PANAS requires only 1 or 2 minutes. Patients indicate using a 5 point Likert scale (1 = very slightly or not at all; 5 = extremely) the extent to which they felt each emotion during the past week. The PANAS can be used over a wide range of intervals. I generally use a 1-week interval to correspond to the interval between therapy sessions. The PANAS is sensitive to change in treatment and can be used to monitor progress during treatment.

To collect information for a conceptualization of a phobia or anxiety disorder based on Lang's bioinformational model, the therapist can use the typical assessment strategies used to develop conditioning conceptualizations of anxiety disorders in preparation for behavioral exposure treatments, including obtaining a fear hierarchy and identifying avoidance, escape, and safety behaviors. In addition, to collect information about the meaning propositions of the fear memory network and their links to the stimulus and response elements, the therapist can use the clinical interview and the tools described in Chapter 2 to assess cognitions. Accurate assessment typically requires activation of the memory network. Thus, I often find that I do an initial assessment in the office to get a lay of the land of the patient's fear memory network but do not learn all the details of the elements of the network and their links until exposure begins and the network is activated.

Intervention Guided by Emotion Theory

The emotion models presented in this chapter can provide useful ideas and lead to useful intervention strategies for many patients. The therapist using these models can select interventions from the available ESTs, especially those that rely on emotion theory (e.g., DBT; Linehan, 1993a), Strauman's self-system therapy (Strauman et al., 2006), exposure-based therapies for anxiety disorders (Foa & Kozak, 1986), and emotion regulation therapy for generalized anxiety disorder (Mennin, 2004). Interventions can strive to change the mechanisms that are causing the symptoms and/or to teach compensatory strategies.

Treatment Targets and Mechanism Change Goals

The formulation identifies the treatment targets and the mechanisms linking them that need to be changed in the therapy. The formulation's identification of the *treatment targets* and the *mechanism change goals* of the therapy (that is, the psychological mechanisms the therapy is designed to change) provides useful guides to intervention. If the therapist is conceptualizing the case as resulting from deficits in the core and control discrete emotion model, then the treatment targets are the core and control system activities that are described in the conceptualization as contributing to the patient's problems. The mechanism change goals of the therapy are to modify or prevent core system activation, to decrease or stop the use of maladaptive emotion regulation strategies, and to teach and increase the use of adaptive emotion regulation strategies.

If the therapist is conceptualizing the case as resulting from malfunctions of the approach and withdrawal systems, the treatment targets are the activities of the BAS, BIS, and/or FFS that are identified in the formulation as contributing to the patient's problems. The mechanism change goals of the therapy are to modulate the excessive or deficient activity of the BAS, BIS, and/or FFS and to unhook systems that appear linked (e.g., the patient appears to alternate between states of excessive and deficient BAS).

If the therapist is conceptualizing the case as resulting from pathological fear networks as described in Lang's bioinformational model, the treatment targets are the problematic connections in the memory network that are causing the patient's symptoms. The mechanism change goal of the therapy is to achieve full emotional processing. This is done by activating the fear networks and presenting the patient with information that allows him or her to create new response and meaning elements for the stimulus elements in the feared situation. Foa & Kozak (1986) propose that exposure-based treatments, perhaps combined with some cognitive restructuring (Bennett-Levy et al., 2004; Foa et al., 2007), can accomplish this goal. The behavioral experiments by Bennett-Levy et al. (2004) and the work by Anke Ehlers and David Clark on PTSD (Ehlers & Clark, 2000) also seem designed to promote emotional processing.

* * *

This description of emotion models concludes the conceptual chapters of the book. With the next chapter I shift from conceptual to practical and begin describing how to use the basic theories of cognition, learning, and emotion (described in Chapters 2, 3, and 4) to develop an individualized case formulation and treatment plan.

FIVE

Beginning the Therapeutic Relationship and Obtaining a Problem List and Diagnosis

The clinician is now armed for battle, as it were. She understands the model of case formulation-driven CBT (presented in Chapter 1) and the main propositions and clinical implications of the cognitive, learning, and emotion theories (presented in Chapters 2, 3, and 4) that underpin most of the cognitive-behavior ESTs. It is helpful if she is also familiar with the details of several ESTs (and the formulations underpinning them) for the most common disorders she sees. Now the patient—or rather, the potential patient—arrives on the scene and the clinician must translate all this general knowledge into case-specific action.

Treatment itself, however, does not start in the first session. Instead, the therapist conducts a series of pretreatment sessions. This pretreatment or consultation phase is time-limited. A maximum of four sessions is a good general rule. If pretreatment is open-ended or too long, the distinction between pretreatment and active treatment is difficult to maintain.

This chapter and the next two describe pretreatment. I begin this chapter by discussing the need for demarcating a pretreatment phase (see also Linehan, 1993a; Persons & Mikami, 2002) and briefly describing the tasks of pretreatment. Then I offer detailed descriptions and an example that illustrate the first pretreatment tasks, which are to begin to build a therapeutic relationship and to develop a Problem List and diagnosis.

THE NEED FOR A CLEAR BOUNDARY BETWEEN ASSESSMENT AND TREATMENT

Establishing a clear boundary between assessment and treatment is an ethical obligation of mental health professionals (American Psychological Association, 1992). It is not ethical to provide treatment before providing patients with information about the proposed treatment and obtaining their consent to proceed. Obtaining full informed consent is particularly important for the therapist doing case formulation-driven treatment because the therapist is often modifying and combining ESTs or drawing on basic theory to develop a formulation and treatment plan to address problems and disorders for which no EST is available.

Initiating treatment without informing the patient about what is needed to get a successful outcome can be dangerous, much as embarking on a hike in the desert without taking water is dangerous. It is the therapist's job, as leader of the expedition, to make sure the patient is adequately prepared. Many of the interventions of CBT are stressful and demanding and this heightens the importance of taking some time to prepare patients and get their agreement to proceed. Linehan (1993a) uses a pretreatment phase in DBT for borderline personality disorder. This is when she asks, as a condition of providing treatment, that the patient agree to goals of stopping suicidal and self-harming behaviors. Therapists who neglect this task can find themselves attempting to prevent the suicide of a patient who has not agreed that stopping suicidal behaviors is a goal of treatment.

The conditioning and emotion theories described in Chapters 3 and 4 alert us to the usefulness of a pretreatment phase. When patients first come to us they are often quite uncomfortable and eager to get some help. Principles of operant conditioning tell us that they are more likely to sign on to a more aggressive treatment plan at this point than they will agree to later, after they have obtained some relief. The therapist can (benevolently) capitalize on this by asking for a commitment to a comprehensive treatment package as a condition of beginning treatment. Emotion theory tells us that the patient's distress is likely to elicit complementary emotional responses from the therapist that prompt him or her to begin to offer interventions without first carrying out a complete assessment or obtaining the patient's agreement to the needed treatment. Installing an explicit pretreatment phase prior to the formal beginning of treatment helps the therapist avoid this trap.

The Trevose behavior modification program (described in Figure 5.1) provides a fascinating example of how requiring potential patients to jump through big hoops before they can enter (or stay in) treatment can contribute to change. I keep this example in mind to help me be assertive in asking patients for what is needed to accomplish the changes they want. Instead of agreeing quickly to a treatment plan that the patient is asking for and feels comfortable with, I encourage therapists to think through carefully what is actually needed and to use motivational interviewing (W. R. Miller & Rollnick, 2002) and other strategies (described in Chapter 7) to help the patient understand this and agree to it (Gruber & Persons, 2008).

The Impossibility of Completely Separating Assessment and Treatment

Despite the importance and advantages of demarcating assessment from treatment, it is not completely possible or even desirable to do this for several reasons. First, assessment often functions like an intervention. For example, monitoring a behavior typically causes it to change in the desired direction (Korotitsch & Nelson-Gray, 1999).

Second, one very useful way to inform patients about the treatment and help them determine whether they want to go forward is to demonstrate some of the interventions in order to provide them with both intellectual and experiential information about the therapy. For example, to teach the cognitive model and give the potential patient infor-

The Trevose behavior modification program (Latner, Wilson, Stunkard, & Jackson, 2002) provides a fascinating example of the way in which requiring a demanding treatment plan can lead to impressive outcomes. The program also illustrates the therapeutic use of principles of operant learning. The Trevose behavior modification program is a self-help group that uses behavioral strategies to treat obesity and has been shown to produce large weight losses that are sustained over long periods of time. Latner et al. (2002) reported that 47.4% of members remained in treatment at 2 years and had lost 19.3% of their body weight. At 5 years, the 21.6% who remained had lost 17.3% of their body weight.

Participants are eligible for the Trevose program if they are between 25 and 100 pounds above insurance industry standards for normal weight, have no history of diabetes, and have never been a member of the Trevose program. To be admitted to the program, participants must, during their first 5 weeks of participation, log their food intake, bring their food records to a weekly meeting, and lose 15% of their total assigned weight loss goals (unless they have a weight loss goal of 80 or more pounds, in which case they are required to lose exactly 12 pounds during the screening phase). Those who pass all of these requirements are accepted as "members," and those who do not are permanently dismissed from the group.

Members must also meet stringent standards in order to continue their membership. They must attend weekly groups, monitor their food intake, and meet specific weight loss goals each month. In order to take a vacation, members must provide 2 weeks advance written notice, and when they are on vacation members must weigh themselves and mail a record of their weight to their group leader on the day of their usual meeting. Members who fail to meet these requirements are asked to leave the group and are not permitted to rejoin. After members have participated for a certain length of time, they are no longer vulnerable to being asked to leave the program, but if they fail to meet participation requirements, they are penalized by being placed on "Parole," which gives them an extra 2 months in which to meet their goals. Successful members are encouraged to volunteer as group leaders or office workers for the Trevose program. When they have maintained their weight loss goals for 12 months, meeting attendance is no longer mandatory, but members must mail in their weight records monthly.

FIGURE 5.1. Trevose behavior modification program. From Jacqueline B. Persons (2008). Copyright by The Guilford Press. Permission to photocopy this figure is granted to purchasers of this book for personal use only (see copyright page for details).

mation about the therapy process, the therapist can work through a Thought Record addressing one of the patient's current concerns.

Third, occasionally the patient arrives at the therapist's office in a crisis that requires immediate intervention. When that happens, the therapist makes a contract with the patient to suspend pretreatment to address the crisis and then return to pretreatment when the crisis has been resolved.

In addition, the problems for which patients seek treatment often impede them from agreeing to a good treatment plan to address them. For example, the person who has difficulty making decisions can find it difficult to make the decision to go forward to treat his indecisiveness!

Finally, people are often ambivalent about change (Prochaska & DiClemente, 1992). Thus, although patients must give informed consent before treatment begins, some interventions are often needed to inform patients about treatment and help them overcome reluctance to accept a good plan (W. R. Miller & Rollnick, 2002). The pretreatment phase, a term I borrow from Linehan (1993a), helps resolve this tension.

THE TASKS OF PRETREATMENT

The tasks of pretreatment are (1) beginning to build a therapeutic relationship; (2) obtaining a diagnosis; (3) developing an initial case formulation; (4) developing an initial treatment plan; and (5) informing the patient about the results of the assessment and reaching agreement about how to proceed. Although I describe these tasks in order, in fact the therapist works on all of them simultaneously. That is, at the same time he is collecting information to obtain a diagnosis and initial formulation, the therapist is working to build a relationship with the patient, generate ideas about the treatment plan, and inform the patient about his thinking. For that reason, I recommend reading all of the pretreatment chapters (Chapters 5, 6, and 7) in their entirety before beginning to carry out any of the pretreatment tasks with your patient.

Beginning to Build a Relationship

Relationship building is a key task of pretreatment. The patient is unlikely to accept even an outstanding empirically supported treatment plan if he does not like and trust the therapist and believe that the therapist truly understands his struggles. For that reason, I discuss the relationship first. It is a foundation upon which everything else rests. However, this is not to say that the therapist first works to develop a relationship and after that is done approaches the other pretreatment (and treatment) tasks. Instead, working collaboratively with the patient to accomplish the pretreatment tasks of obtaining agreement on a diagnosis, formulation, and treatment plan, as described in these pretreatment chapters, is a key part of the process of building a strong therapeutic relationship (Bordin, 1979).

Thus, the main relationship-building tasks during pretreatment are the collaborative ones undertaken to develop a shared formulation and treatment plan. In addition, patient and therapist use the pretreatment phase to assess how well they work together at these tasks in order to evaluate whether they are a good match to work together in treatment.

Diagnosis

Why diagnose? Many clinicians see diagnosis as irrelevant and are reluctant to conduct a formal diagnostic assessment. They don't want to interrupt the patient's "telling his story," they fear the patient will have a negative reaction to diagnosis, and they note that diagnostic classification and cognitive-behavior theories are difficult to reconcile conceptually (Follette, 1996). Despite the validity of these and other concerns, diagnosis yields information that is helpful in treatment. One key example is the important implications for both psychotherapy and pharmacotherapy of distinguishing between unipolar and bipolar mood disorders. In addition, the treatment efficacy literature and even the epidemiological and psychopathology literatures are organized by diagnosis and effective clinicians will want to draw on those literatures in their clinical work. In fact, one of the main methods (described in the next chapter) for developing an individualized case conceptualization and treatment plan calls for the therapist to rely on evidence-based formulations and treatment protocols; these usually target a DSM disorder. Diagnosis can provide the therapist with some immediate formulation hypotheses. For example, a diagnosis of panic disorder suggests the formulation that panic symptoms result from catastrophic interpretations of benign somatic sensations (Clark, 1986).

Initial Case Formulation

A key task of pretreatment is to develop an initial case formulation. The elements of the case-level formulation are (1) *a complete list of all the patient's problems and disorders*, (2) the *mechanisms* (e.g., schemas or CRs) maintaining all of the patient's problems and disorders, (3) the *precipitants* that are triggering the mechanisms to cause the problems, and (4) the *origins of the mechanisms* (e.g., how the schemas or the conditioned responses were acquired). The formulation describes the relationships among all of these elements.

The goal in pretreatment is to obtain enough of a formulation to identify the key features of the treatment plan and to give the patient enough information about it to allow him to make an informed choice about whether to accept the therapist's treatment plan. That is, the goal is to avoid learning in the fifth—or twenty-fifth!—session that the patient uses self-harming behavior to regulate painful emotions and refuses to agree on a goal to stop it. A formulation (and the process of collaboratively developing it) also helps build the alliance by assuring the patient that the therapist understands his situation. Nevertheless, the case formulation that the therapist obtains during the pretreatment phase is preliminary, for two reasons.

One is that in pretreatment therapists usually don't get all the information they need to get a complete and fully detailed case formulation. Thus, the therapist may find out in pretreatment that the patient has a panic disorder and may conceptualize it as resulting from irrational fears of panic sensations. However, the therapist will probably not have time during pretreatment to collect all of the idiographic details of the catastrophic thoughts, the feared disastrous consequences, the exact somatic sensations, and their sequence that are part of a detailed and fully elaborated formulation. Much of this information will be obtained later, during treatment.

Second, the case formulation developed during pretreatment is preliminary because it is likely to be modified as treatment proceeds. Often during the course of treatment, as some problems are solved, new ones emerge and the therapist obtains new information that leads to a new case formulation.

Finally, remember that the case-level formulation is just one of many formulations that help guide treatment. Symptom-level formulations (described further in Chapters 2, 3, 4, and 10) and disorder-level formulations also guide the clinician's decision making during treatment.

Treatment Planning

The treatment plan flows out of the formulation of the case. For example, if the formulation proposes that the patient's panic symptoms result from catastrophic fears of benign somatic sensations, then the treatment plan will entail interventions to help him overcome his fears of those somatic sensations. As already mentioned, in pretreatment the therapist will probably not have the information needed to flesh out every detail of a treatment plan but must provide enough information to allow the patient to make an informed consent about whether to proceed. At a minimum the therapist must make some recommendations about what treatment modality (that is, individual, group, or couple), frequency, and adjuncts (e.g., pharmacotherapy or pharmacotherapy consult) are needed and what sorts of interventions the psychotherapy will entail. For example, patients who want to overcome phobias and anxiety disorders must be informed that CBT will entail approaching feared situations to some degree or another. The therapist may also ask the patient to agree to certain treatment goals. DBT for borderline personality disorder, for example, typically requires the patient to agree to goals of stopping suicidal and self-harming behaviors as a condition of treatment.

A major challenge of pretreatment is that patients are usually quite uncomfortable and wish to begin treatment immediately but the therapist wants to accomplish all of the pretreatment tasks before beginning treatment. To address this dilemma, remember that assessment and treatment planning and relationship building are themselves interventions. In addition, the therapist can assign homework during pretreatment, including psychoeducational reading, which facilitates the assessment process and may provide the patient with some symptom relief.

Obtaining Informed Consent

Before going forward with treatment, the therapist summarizes her hypotheses about diagnosis and formulation, describes the treatment plan she recommends and other options that are available to the patient, and obtains the patient's permission to the proposed treatment plan. Some interventions (described in Chapter 7) may be needed to obtain the patient's permission.

Unless the patient and therapist can agree on a treatment plan, they do not go forward. Thus, as she carries out all the tasks of pretreatment described in this chapter and the next two, the therapist keeps in mind and reminds the patient that no decision to work together in treatment has yet been made. After collecting information in pretreatment, the therapist may conclude that she does not have the expertise to treat the patient. Or the patient may not agree to the treatment plan the therapist recommends. In these cases, the clinician must refer the patient to another treatment provider.

To summarize, the therapist works in pretreatment on five tasks: relationship building, diagnosis, formulation, treatment planning, and obtaining the patient's informed consent to the treatment plan proposed by the therapist. In the balance of this chapter I focus on three of these tasks: relationship building, diagnosis, and obtaining the first part of the formulation—the Problem List. Although I focus on these pieces here, the therapist works simultaneously on all elements of pretreatment. Thus, while working on the relationship, diagnosis, and the Problem List, the therapist is also collecting data to develop mechanism hypotheses and taking advantage of opportunities to inform the patient about what the treatment plan the therapist is contemplating looks like.

BEGINNING TO BUILD A THERAPEUTIC RELATIONSHIP

The task of building a relationship starts right away, with the first contact on the telephone. A good relationship is as necessary to successful pretreatment as to treatment.

As already noted, patient–therapist agreement on diagnosis, formulation, and treatment plan are key elements of a strong therapeutic relationship (Bordin, 1979).

To promote this agreement, the therapist works collaboratively to educate the patient about what he is learning at each step as he collects information to obtain a diagnosis, formulation, and treatment plan. Padesky (1991) uses the term "shoulder-to-shoulder case conceptualization" to capture this point. By the time the therapist presents the diagnosis, formulation, and proposed treatment and asks for the patient's permission to go forward, he is simply presenting a summary of things that the patient and therapist have already discussed.

Unless a good, trusting relationship is present, it is difficult for the therapist to collect the assessment information needed to obtain a formulation. At the same time, having a formulation hypothesis about the patient's vulnerabilities will help the therapist establish a good relationship. The solution to this dilemma is to begin to develop formulation hypotheses very early and use them to guide the development of the relationship. In fact, the therapist's work in pretreatment requires a kind of bootstrapping approach, where each step on one task (formulating the case, establishing the relationship) helps with the other. So, for example, a skilled therapist might quickly identify that the patient is hypersensitive to criticism and use that awareness to guide careful and supportive questioning during the assessment process that will allow the therapist to both get the information needed and build a trusting relationship. In fact, part of the purpose of pretreatment is for both therapist and patient to gauge whether they are successful in this balancing act and would work well together in treatment.

STARTING CASE FORMULATION: THE COMPREHENSIVE PROBLEM LIST

Rationale for Developing a Comprehensive Problem List

It is important to develop a comprehensive list for three reasons. First, the import of any symptom, problem, or diagnosis is dependent on the patient's other problems and diagnoses. Thus, for example, a symptom of derealization may have different implications for a person with panic disorder than for a person who is abusing substances. To understand the case fully, the therapist must know what *all* the problems are. The problems on the list are like pieces of furniture in a room. Adding or removing a piece makes the other pieces look different and can even lead to rearranging all the furniture.

Second, if the therapist does not make a comprehensive Problem List and instead simply focuses on the problems the patient wishes to focus on or that are in plain view, important problems can be missed. Patients frequently wish to ignore serious problems like substance abuse, self-harming behaviors, and others that, if ignored, can prevent successful treatment of the problems that the patient does want to focus on.

Third, a review of a comprehensive Problem List often reveals common elements or themes that cut across problems. An awareness of these common elements can be helpful in generating initial mechanism hypotheses. This was true for the case of Angela, described later in this chapter.

The Context of Obtaining the Problem List

A first systematic step to developing a case formulation is to obtain a comprehensive list of all of the patient's problems. While working to do this, the therapist keeps her eyes and ears open for information relevant to the other elements of the case-level formulation: origins, precipitants, and mechanisms. The therapist also works on the other tasks of pretreatment (building a relationship, diagnosis, treatment planning, and obtaining informed consent).

In addition, frequently the therapist diverges from the task of drawing up the comprehensive Problem List in order to collect information for the formulation of a key problem or symptom. This digression makes most sense in three situations. First, if a beautiful opportunity presents itself to work collaboratively with the patient to develop a formulation of a particular symptom or problem (especially one of the problems that is most troubling to the patient), it is often wise to seize on it. Working with the patient on a problem-level formulation helps build the alliance and inform the patient about how CBT conceptualizes and treats problems. This sort of digression is typically brief (e.g., 10 minutes). Second, if the patient presents with a high-risk problem (e.g., suicidality), the therapist must immediately shift to the task of conceptualizing and intervening to address that problem. Third, if the therapist encounters a key behavior, symptom, or problem that is likely to interfere with the patient's ability or willingness to agree to an effective treatment plan, it is important to develop a formulation of that problem that can lead to some interventions to address it. To develop a formulation at the level of a symptom or problem, the therapist uses the methods described in Chapters 2, 3, and 4 and illustrated below and in the next chapter in the discussion of the case of Angela.

In this context, the therapist focuses in the first session on the task of obtaining a comprehensive Problem List.

Contents of the Problem List

To obtain a comprehensive list, the therapist assesses the following domains: psychiatric symptoms, interpersonal, occupational, school, medical, financial, housing, legal, leisure, and difficulties with mental health or medical treatment.

The Problem List overlaps considerably with Axes I–IV of a DSM diagnosis. However, in the Problem List the therapist begins to translate diagnostic information into terms that facilitate conceptualization and intervention from a cognitive-behavior point of view. One way the Problem List facilitates cognitive-behavior treatment planning is by giving higher priority to problems in functioning than does the DSM diagnosis format, which places those problems down the list in Axis IV. Another way the Problem List does this is by detailing the symptoms of the particular Axis I and II psychiatric disorders the patient is experiencing.

In addition, a good Problem List includes counts or severity ratings for at least some of the problems (e.g., a count of the number of panic attacks per week or a Beck Depression Inventory [BDI] score). Stating problems in this way facilitates setting treatment goals in terms that allow for measurement of change.

The Problem List also includes Axis III disorders. Identifying medical problems is important for several reasons. Cognitive-behavior skills can often be useful in the treatment of medical problems, especially the chronic medical problems like obesity and cardiac disease that often require, as part of their management, behavioral change. In addition, many medical disorders cause problems and symptoms that mimic or exacerbate mental disorders (e.g., thyroid dysfunction can exacerbate mood disorders) and the therapist must be aware of these interplays. Finally, medical problems can constrain interventions. The diabetic graduate student cannot reward himself with an ice cream cone for work on his dissertation.

As already noted, psychosocial problems (Axis IV) such as financial, housing, and legal problems also belong on the Problem List. In fact, patients, even those who have significant Axis I disorders, often come to therapy for help extricating themselves from an abusive relationship or handling a series of stressful life events. They often have not identified and are not seeking treatment for the Axis I disorders. In addition, Axis IV problems can weaken or even destroy a therapy that is targeting an Axis I disorder—especially if they take the therapist by surprise. A depressed young man came to his therapy session and told me, "I can't pay my rent, so next month I'll be living out of my car—that's not a problem really, but I just wanted you to know about it." This young man had two problems: a housing problem and poor insight about the seriousness of his housing problem.

Not all of the problems on the Problem List will be addressed in psychotherapy. For example, treating a broken leg will obviously not be a goal of CBT. However, it is useful for the cognitive-behavior therapist to place the broken leg on the Problem List because it may have implications for the diagnosis, formulation, and/or the Treatment Plan (e.g., the broken leg may have resulted from impulsive behavior and means that exercise cannot be used to treat the patient's depressed mood).

The next section describes the process of collecting the information needed to obtain a Problem List and diagnosis. As noted above, as the therapist does this, he or she also takes advantage of opportunities to accomplish other pretreatment tasks, including building the relationship and informing the patient about treatment.

The Process of Obtaining a Problem List and Diagnosis

The therapist relies on multiple sources of information to develop a Problem List and diagnosis, including the clinical interview, paper-and-pencil measures, structured interview protocols (e.g., diagnostic interview protocols), and previous and concurrent treatment providers. Family members can often provide useful information as well. For example, it is not uncommon for the wife of a patient who has OCD to be more aware than the patient of how his rituals interfere with the normal functioning of their household. Information from family members is especially useful when patients have disorders or problems in which minimization of symptoms or lack of insight is part of the problem (e.g., bipolar disorder, schizophrenia, hoarding).

I describe here the process of using many of these sources to obtain a Problem List and diagnostic hypotheses for "Angela." In addition to focusing on obtaining a Problem List and diagnosis, I took advantage of opportunities to collect other information as well, including elements of the case-level formulation (mechanisms, precipitants) and information about some key problems and symptoms. I also worked to build our relationship and to give her some information about CBT. Details of Angela's case are modified and she reviewed this material and gave me permission to use it here.

Telephone Contact prior to the First Session

The patient's first words on the telephone often yield valuable diagnostic and formulation information and hypotheses. Angela's first words to me when she called were "I'm desperately miserable, but I'm skeptical about whether therapy can help." Angela had been referred by her psychopharmacologist, who had already called and provided a thumbnail sketch of Angela's situation. I knew that Angela was an attorney and that a physical assault by a client had precipitated symptoms of anxiety and depression that were so incapacitating that she had taken a leave of absence from work. Thus, even before Angela called, I was entertaining diagnoses of PTSD and some type of mood disorder.

What particularly caught my attention in Angela's first words to me was her skepticism about treatment. This is a top-priority problem because it fits into the category of "problems that can undermine or jeopardize the therapy itself." Because of its importance, even as I embarked on the process of collecting a Problem List and diagnosis, I immediately began developing symptom-level formulation hypotheses about Angela's skepticism. I hypothesized that it might be a symptom of PTSD, which frequently leads to a sense that all the rules have changed and nothing makes sense anymore. The hopelessness could be a symptom of depression. It could, using A. T. Beck's (1976) cognitive model, result from schemas of others as unhelpful, the future as hopeless, and herself as helpless. It might be a specific negative belief about mental health professionals obtained from our culture or from Angela's personal experience or that of people around her. I would need to assess further to determine which of these hypotheses best accounted for Angela's skepticism and decide how to address it. My use of the first bit of information from the patient is consistent with studies of the decision-making process of competent physicians; they develop diagnostic hypotheses very early in the decision-making process (Elstein, Shulman, & Sprafka, 1978).

During my initial telephone interaction with Angela, I also used my interpersonal skills to begin to build an alliance. I wanted to build an early strong interpersonal connection and to convey competence and confidence that I could help in order to engage her in treatment. I also wanted to give her some information about what it would be like to work with me. To accomplish these goals, I balanced empathic statements with actively structuring the time to carry out a brief assessment. I asked her to give me a brief description of her problems "so I can be sure that it is a good use of your time to meet with me for a consultation." I also asked whether she was feeling suicidal or felt she was in crisis, to help determine how soon I needed to meet with her. After a brief discussion in which I learned that she was not in a crisis and had problems that appeared to fall within my areas of expertise, I let Angela know that I would be happy to meet with her for a consultation that would take a minimum of two sessions and might take three or even four sessions to complete. I explained that I would collect a lot of information to assess her situation and then give her my ideas about what was going on and my treatment recommendations, which might or might not include me. We would leave all options open at the beginning. Similarly, she would assess whether my recommendations made sense to her and, if I recommended that we work together, whether she felt I could help her. I asked permission to send her a packet of intake questionnaires (described below) that she would complete and bring to the initial interview and that would allow me to collect a lot of information to assess her situation without taking too much time in the session. I let her know that the packet would include a copy of my Treatment Agreement (Figure 5.2), which describes the business and clinical policies of my practice. I asked her to review the agreement and, if she was comfortable with it, to

(text continues on page 103)

This document contains important information about the professional services and business policies of Jacqueline B. Persons, PhD, and the San Francisco Bay Area Center for Cognitive Therapy. Please read it carefully and discuss any questions you have with Dr. Persons.

ASSESSMENT AND TREATMENT: Dr. Persons will provide an assessment of your difficulties and available treatment options. If she recommends and you agree, she will provide cognitive-behavior therapy, which has been shown in controlled outcome studies to provide effective treatment for a number of problems and disorders. (Dr. Persons will review the outcome data most pertinent to your situation upon request.) However, no guarantees can be made regarding the success of treatment. Treatment can be time-consuming and stressful; it can bring on strong feelings, such as anger, frustration, sadness, or anxiety, and may result in changes that were not originally intended (such as divorce or remaining in a relationship you believed you would leave). For people in some professions (e.g., politics, law enforcement), the fact of being in treatment may negatively affect their career. There is a small risk that your condition will worsen due to treatment. After meeting with you to assess your situation, Dr. Persons will offer, if you would like, an estimate of the number of sessions of treatment she recommends for you. For most patients, this ranges between 5 and 40 sessions. Dr. Persons's estimate of the duration of treatment is only an estimate, and no guarantees can be made as to the length of treatment required.

ALTERNATIVE TREATMENTS: Many options to the cognitive-behavioral treatment that Dr. Persons can provide are available, including other types of psychotherapy, group, couple, or family therapy, and, in many cases, medications. Testing and other formal evaluation procedures can be helpful in some cases and if Dr. Persons recommends this in your case, she will let you know what her recommendation is and the reasons for it.

You are entitled to ask questions about all aspects of treatment. Dr. Persons will help you secure a consultation with another mental health professional whenever you request it or she recommends it.

TRAINING AND EXPERIENCE: Dr. Persons is a psychologist licensed to practice in California. She graduated from the University of Pennsylvania with a Ph.D. in Clinical Psychology in 1979. She is Clinical Professor in the Department of Psychology at the University of California at Berkeley. She has been trained to provide and has 25 years of experience conducting cognitive-behavior therapy to treat depression, anxiety, and related problems in adults; she does not have extensive training or expertise in treating couples, families, or children.

THE PATIENT'S ROLE: You are expected to play an active role in your treatment, including working with Dr. Persons to outline treatment goals and completing questionnaires at the beginning of treatment and periodically during treatment to assess progress. You will be asked to complete homework assignments between sessions. If at any point you are unhappy about the progress, process, or outcome of the treatment, please discuss this with Dr. Persons in an attempt to resolve any difficulties that have arisen and to arrive at a treatment plan that better meets your needs.

THE PATIENT'S RIGHTS: A document entitled *Patient's Bill of Rights,* adapted from a publication by the California Department of Consumer Affairs, is attached. Please read it carefully and raise with Dr. Persons any questions you have about it.

FIGURE 5.2. Treatment/Evaluation Agreement. Copyright 2008 by the San Francisco Bay Area Center for Cognitive Therapy. Reprinted by permission in Jacqueline B. Persons (2008). Permission to photocopy this figure is granted to purchasers of this book for personal use only (see copyright page for details).

HOURS/AVAILABILITY: Dr. Persons is usually available in the office from 8 A.M. until 6 P.M. Monday through Friday. Therapy sessions are usually scheduled as 50-minute sessions weekly, or as your treatment needs dictate and you and Dr. Persons agree. In the event of an emergency, Dr. Persons is available by pager at 510-448-2764. In addition, in a crisis, you can call 911, contact your primary care physician, the local emergency room, or crisis intervention services. When Dr. Persons is out of town, she will let you know and will give you the name and telephone number of another therapist who will be available.

CONFIDENTIALITY: The confidentiality of communications between the patient and therapist is important and, in general, is legally protected. Dr. Persons will make every effort to keep the results of all your evaluation and treatment strictly confidential, as is required by law. Information regarding your evaluation and treatment may be disclosed to personnel of the Center for Cognitive Therapy unless you specify to the contrary in writing. Information about you will be released by Dr. Persons only with your written permission, with the following exceptions:

- when there is suspected elder, dependent adult, or child abuse or neglect.
- when, in Dr. Persons's judgment, you are in danger of harming yourself or another person, or are unable to care for yourself.
- If you communicate to Dr. Persons a serious threat of physical violence against another person, Dr. Persons is required by law to inform both potential victims and legal authorities.
- if Dr. Persons is ordered by a court to release information as part of a legal proceeding.
- as otherwise required by law.

In the event that group therapy services are provided, you are expected to keep materials shared in the group confidential. Dr. Persons cannot be held responsible for a breach of confidentiality on the part of group members.

If you elect to seek reimbursement from an insurance company for your treatment, Dr. Persons will provide you with a monthly statement you can submit to your insurance company. Most insurance companies require information about your diagnosis, the type of service provided (e.g., 50-minute individual psychotherapy session), the date of the session, and the fee, and Dr. Persons will include this information on your statement upon your request. Dr. Persons will generally send this statement to you directly. When it is unavoidable and upon your request, Dr. Persons will bill your insurance company directly. Please be aware that when information is sent to an insurance company, Dr. Persons has no control over who sees it. Almost all insurance companies state that they will keep the information confidential, but Dr. Persons cannot assure that they will do so. Some share information with a national medical information data bank for the purposes of deciding eligibility for life, disability, health, and other insurance. Before Dr. Persons sends any information to an insurance company, she will talk with you about what she has written and she will obtain your written permission to provide information to your insurance company. You do have a choice about whether to release the information requested by an insurance company, but if you refuse to consent to releasing it, most insurance programs will not pay for any services.

RECORD KEEPING: Dr. Persons maintains a clinical chart for each patient. Information in the chart includes a description of your condition, your diagnosis, treatment goals, treatment plan and progress in treatment, dates of and fees for sessions, and notes describing each therapy session. Dr. Persons also keeps records of any consent, release, assessment, or other forms completed in the course of your treatment. Clinical records are kept in a locked file cabinet and on the computer in Dr. Persons's office. The hard drive that includes the material from your clinical record is stored in a locked file cabinet when Dr. Persons is not in the office. When your treatment is over, the hard copy of the medical record is sent to an off-site medical record storage facility.

(continued)

FIGURE 5.2. *(page 2 of 3)*

AUDIOTAPING: You may wish to audiotape therapy sessions so you can review them at a later date. If so, you may bring a tape to the session.

RESEARCH, WRITING, TEACHING, CONSULTATION: Dr. Persons conducts research, training, and supervision, and she writes for professional and lay audiences. Dr. Persons may wish to consult with other professionals, especially her colleagues at the San Francisco Bay Area Center for Cognitive Therapy, about treatment planning for your case. Your signature below gives Dr. Persons permission to use information about you and your treatment in any of these ways, provided that she takes reasonable efforts to protect your identity.

FEES: Dr. Persons's fee is $____ per 50-minute session. Longer or shorter sessions are generally prorated from this fee. If you meet with Dr. Persons on the telephone, you will be charged the standard fee, prorated according to the length of the call. Of course, there will be no charge for brief telephone calls, such as those made to schedule appointments.

PAYMENT: Payment is due at the time of the session unless another arrangement has been made. Dr. Persons will send you a monthly statement if you request one.

CANCELLATIONS AND MISSED APPOINTMENTS: If an appointment is missed or cancelled without 24 hours notice, you will be charged for the session. Please be aware that insurance companies will not generally reimburse for a cancelled session.

REIMBURSEMENT: You are responsible for collecting reimbursement from your insurance company or other source.

ENDING TREATMENT: You may withdraw from treatment at any time. Dr. Persons recommends that you discuss your plan to terminate treatment with her before taking action, so that she has an opportunity to offer her recommendations and to offer referral options if they are needed.

If you discontinue meeting with Dr. Persons for a period of 4 weeks or more, she will attempt to contact you. If she is unable to reach you, she will assume (unless other arrangements have been made) that you have elected to terminate your treatment and she will close your case. Of course, should you wish to resume your treatment, she will be happy to discuss that option with you at any time.

Should Dr. Persons become incapacitated or die, one of her colleagues at the San Francisco Bay Area Center for Cognitive Therapy will know how to access her medical records and will contact you to let you know of her incapacitation or death and to help you make arrangements for continuing your care with another provider if needed, and to discuss arrangements for handling your medical record.

* * * * *

I have read and understood this agreement and the *Patient's Bill of Rights* and I have had my questions answered to my satisfaction. I accept, understand, and agree to abide by the contents and terms of this agreement and consent to participate in evaluation and/or treatment.

Name of patient (please print): _____

Signature of patient: _____

Date: _____

FIGURE 5.2. (page 3 of 3)

sign it and bring it with her so I could place it in the clinical record, and if she had any questions, to raise them when we met. I informed her about my fee and that I like to be paid at the time of the session. Angela was agreeable to meeting and seemed not to have any reservations about anything I proposed, so we made a plan to meet about a week later.

Collecting Data in the Pretreatment Session(s)

In the pretreatment sessions, especially the first one, the therapist must handle powerful emotional pulls. One is to immediately move into treatment. It is always a good idea to begin the initial interview by reminding the patient (and the therapist!) that this session is a consultation for the purpose of assessing the patient's situation and beginning the process of developing a treatment plan and to reissue this reminder at the beginning of each consultation session. Without these reminders, it is amazingly easy to slide from assessment into treatment without demarcating the transition.

Another pull is to focus in detail on the problems that are most distressing to the patient. The patient tends to be preoccupied with one or two problems and wants to immediately plunge into them in depth. The therapist must spend some time on these problems or he will not get the needed information and the patient will not feel heard and believe that the therapist can help. At the same time, it is risky for the therapist to dive too deeply into one or two problems before getting an overview of all of the patient's problems and situation. I have done this at times, focusing in detail on a person's distress about a relationship rupture, only to learn later that he has a significant substance abuse problem or psychotic symptoms that require immediate attention and that the patient and I are not in agreement about how to treat.

Another pull is to conceptualize problems the same way the patient does. Instead, the therapist must carry out a delicate balancing act, understanding the patient's view of his situation and problems and conveying to the patient that he understands these things without getting so pulled into the patient's view that he loses his judgment and perspective. Often patients have unhelpful formulations or worldviews that contribute to their problems or their failure to solve their problems. Examples include the person who views losing weight as the linchpin that will change her life completely and the individual who views herself as helpless and hires the therapist to take care of her (rather than to teach her to take care of herself).

Another pull is to ignore topics that the patient doesn't perceive as problems or want to discuss, such as substance abuse. Although the therapist must use clinical judgment and will appropriately elect to postpone assessing certain topics in detail, in general it is important that the therapist strive to open during pretreatment any and all topics that are important and relevant to the patient's situation. Failing to do so can get the therapy and the therapist's relationship with the patient off on the wrong foot from the very beginning.

The pretreatment format and a funnel approach to assessment (Mash & Hunsley, 1993) help address all of these pressures. In the pretreatment format, the therapist strives to gather all of the information in all domains needed to understand the patient's situation and advise him or her about treatment. In a funnel approach, the therapist first carries out a broad-band assessment to determine which areas require more detailed assessment. Paper-and-pencil or online assessment tools that the patient completes and provides to the therapist before the initial interview can help with such an approach because they give the therapist information about many problem domains quickly. In addition, to address the patient's usual urgency to complete the assessment and start treatment, the therapist may want to schedule consultation sessions at a twice-weekly pace and/or to meet for 90-minute sessions.

I used all of these tools with Angela. When she sat down in my office, I began the interview by reminding Angela of our pretreatment agreement, that is, that the goal of the session was for me to collect information that would allow me to assess her situation and, after two or three or perhaps even four sessions, to make some treatment recommendations. Then I asked her permission to take the first 5 minutes of the session to review the intake packet, offering the rationale that doing this would make for a more efficient use of our time.

The intake packet I had sent to Angela and that she had completed and brought to the session is the one we use at the San Francisco Bay Area Center for Cognitive Therapy (see Figure 5.3). It includes the Symptom Checklist-90—Revised (SCL-90R; Derogatis, 2000), the BDI (A. T. Beck et al., 1979) or the Quick Inventory of Depressive Symptomatology (QIDS; Rush et al., 2003), the Burns Anxiety Inventory (Burns AI; Burns, 1997), and our own Functioning and Satisfaction Inventory (Davidson, Martinez, & Thomas, 2006). Also included is our Adult Intake Questionnaire (Figure 5.4), which asks questions about previous and concurrent treatment, substance use, trauma, family and social history, and legal and other problems.

Based on the information obtained in the brief telephone screen, I sometimes add scales to this standard packet to assess other symptoms and problems, such as the Yale–Brown Obsessive—Compulsive Scale (Y-BOCS; Goodman et al., 1989), the Penn State Worry Questionnaire (Meyer, Miller, Metzger, & Borkovec, 1990), the Mobility Inventory for Agoraphobia (Chambless, Caputo, Jasin, Gracely, & Williams, 1985), or the Body Sensations and the Agoraphobic Cognitions Questionnaires (Chambless, Caputo, Bright, & Gallagher, 1984). Readers will want to develop their own packet that assesses the typical presenting problems of the patients they see; Figure 5.5 provides a list of useful sources of measures. Much of this information is important to consider not only for formulating the case but for treatment planning, which I discuss in Chapter 7. In addition to scales that assess symptoms, the therapist can also include scales to assess mechanisms, such as dysfunctional attitudes (e.g., using the version of the Dysfunctional Attitude Scale published in Burns [1999]), perfectionism (Frost, Martin, Lahart, & Rosenblate, 1990), or thought–action fusion (Shafran, Thordarson, & Rachman, 1996).

I scanned the SCL-90R and noted that Angela had given high scores on many items, indicating that she was quite distressed. I highlighted the items she had high scores on (especially those that did not reflect the symptoms of depression and PTSD that I was expecting her to report) to remind myself to follow up on them in the interview. Angela had endorsed several items related to anger and irritability, including "feeling easily annoyed or irritated," "temper outbursts that you could not control," "getting into frequent arguments," and "feeling critical of others." Because an angry physical altercation was involved in the event that appeared to have precipitated her symptoms, I made a note to be sure to assess this area in some detail and to make sure there was no domestic violence, homicidality, or other big-ticket problem in this area.

(text continues on page 113)

Broad-Band Measures

The Symptom Checklist-90—Revised (SCL-90R; Derogatis, 2000) is a 90-item self-report instrument. Because it includes items that assess phenomena that might not otherwise be assessed in the clinical interview (including auditory hallucinations and hostility, and paranoia), the SCL-90R is useful as a broad-band screen to identify areas needing further assessment. Subscale scores can be calculated (to assess anxiety, depression, somatization, interpersonal sensitivity, OCD, phobic anxiety, psychoticism, and paranoid ideation). However, their utility is limited because they are highly intercorrelated (Nezu, Ronan, Meadows, & McClure, 2000). The SCL-90R is copyright protected and available from Pearson Assessments at *www.pearsonassessments.com*.

The Functioning and Satisfaction Inventory (Davidson et al., 2006) is a self-report questionnaire that assesses functioning in eight life domains (work or school, love relationship, relationships with relatives, friendship, recreation, health, standard of living, and home) and is available at no cost at *www.sfbacct.com*. Convergent validity with the general activities items of the short form of the Quality of Life Enjoyment and Satisfaction Questionnaire (Endicott, Nee, Harrison, & Blumenthal, 1993) is excellent. In fact, the correlation of the two scores disattenuated for measurement error slightly exceeds 1.0, supporting the position that these scales measure nearly identical constructs.

The Adult Intake Questionnaire (Figure 5.4) assesses the patient's report of previous and concurrent treatment, substance use, trauma, family and social history, and legal and other problems.

Depressive Symptoms

We have been using the original Beck Depression Inventory (BDI; A. T. Beck et al., 1979) for many years, and are currently experimenting with the self-report version of the Quick Inventory of Depressive Symptoms (Rush et al., 2003)

The BDI and BDI-II (A. T. Beck, Steer, & Brown, 1996) are 21-item self-report instruments that assess the presence and severity of symptoms of depression. The BDI-II is the successor to the original BDI. Both measures calculate a total score by summing the scores on the 21 items. The BDI-II differs from the BDI in that on two items (16 and 18) there are options to indicate either an increase or decrease of appetite and sleep. Another difference is that on the BDI-II patients are asked to consider each statement as it relates to how they have felt for the past 2 weeks, to more accurately correspond to the DSM-IV criteria for major depressive disorder (MDD). The BDI-II is copyright protected and available from PsychCorp at *www.psychcorp.pearson assessments.com*.

The original BDI is superior to the BDI-II for monitoring change, as it asks patients to report symptoms over the past week (the typical interval between therapy sessions), whereas the BDI-II asks patients to report symptoms over the past 2 weeks (to aid in assigning a DSM diagnosis of major depression). However, the original BDI is difficult to obtain, as the Psychological Corporation, which sells the BDI-II, does not sell the original measure.

FIGURE 5.3. Intake questionnaires used at the San Francisco Bay Area Center for Cognitive Therapy. From Jacqueline B. Persons (2008). Copyright by The Guilford Press. Permission to photocopy this figure is granted to purchasers of this book for personal use only (see copyright page for details).

Strengths of the BDI and BDI-II include their wide use in research, extensive reliability and validation and normative data, clinical utility, and sensitivity to change. Drawbacks of the BDI-II are its expense (over $1.50 per copy) and the fact that the publisher requires purchasers to have a PhD or be a licensed mental health professional.

The Quick Inventory of Depressive Symptomatology-Self-Rated (QIDS-SR; Rush et al., 2003) is a 16-item self-report measure that is designed to assess the severity of depressive symptoms. The scale evaluates all the criterion symptom domains in the DSM-IV criteria for MDD. The QIDS-SR total score ranges from 0 to 27. Severity thresholds are defined as follows: No depression (QIDS score 0–5), Mild (6–10), Moderate (11–15), Severe (16–20), and Very Severe (21–27). The QIDS-SR is a shortened version of the 30-item Inventory of Depressive Symptomatology (IDS-SR).

The IDS-SR, in addition to assessing depressive symptoms, differs from the QIDS in that it also assesses many symptoms of anxiety. The QIDS-SR and IDS-SR are adaptations of clinician-rated versions of the IDS and QIDS. Both the QIDS and the IDS were designed to be maximally sensitive to symptom change. The norming, reliability, and validity of the QIDS-SR are excellent. Lamoureux et al. (2007) conducted ROC (receiver operating characteristic) analysis in a sample of 125 primary care patients who completed the QIDS-SR and the SCID and concluded that a score of 11 on the QIDS-SR provided the best balance of sensitivity (Sn = .81) and specificity (Sp = .72) and correctly classified 75% of the sample as to their MDD status. The clinician-rated and self-rated versions of the IDS and QIDS as well as copious psychometric information about the scales are available free for download from the Internet (*www.ids-qids.org*). The measures are available in 13 languages.

Strengths of the QIDS and IDS are that they are free and supported by extensive psychometric data, including data that calibrate their scores with the well-established BDI. The measures do a good job of assessing DSM symptoms for depression, including suicidality.

Anxiety Symptoms

The Burns Anxiety Inventory (Burns AI; Burns, 1997) is a 33-item scale of anxiety symptoms. The Burns AI is useful for weekly outcome monitoring because it assesses three groups of anxiety symptoms (feelings, thoughts, physical symptoms) that map well onto cognitive-behavioral models of anxiety (although unfortunately it does not measure avoidance and safety behaviors). The measure is also sensitive to changes during treatment. Some validation data are available (Burns & Eidelson, 1998; Persons et al., 2006), and it is inexpensive. David Burns sells a license that allows the clinician to make unlimited copies of the scale. The measure (together with many others) is available at *www.feelinggood.com*.

The *Yale–Brown Obsessive–Compulsive Scale* (Y-BOCS; Goodman et al., 1989) is widely used to assess obsessive–compulsive symptoms, including in the randomized controlled trials. It is sensitive to change during treatment (Franklin, Abramowitz, Kozak, & Foa, 2000) and is available at no cost online from multiple sources (just go to the Internet and search for Y-BOCS).

FIGURE 5.3. *(page 2 of 2)*

Your Name: _____

Address: _____

Phone: (Home) _____ (Work) _____

       (Cell) _____ (Other, please specify) _____

Emergency Contact: (Name) _____

                        (Phone) _____ (Relationship) _____

Referred by _____ Phone _____

REIMBURSEMENT If you would like us to send you a monthly statement which you can forward to your insurance company to request reimbursement, please indicate below:

Monthly statement (circle one):   Yes   No

Please mail the monthly statement to the following address (circle one):   Home Business Other

_____

_____

Age: _____ Gender: _____ Date of birth: _____

Ethnicity (circle one):   Caucasian   African American   Hispanic   Asian
                      Other: _____

Religious background: Protestant Catholic   Jewish Muslim Buddhist   No affiliation
(circle one)   Other: _____

Marital status: Single, never married   Married   Separated   Divorced
(circle one)   Widowed   Cohabiting

       If you are divorced, when did you divorce your previous partner? _____

             How long were you married? _____

       If you are widowed, when did your spouse die? _____

Education: (number of years completed) _____

Occupation: _____

Are you working now?   No   Yes (circle one)   If yes, circle one: Full-time   Part-time

Are you going to school now?   No   Yes (circle one)   If yes, circle one: Full-time   Part-time

Names of persons living in your home and your relationship to them:

Name   Relationship

_____   _____

_____   _____

_____   _____

_____   _____

Spouse/partner's occupation, if applicable:_____

(continued)

FIGURE 5.4. Adult Intake Questionnaire. Copyright 2008 by the San Francisco Bay Area Center for Cognitive Therapy. Reprinted by permission in Jacqueline B. Persons (2008). Permission to photocopy this figure is granted to purchasers of this book for personal use only (see copyright page for details).

Please provide the following information about your family:

<u>Mother</u> Name: _____

    If deceased, year and cause of death: _____

    If living, age and health status: _____

    If living, where does she live now? _____

    Her occupation (past and/or present): _____

<u>Father</u> Name: _____

    If deceased, year and cause of death:_____

    If living, age and health status: _____

    If living, where does he live now? _____

    His occupation (past and/or present): _____

Siblings:

<u>Name</u>	<u>Age</u>	<u>Occupation</u>	<u>Where does s/he live?</u>

Where did you grow up?_____

Were your parents ever separated?   Yes   No (circle one) If yes, when?_____

Did your parents get divorced?   Yes   No (circle one) If yes, when? _____

Did they remarry?   Yes   No (circle one) If yes, when? _____

At what age did you move out of your parents' home? _____

What is the highest degree you earned in school? _____ When? _____

Did you ever leave a school you were enrolled in prior to completion?   Yes   No (circle one)

If yes, give details: _____

Did you ever receive any special education services (e.g., academic tutoring, IEP, classroom accommodations, etc.)?   Yes   No (circle one) If yes, give details: _____

_____

If you were physically disciplined as a child, were you ever injured as a result?   Yes No (circle one)

Did your parent or a person taking care of you ever purposefully injure you in other circumstances (that is, when you were not being disciplined)?   Yes   No (circle one)

Did you ever have sexual contact with someone else that you did not want? Yes No (circle one)

Have you experienced or witnessed any traumas (events that felt life-threatening)? Yes No (circle one)

Have you experienced physical or sexual abuse or assaults? Yes No (circle one)

(continued)

FIGURE 5.4. *(page 2 of 6)*

108

Please provide some general information on your work history:

Type of job held   How long?

_____

If you have a partner or spouse, how long have you been together? _____

Please list names and ages of your children, if applicable:

Name	Age	Biological?	Name	Age	Biological?
_____		Y / N	_____		Y / N
_____		Y / N	_____		Y / N

Please describe, briefly, the problem(s) that bring you in to see me.
 What are the symptoms, how intense are they, and how often do they occur?

_____

_____

_____

_____

 Have there ever been problems like this before? Yes No (circle one)

 If yes, when? _____

Are you presently seeing another therapist? Yes No (circle one)

If yes, please give us the following information:

 Therapist's name: _____ Date treatment began: _____

 Therapist's address:_____

 Therapist's phone number: _____

Have you previously been in psychotherapy or counseling, including individual, group, marital or family therapy?

Yes No (circle one)

If yes, please give us the following information:

 Therapist's name(s), phone number(s) and address(es): _____

 _____

 _____

 Date(s) of treatment : _____

 Problem for which treatment was sought:_____

If you have been in psychotherapy before, was it helpful? Yes No (circle one)

 If yes, in what way was it helpful? _____

 If not, in what way was it unsatisfactory? _____

(continued)

FIGURE 5.4. *(page 3 of 6)*

Has hospitalization or partial hospitalization for mental or emotional difficulties ever been recommended for you?

Yes   No (circle one)   If yes, when and why? _____

Have you ever been hospitalized or participated in a partial hospitalization program for mental or emotional difficulties?   Yes   No (circle one)   If yes, when and why? _____

_____

Was the hospitalization voluntary?   Yes   No (circle one)

Has a physician/psychiatrist ever recommended that you take medication for mental or emotional difficulties (e.g., Prozac, Xanax, etc.)?   Yes   No (circle one)

If yes, what medications were recommended, when, and for what symptoms?

_____

Have you ever taken medications for mental or emotional difficulties prescribed by a physician/ psychiatrist?

Yes   No (circle one)

If yes, what medications were prescribed, when and for what symptoms?

_____

Are you currently using any prescribed medications?   Yes   No (circle one)
Please indicate what medications you are taking:

Medication	Dosage	When started	Prescriber

Have you ever used any drugs or medications other than as prescribed? This includes prescription medications, marijuana, PCP, LSD, amphetamines, barbiturates, cocaine, opiates, prescribed drugs (e.g. valium), Ecstasy, and others.

Yes   No (circle one)   Are you currently using?   Yes   No (circle one)

If yes, please check which ones and fill out the requested information:

Type	Frequency/amount	Duration	How taken

If you have used any substances listed above, do you feel they have caused any problems in your work, school, or relationships?   Yes   No (circle one)

If yes, please explain: _____

_____

(continued)

FIGURE 5.4. *(page 4 of 6)*

Do you drink alcohol?   Yes   No (circle one)

How much alcohol do you drink? _____ drinks per _____

Do you feel your drinking has caused any problems in your work, school, or relationships?
    Yes   No (circle one)

    If yes, please explain: _____

    _____

Has treatment for drug or alcohol abuse ever been recommended to you?
    Yes   No (circle one)

    If yes, please describe the circumstances and give dates.

    _____

    _____

Have you ever been treated for drug or alcohol abuse?
    Yes   No (circle one)

    If yes, please describe the provider and program, give dates, and describe the outcome.

    _____

    _____

Have you ever had a physical fight with anyone, including your spouse or partner
(including throwing things, hitting, shoving, etc.)? Yes   No (circle one)

Do you currently have, or have you had in the past, any serious, chronic, or recurrent health
problems or disabilities? Yes   No (circle one)

    If yes, please describe: _____

List dates of any hospitalizations you have had for physical problems:

    Date   Problem

    _____

    _____

    _____

When was your last physical examination by a doctor? _____

What was the outcome? _____

Do any biological relatives have any history of psychiatric or emotional problems?   Yes   No

    If yes, which family members and what types of problems?

    _____

    _____

Have you ever been involved in a lawsuit?

    Yes   No (circle one)

    If yes, please describe the circumstances and give dates.

    _____

    _____

(continued)

FIGURE 5.4. *(page 5 of 6)*

Have you ever been arrested for a crime?

       Yes   No (circle one)

       If yes, please describe the circumstances and give dates.

_____

_____

Have you experienced any particular sources of stress in the last year?

       Yes   No (circle one)

       If yes, please explain: _____

Are there any other health care professionals (e.g., physicians, psychotherapists, etc.) whom you feel might have information that would help in your treatment?

       Yes   No (circle one)

       If yes, please give details: _____

_____

_____

_____

Is there any other background information you think would be helpful for me to know?

       Yes   No (circle one)

       If yes, please explain: _____

_____

_____

_____

_____   _____

Signature   Date

FIGURE 5.4. *(page 6 of 6)*

Antony, M. M., & Barlow, D. H. (Eds.). (2002). *Handbook of assessment and treatment planning for psychological disorders.* New York: Guilford Press.

Antony, M. M., Orsillo, S. M., & Roemer, L. (Eds.). (2001). *Practitioner's guide to empirically based measures of anxiety.* New York: Kluwer Academic/Plenum Publishers.

Burns, D. D. *Therapist's Toolkit.* Available at www.feelinggood.com.

Fischer, J., & Corcoran, K. (2007). Measures for clinical practice and research: A sourcebook (Vol. 2, Adults). Oxford: Oxford University Press.

Hunsley, J., & Mash, E. J. (Eds.). (2008). *A guide to assessments that work.* New York: Oxford University Press.

Nezu, A. M., Ronan, G. F., Meadows, E. A., & McClure, K. S. (Eds.). (2000). *Practitioner's guide to empirically based measures of depression.* New York: Kluwer Academic/Plenum Publishers.

Rush, J. A. Jr. (2000). *Handbook of psychiatric measures.* Washington, DC: American Psychiatric Association.

Sederer, L. I., & Dickey, B. (Eds.). (1996). *Outcomes assessment in clinical practice.* Baltimore: Williams & Wilkins.

FIGURE 5.5. Sources of outcome measures for use in clinical practice. From Jacqueline B. Persons (2008). Copyright by The Guilford Press. Permission to photocopy this figure is granted to purchasers of this book for personal use only (see copyright page for details).

I reviewed the BDI and saw that Angela had endorsed anhedonia, feeling she may be punished, self-criticism, and a number of other symptoms, with a total score of 14. Hopelessness was present, but not severe; she scored 1 (scores on BDI items range from 0 to 3), endorsing, "I feel discouraged about the future." She scored 0 on the suicide item. A BDI score of 14 is in the mild range. Given the disruption to her functioning (she had taken a leave from work), I had expected a higher score, so I made a note to ask about that.

On the Burns Anxiety Inventory (Burns AI), Angela scored 24, in the mild to moderate range (Persons et al., 2006). This score, like the BDI, was a bit lower than I had expected.

On the Adult Intake Questionnaire, Angela reported drinking less than one glass of wine per week and she denied current or past use of illicit substances, a history of lawsuits, current or past medical problems, unwanted sexual contact, and assaults or traumas other than the one that had precipitated her current symptoms. Angela did give an affirmative response to the item "If you were physically disciplined as a child, were you ever injured as a result?" and I made a note to ask some follow-up questions about this.

The referring psychiatrist had told me that Angela had taken a leave of absence from work. The Functioning and Satisfaction Inventory revealed that Angela was struggling in other domains as well. She was having particular difficulty in her relationship with her husband, where she indicated that she was functioning "somewhat poorly," and in the areas of finances and leisure, where she also reported doing "somewhat poorly."

After reviewing the measures, I thanked Angela for all the information she had given me in the questionnaires. I asked her to tell me in her words what was bringing her to the office now. Angela stated tearfully, "I feel as though I have fallen off a cliff and smashed to smithereens at the bottom." She described feeling devastated by her current situation, crying a lot, sleeping a lot, and unable to function. She spontaneously gave a brief account of the trauma, which had happened nearly a year previously. A client who had come to her office to discuss a case had verbally attacked her and pushed her to the floor. An investigation had ensued and the managing partner of the firm had found Angela, who was an associate in the firm, to be at fault, and had docked her pay and put her on probation. Angela was angry and resentful about the way she had been unfairly blamed for the assault by her colleagues and superiors rather than offered support and assistance. She felt she had been "stabbed in the back" by the managing partner and undermined by others that she had expected would be supportive. Although she had returned to work on a part-time basis for several months after the trauma, Angela had recently found herself unable to go to work at all, reporting that she experienced bursts of panic whenever she encountered any of the people who had been involved in the assault or its aftermath.

As Angela talked, with her permission, I began working with her to construct a Problem List, making notes on the Case Formulation Worksheet (Figure 5.6). I began by asking Angela some questions about the symptoms she had developed after the trauma. I learned that, as I had expected, she was reporting many symptoms of PTSD and depression, and I pointed that out to Angela and wrote those two problems on the worksheet. I then asked if, instead of pursuing all the details of those problems at that moment, we might take a broad view and examine whether other problems were present in other domains. Angela was agreeable to doing this.

I asked her to give me more information about some of the items on the SCL-90R relating to anger that she had endorsed. Angela reported feeling very angry and resentful about how her colleagues and superiors in her workplace had responded to the trauma she had experienced. She also reported she was blowing up and yelling at her kids and her husband several times a week and was quite unhappy about this. She denied any physical violence, either now or in the past, with the exception of the recent assault she had experienced.

Work was a major problem. Angela reported that she had previously enjoyed and been quite successful at her work but now felt simply unable to function there and had arranged for a leave of absence. She was scheduled to return to work in 90 days. She reported feeling resentful and frustrated about her colleagues' response to her situation and felt on edge and frightened and tense in the workplace. She was also experiencing "mini panic attacks" whenever she encountered a reminder of the assault or its sequelae, especially colleagues who had "stabbed her in the back" after the trauma.

Angela was also experiencing strains in her relationship with her husband. He was an engineer and worked for a start-up company in the Silicon Valley. He had a long commute and worked long hours. Angela reported that when she put pressure on him to provide more help and support at home he flared up and got angry with her, saying, "I have no choice. This is what working for a start-up involves and you knew that when I took this job."

Angela was also having trouble coping at home, where she felt overwhelmed and demoralized. A leak in the roof had caused significant damage to a part of the house and insurance hassles were disrupting the repair process. In addition, one of her two

(text continues on page 117)

Name _____   Date _____

Problem List

1.

2.

3.

4.

5.

6.

7.

8.

Mechanisms

Precipitants of the problems

Origins of the mechanisms

The case formulation (origins, mechanisms, precipitants, problems):

FIGURE 5.6. *(page 2 of 2)*

116

children had been diagnosed with diabetes and Angela was exhausted and frustrated by her efforts to manage her daughter's symptoms, especially because she received little support from her husband in carrying out all of these tasks. She reported that she was coping by "doing the minimum to get by."

I asked Angela for a bit more information about the financial strains she had identified on the Functioning and Satisfaction Inventory. This issue is a delicate one and can be hard for mental health professionals to approach. However, I've learned (the hard way!) that if I ignore this issue, it can interfere with or even destroy treatment. Angela said that although she was receiving some short-term disability income during her leave and workers' compensation was reimbursing her for her treatment expenses, these sources of income were not up to what she was used to getting so the family was experiencing a bit of a strain. I checked to be sure that she could afford my fee and she reported that workers compensation would pay the bill. I described to her the limits of confidentiality arising from being involved with the workers compensation and disability systems.

In addition to collecting information via the intake questionnaires, the referring psychiatrist, and the interview, I paid particular attention to Angela's interactions with me. The fact that she had experienced a trauma flowing out of an altercation with a client and was having interpersonal problems both at work and at home raised a question about whether she might have social skills deficits that might have contributed to the assault. As I interacted with Angela in the session, I did not note any problems. She was pleasant, collaborative, and cooperative. Of course, I was aware that an individual interview with a therapist was a very different situation from the one (conflict with a client) that had been problematic for her. I elected not to question Angela about this issue at this point, as I knew that she was feeling very blamed by others for the trauma and I certainly did not want her to feel blamed by me. I made a note to follow up on this issue at a later point when our relationship was solid and Angela was ready to address this piece of the puzzle.

I asked Angela about her skepticism about treatment. As we discussed it, we determined that at least part of it arose from a general sense of confusion, powerlessness, futility, and hopelessness that seemed to be symptoms of her PTSD and depression. She felt overwhelmed by her symptoms and problems and had no idea how to address them. I asked her directly if she felt this skepticism would interfere with her ability to engage in treatment. She said no, that she was relieved to be in a therapist's office, felt comfortable with me, and was eager to get some direction about what she needed to do to solve her problems. This statement told me that her skepticism did not appear to be a major impediment to treatment.

I reviewed with Angela the Problem List we had made. I had identified seven problems: depressive symptoms, PTSD symptoms, anger and irritability, work problems, marital problems, difficulty coping at home, and financial problems. Although the list was long, Angela stated, in response to my question, that it seemed manageable and that in fact she felt relieved to have gotten started on the process of getting her life back.

I returned to collect more detailed information about some of the problems. I focused on the depression and I pointed out the discrepancy between her verbal report of desperation and complete misery and immobilization, her tears and obvious distress, her need to take a leave of absence from work, and her BDI score of 14, in the mild to moderate range. Angela was at first unable to explain this, but as we talked about it, she acknowledged that her family members had repeatedly pointed out to her the way she tended to minimize her difficulties and distress and to "keep a stiff upper lip" and just keep plodding along, no matter how miserable she was. She speculated that ignoring noticing how she was feeling was one of her (avoidant) strategies for coping with unpleasant emotions and problems. I took that opportunity to offer my observation that avoidance and withdrawal seemed to be a theme that cut through many of her problems and was one of her major coping strategies right now. She agreed and was receptive to my suggestion that one focus of her treatment would be to help her learn more effective strategies for managing emotional and real-life problems.

Obtaining a Diagnosis

At this point in the interview, I began working to obtain a diagnosis. One way to do this is to allocate time to carry out a formal diagnostic interview. The two best-known are the Anxiety Disorders Interview Schedule, Lifetime Version for DSM-IV (ADIS-IV-L; T. A. Brown, DiNardo, & Barlow, 1994) and the Structured Clinical Interview for DSM-IV-TR (SCID; First, Spitzer, Gibbon, & Williams, 2002). The ADIS is a semistructured interview for the diagnosis of DSM-IV anxiety, mood, somatoform, and substance-related disorders and it is available from Graywind/Oxford University Press (*www.oup.com*). The SCID allows the clinician to identify current and lifetime Axis I and Axis II disorders. A streamlined clinician version of the SCID is available from American Psychiatric Publishing (*www.appi.org*). The research version is available from the New York State Psychiatric Institute (*www.scid4.org*) in an unbound paper version or an electronic version that allows the clinician to evaluate just the diagnostic modules that are most relevant to his or her clinical setting. Each of these interviews requires 60 to 90 minutes to administer.

An alternative strategy, and the one I used with Angela, is to begin by obtaining a Problem List and then to rely on modules of the ADIS (the SCID can also be used in this way) to fine-tune diagnostic hypotheses that arose from the Problem List. Whichever method is used, it is a good idea to carry out the process of developing and evaluating diagnostic hypotheses collaboratively and transparently with the patient. Informing the patient about diagnosis can be a particularly challenging part of the process. Mental health professionals have not typically been trained to provide their patients with diagnostic information. I encourage readers to introspect about how they would feel if they learned their physician was providing treatment for a disorder they had not been informed about.

That said, the process of offering a diagnosis must be handled carefully. The therapist can use skillful interviewing, psychoeducation, and a slow pace to give the patient diagnostic information in a helpful way. To address the fact that the names of many of the personality disorders are pejorative, the therapist might elect to not name the disorder but instead to describe the concept of a personality disorder and the symptoms the patient is experiencing. This approach has the advantage that it is consistent with CBT, which will target symptoms. Occasionally the clinician will judge that it will be more harmful to offer a diagnosis than not.

I began the diagnostic process with Angela by letting her know that I suspected she met criteria for PTSD and used the ADIS (T. A. Brown et al., 1994) to verify that she did indeed meet PTSD criteria. The assault she experienced met DSM criteria for a trauma and she had all three types of PTSD symptoms (reexperiencing, avoidance/numbing, and hyperarousal). I let Angela know that she appeared to have some sort of mood disorder, probably major depressive disorder (MDD), and that I would return in the next consultation session to flesh out the details of her depression diagnosis. I did not see any flagrant evidence of an Axis II disorder, so I did not pursue any formal assessment of Axis II pathology at that time. When patients have severe Axis I disorders, it can be difficult to tease out whether Axis II disorders are present until Axis I disorders, especially severe ones, have remitted at least in part.

Concluding the First Pretreatment Session

My initial interview with Angela ended with a Problem List that I felt was nearly complete, two tentative DSM diagnoses (MDD and PTSD), and information about some of the elements of the case formulation (see Figure 5.7). I had a good start to a positive therapeutic relationship as well. Angela had a direct, frank, straightforward type of style that I appreciated and we took an immediate liking to each other and seemed to be on the same wavelength. We agreed to meet for another consultation session.

As we ended the first session, I asked Angela to do homework in preparation for our next session. Assigning homework during pretreatment serves multiple purposes. It allows the therapist (and patient!) to collect some detailed assessment data, including about the patient's homework compliance. It gets the patient started working on his or her problems, even if only by collecting more information about them. It informs the patient about what treatment will be like, including that it will involve homework and a here-and-now problem-solving approach. And it can also involve some psychoeducation that begins to teach the patient something about his symptoms and about CBT.

It is always a good idea to ask the patient in the first session to begin self-monitoring one or more of the problem behaviors and/or mechanisms that the therapist suspects is playing a major role. The therapist will want this information to assist in the process of identifying problems and developing mechanism hypotheses of the initial case formulation. Useful logs for this purpose were described in Chapters 2, 3, and 4 and include the Activity Schedule (Figure 2.2), Thought Record (Figure 2.3), Event Log (Figure 3.5), Daily Log (Figure 9.5), and Mood Chart (Figure 4.3), and others can be obtained from the resources provided in Figure 5.5. I also ask the patient to repeat any of the measures of depression, anxiety, or OCD from the intake packet that had elevated scores. Other possible homework assignments include reading some psychoeducational materials or taking 15 minutes to write down a list of goals the patient might want to accomplish in therapy.

I asked Angela to read the first three chapters of *Feeling Good* (Burns, 1999). One of my goals in recommending this book to Angela was to reduce her skepticism by giving her some information that would help her see her problems as solvable. In addition, because I was beginning to hypothesize that Angela's behavioral avoidance, which could be seen as a symptom of PTSD or depression or both or as a mechanism, was central to her problems, I asked her to complete an Activity Schedule (Figure 2.2). I also asked her to come 5 minutes early to the session so she could complete a BDI and Burns AI in the waiting room so I could track her symptoms of depression and anxiety.

Name <u>Angela</u>   Date _____

Problem List

1. Depressive symptoms (BDI = 14), symptoms of feeling discouraged about the future, not enjoying things she used to; feeling she may be punished, feeling disappointed in herself, crying more than usual, loss of interest in others, worry about looking old or unattractive, difficulty getting started doing things, early morning awakening, fatigue, and loss of libido. Denies suicidality. Cognitions include: "I don't know where to start to get my life back," "there's no use complaining," "no one will help me." Behaviors include excessive sleeping, not exercising, avoiding going to work or speaking to her employer. Emotions include irritability, anhedonia, sadness, and guilt.

2. PTSD symptoms. Intense fear reaction to physical assault by client followed by re-experiencing symptoms (panic and intense distress whenever she encounters work colleagues or other reminders of the event), avoidance (she is doing a lot of sleeping and has taken a leave of absence from work), and hyperarousal (irritability, insomnia). Cognitions include: "I can't cope," "My boss stabbed me in the back," behaviors include avoidance of work and sleeping, and emotions include panic and irritability.

3. Anger and irritability. Angry and resentful about being blamed by colleagues and supervisors for an act of violence against her. Has difficulty disciplining her kids without losing her temper. Resentful with husband, who is "never at home." She blows up at her kids about 3 times/week, at her husband about twice weekly.

4. Work problems. Recently took leave of absence b/c was having so many re-experiencing symptoms and resentment at work that she felt unable to function. Very distressed at loss of a previously rewarding professional life. She states, "I do not have any confidence that I will ever have energy and enthusiasm for my job again."

5. Marital problems. The marriage is "strained." Problems are chronic but exacerbated by her recent difficulties. Husband has a long commute and high pressure at work in a startup. Does not earn much money. "He's a good man but he's never at home and when he is he yells a lot."

6. Difficulty coping at home. Ongoing conflict with roof contractor, daughter with diabetes. "It's too much. I can't do it all." Coping style is do "do the minimum needed to get by."

7. Financial stresses due to loss of income from Angela's leaving work and husband's low-paying job.

Mechanisms

Precipitants of the problems
Assault at work

Origins of the mechanisms

The case formulation (origins, mechanisms, precipitants, problems):

FIGURE 5.7. Case Formulation Worksheet for Angela after the first session.

It is always a good idea to check in with the patient at the end of the initial session to get some feedback about how the interview went. Angela reported the interview had gone well and she felt encouraged. I was especially glad to hear that she felt hopeful that treatment could help her.

Tips for Constructing a Problem List

Restrict the Length

A good Problem List is comprehensive. However, it is also important to keep the list to a manageable length: a maximum of five to eight items. Angela's Problem List (see Figure 5.7) had seven items. If the list is too long, the therapist can group some of the problems together to shorten the list (e.g., including unassertiveness as an aspect of a social anxiety problem).

Classification of problems is sometimes a dilemma. For example, if the patient has a fear of public speaking that interferes with performance at work, is this best listed as an anxiety symptom or as an aspect of a work problem? The best answer to this question is to classify the problem in the way that is most useful in guiding treatment (S. C. Hayes et al., 1987). The therapist may even choose to describe the problem in more than one way. This strategy is useful when the problem is a high-priority one. Thus, suicidality might appear on the Problem List twice: once as a part of a problem of depression, and once as a problem in its own right.

Describe Problems in Cognitive-Behavioral Terms

In addition to naming problems, it is also useful to describe some of the typical behaviors, cognitions, and emotions that make up the problem. For example, describe depressive symptoms in terms of behaviors (e.g., skipping class), cognitions (e.g., "I'm a worthless piece of crap"), and emotions (e.g., sadness, anhedonia, and hopelessness). Describing problems in these terms facilitates conceptualization and treatment from a cognitive-behavior point of view. Of course, some problems (cancer or legal problems, for example) are not readily described in terms of cognitions, behaviors, and emotions.

Strive for Agreement

Obviously it is ideal if patient and therapist agree on the Problem List. However, complete agreement is not always possible. Common areas of disagreement include substance abuse, suicidality, and self-harm (therapists tend to see these as problems when patients do not). When a comprehensive and mutually-agreed-upon Problem List cannot be obtained, comprehensiveness trumps agreement. Thus, if the therapist identifies a substance abuse problem that the patient denies is a problem, the therapist includes the problem on the Problem List, noting the patient–therapist disagreement about the problem as an aspect of the problem or even as a distinct problem.

When disagreement exists, the therapist will likely want to use motivational interviewing and other strategies described in Chapter 7 to attempt to get agreement. When it comes time to offer a treatment plan, the therapist will need to make a judgment call as to whether the disagreement between therapist and patient about the Problem List is so large as to prevent the patient from accepting adequate treatment or succeeding in treatment.

Observe Carefully

The therapist who is collecting a Problem List cannot simply ask the patient what problems she is having and write them down. He must also pay careful attention to all the other information that comes his way. Careful observation can alert the therapist to problems that patients may not acknowledge, recognize, or verbalize, such as a disheveled appearance, disorganized thinking, delusional thinking, or social skills deficits such as poor eye contact, failure to participate in a back-and-forth dialogue, or untruthfulness. These behaviors and phenomena yield valuable information about problems and even suggest hypotheses about underlying mechanisms.

Many of these difficulties (e.g., disheveled appearance) can be very awkward to discuss and the therapist may be tempted to put them off for later. Sometimes it does make sense to put off sensitive issues until a trusting therapeutic relationship can be established. Sometimes, however, I make a point of raising this type of issue during pretreatment assessment, for several reasons. One, the longer I avoid talking about the elephant in the living room, the harder it gets. Second, I want to give the patient now the information that I won't ignore the elephant in the living room and some information about how I will approach the topic of the elephant so the patient will have this information when deciding if he or she wants to work with me. Third, I need to know how the patient responds to my raising the topic of the elephant in order to know whether I believe I can work well with and help the patient and what treatment plan is needed.

When raising a delicate issue I try to protect the patient from shame a bit by beginning with a piece of genuine support or validation, saying, for example, "I can see that you are really are working hard to answer my questions. However, I also notice that once you get started talking it is hard for you to pause and let me interrupt or have a back-and-forth dialogue with you. Have you noticed that?" Also helpful is a matter-of-fact and nonjudgmental tone: "You know, as I try to understand your situation, I notice that one piece you are having trouble with right now is keeping your clothes clean and laundered. Could we talk about that for a moment?"

List Problems in Priority Order

Ordering problems by priority helps the patient and therapist make decisions about the order in which to tackle them. The following questions are helpful in prioritizing problems on the Problem List:

- Is there a threat to life and limb of the patient or another person?
- Do any problems undermine or jeopardize the therapy itself?
- Is there a problem that, if it is not solved, will prevent solution of any other problem?
- What problem does the patient have the biggest emotional commitment to solving?
- What problem is interfering most with the patient's functioning?

- What problem, if solved, will solve many or most of the patient's other problems?
- What problem, when treated, might destabilize the patient? (this problem is a lower priority problem, to be addressed later)
- Is there a problem that can be quickly and easily solved?

I address each of these criteria in turn below.

IS THERE A THREAT TO LIFE AND LIMB OF THE PATIENT OR ANOTHER PERSON?

Treating suicidality is always the top-priority treatment goal for the simple reason that psychotherapy is not helpful to dead people (Linehan, 1993a, p. 124, citing Mintz, 1968). Even when there is no imminent threat, suicidal behavior is always a top-priority treatment target. Related, parasuicidal behaviors (nonfatal self-harm, which includes both failed suicide attempts and self-harming behaviors that are not intended to cause death) are also high on the priority list because even when they are not intended to cause death they can have this result. Similarly, if the patient is harming or threatening to harm another person, this problem is top priority.

The fact that behaviors intended to cause death or self-harm are top priority treatment targets may seem so obvious as to not need discussion. However, often patients who have these problems do not wish to focus on them and are skilled at evading these topics and punishing the therapist for addressing them. Often patients do not view suicidal and parasuicidal behaviors as problems. In fact, they view them as solutions. And in the rush of problems presented by a multiple-problem patient, even suicidality can get lost in the shuffle.

DO ANY PROBLEMS UNDERMINE OR JEOPARDIZE THE THERAPY ITSELF?

Linehan (1993a) recommends making problems that jeopardize or undermine therapy the second highest in priority, with the rationale that if the therapy time is wasted or the therapy collapses altogether, no other problems can be solved. Such problems (Linehan labeled these as therapy-interfering or therapy-destroying behaviors) include: agoraphobia so severe that the patient cannot travel to the therapy session, interpersonal problems that impede the patient and therapist from working collaboratively together, intense urges to leave town and start a new life elsewhere, or problems that interfere with the assessment process. Sometimes the patient's presenting problems interfere with collecting assessment data to identify goals and tasks of therapy. Examples include the person who experiences so much shame that she cannot provide an accurate problem list, the one who is so indecisive that he cannot set treatment goals, or the person who is so untrusting and fearful that others will hurt him that he refuses to complete the intake questionnaires and cannot establish a warm and trusting connection with the therapist.

IS THERE A PROBLEM, WHICH IF IT IS NOT SOLVED, WILL PREVENT SOLUTION OF ANY OTHER PROBLEM?

Linehan (1993a) recommends placing problems that she terms "quality-of-life-interfering behaviors" third on the priority list. Examples include homelessness, unemployment, significant substance abuse, homicidality, criminal behavior that may lead to jail, high-risk sexual behaviors, and living with an abusive partner. The rationale here is that unless these problems are solved, the patient is not likely to be able to solve other problems. Again, it is vital for therapists to attend to these. Patients often want to ignore them. For example, a marketing executive who sought treatment for depression had a long-standing habit of drinking a bottle of wine several nights a week despite the fact that it was interfering with his functioning at work. He stated that did this in order to escape his dysphoria. This was not only a quality-of-life-interfering behavior, it was also a therapy-interfering behavior, since it made diagnosis impossible because of the difficulty distinguishing between alcohol-related and mood disorder symptoms. A journalist had a panic disorder and agoraphobia that prevented her from flying on an airplane. She also had anger problems that meant she kept getting fired. Although the patient was more motivated to overcome her fear of flying so she could travel to Europe with friends, the therapist viewed the anger problem as a higher priority because it led to frequent ruptures in the patient–therapist relationship. In addition, it caused her to be repeatedly fired, which jeopardized her ability to pay for rent and therapy.

WHAT PROBLEM DOES THE PATIENT MOST WANT TO SOLVE?

Focusing on problems that are emotionally compelling and important to the patient contributes to a successful therapy. An academic who sought treatment for depression had goals of improving his scholarly productivity and his marriage. I assumed his work problems were of highest priority and I tended to focus on them. In fact, the interpersonal goals were actually more important to him and therapy was more successful when we prioritized them because he was willing to work harder to achieve them.

WHAT PROBLEM IS INTERFERING MOST WITH FUNCTIONING?

A patient with OCD has both washing and checking symptoms. She is spending 5 hours every evening in the shower and as a result is having a hard time getting enough sleep and functioning at work the next day. She is also spending a half-hour at home in the evening checking the doors and windows before she goes to bed. The washing problem is interfering much more with functioning than is the checking problem and therefore deserves a higher priority. Sometimes one problem can exacerbate another problem, and when this happens, the first problem is a high priority treatment target, as in the case of the patient who spends so much time on OCD checking rituals that her sleep is disrupted, which exacerbates her bipolar disorder. In this patient's case, the OCD checking rituals are highest priority because solving that problem will address both the OCD and the bipolar disorder.

WHAT PROBLEM, IF SOLVED, WILL SOLVE MANY OR MOST OF THE PATIENT'S OTHER PROBLEMS?

To answer this question, the therapist must have a hypothesis (formulation) about how the patient's problems are related (see Haynes, 1992). For example, Anita had three problems. Her chief complaint was worry and catastrophic fears that her graphic design business would fail. Her second problem was that her business *was* beginning to fail: her phone was not ringing and she had almost no customers. A third problem was her passivity: she wasn't taking productive action to solve her business problem. Instead, she spent her time reading the newspaper, working out at the gym, chatting online, and waiting for the phone to ring.

To develop an initial treatment plan I relied on my hypothesis (formulation) that Anita's passivity was the problem that, if solved, would solve all the other problems. My formulation proposed that if Anita got more active, she could solve the business problems and this would reduce her worry, both because she would be doing activities (business problem solving) that were incompatible with worry and because she would have less to worry about! Anita accepted the formulation and the plan to focus on the passivity. We worked to help her develop and carry out a marketing plan for her business. As predicted, when she became more active her business improved and her worry decreased.

WHAT PROBLEM, WHEN TREATED, MIGHT DESTABILIZE THE PATIENT?

Treatment of some problems can make things worse before they get getter. For example, exposure-based treatments for anxiety disorders can increase the patient's discomfort in the short run (Foa, Zoellner, Feeny, Hembree, & Alvarez-Conrad, 2002). In cases like this the therapist may elect to begin by increasing the patient's armamentarium of coping tools before tackling tough problems. Or the therapist may elect to address other problems that are easier to solve and will strengthen the patient's coping ability before tackling challenging problems. For example, if a person with PTSD has a minimal or even abusive social support network, the therapist might elect to work to firm up the patient's social support network before tackling the PTSD symptoms (Kimble, Riggs, & Keane, 1998).

IS THERE A PROBLEM THAT CAN BE QUICKLY AND EASILY SOLVED?

Sometimes a quick success in addressing a problem, even if it is not a major one, can help the patient build the confidence and motivation to tackle bigger problems. For example, interventions to overcome panic symptoms or a specific phobia can often be quickly effective and give the patient the impetus to take on bigger problems. This notion can also help the therapist resist starting treatment by taking on goals that are likely to be difficult to achieve, as when a severely depressed person wants to set a goal of stopping smoking.

* * *

This chapter describes the first steps in the pretreatment process, namely the steps of beginning to build a relationship and obtaining a Problem List and diagnosis. The next chapter describes the next steps in the process. These include developing mechanism hypotheses for the problems by using the theories covered in Chapters 2, 3, and 4; identifying precipitants of the current problems and origins of the mechanisms; tying the elements of a formulation together; and using the formulation to set treatment goals.

SIX

Developing an Initial Case Formulation and Setting Treatment Goals

This chapter continues the discussion of pretreatment, describing how to go from Problem List to initial case formulation and how to use the formulation to set treatment goals. As the therapist focuses on these tasks, he or she takes advantage of opportunities that present themselves to address other pretreatment tasks, including building the relationship and informing the patient about the therapist's formulation, diagnostic hypotheses, and intervention ideas.

FORMULATING THE CASE

To review, the case-level formulation proposes hypotheses about the *mechanisms* causing the patient's *problems*, the *precipitants* that are activating the mechanisms, and the *origins* of those mechanisms, and ties all of these elements together into a coherent whole. I discussed strategies for obtaining a list of *problems* in Chapter 5. Here I discuss strategies for developing hypotheses about *mechanisms*, *precipitants*, and *origins*, and tying these elements together into a formulation of the case. I also describe the process I used to develop an initial case formulation for Angela, the patient who was introduced in the previous chapter.

Developing Mechanism Hypotheses

The heart of the case-level formulation is a description of psychological mechanisms that cause and maintain the patient's problems and symptoms. The formulation might also include some biological mechanisms (e.g., low thyroid can cause depressive symptoms) but here I focus primarily on the psychological.

I describe two strategies for developing a mechanism hypothesis. The first strategy is to use a disorder formulation that underpins an EST, such as the formulation of OCD that underpins exposure and response prevention or the formulation of depression that underpins behavioral activation (BA). A second strategy is to use a more general psychological theory such as one of the cognitive, learning, or emotion theories described in Chapters 2, 3, and 4.

Using a Disorder Formulation That Underpins an EST

A key advantage of this strategy is that it is tightly tied to an EST. The therapist identifies the nomothetic formulation that underpins the EST and uses that as a template for the formulation of the case at hand. Then the EST manual (Wilson, 1996a) can serve as a template for the cognitive-behavior treatment plan for that patient.

There are three steps to this strategy for developing a mechanism hypothesis. Because most ESTs target a DSM disorder, the therapist's first step is to identify a DSM disorder that will serve as an "anchor" for the case formulation. Second, the clinician selects an EST for the anchoring disorder and uses the formulation underpinning that treatment as a template for the formulation of the case at hand. Third, the therapist individualizes the formulation template to fit the case at hand and extrapolates to account for all of the problems on the patient's Problem List.

SELECT AN ANCHORING DISORDER

Selecting an anchoring disorder is easy if the patient has a single DSM disorder for which an EST is available. When the patient has more than one disorder, the therapist must decide which disorder to use as an anchoring disorder. The main criterion for selecting an anchoring disorder is treatment utility (S. C. Hayes et al., 1987). That is, which will lead to an effective treatment plan? Of course, this question can be difficult to answer. However, I highlight it to make the point that the therapist is not seeking a correct formulation, just a helpful one.

Often the most helpful anchoring disorder is the one that accounts for the largest number of problems on the Problem List or the one that interferes most with the patient's functioning. Thus, disorders like bipolar disorder, schizophrenia, and borderline personality disorder (disorders that can account for many presenting problems) are often good choices for the anchoring diagnosis. Another way to choose an anchoring diagnosis is to select the diagnosis that provides the simplest or best account of how the problems are related or provides a formulation of the problems the patient most wants to address in treatment.

The strategy of beginning to develop a formulation by selecting an anchoring disorder can be helpful even when the patient's main or only disorder is one for which no EST is available. In any of these situations the therapist can select a DSM disorder for which an EST is available to serve as an anchoring disorder even if the patient does not meet criteria for that disorder. The therapist might select a DSM disorder that captures some of the patient's primary symptoms. Or the therapist can select a disorder that is in the same class of disorders as the patient's main disorder (e.g., another impulse control disorder for a patient who has a problem with skin picking). Again, the main criterion for selecting an anchoring diagnosis is treatment utility.

SELECT AN EST FOR THE DISORDER AND USE ITS FORMULATION AS A TEMPLATE

Locate an EST for the anchoring diagnosis and then identify the nomothetic disorder formulation that underpins the EST. For example, several ESTs for PTSD are available, including cognitive therapy (Ehlers & Clark, 2000), prolonged exposure (Foa et al., 2007), and cognitive reprocessing therapy (Resick & Schnicke, 1993). Each of these ESTs is based on a nomothetic formulation of the disorder, any of which might serve as a template for formulating the case of a patient who meets criteria for PTSD.

INDIVIDUALIZE AND EXTRAPOLATE THE TEMPLATE FORMULATION

To individualize the formulation, first identify the key elements of the nomothetic template's formulation hypothesis. For example, the formulation underpinning Beck's EST for depression states that past early events (origins) cause the patient to learn particular types of dysfunctional schema (mechanism). When triggered in the present (precipitants), these schema produce painful emotions, automatic thoughts, and maladaptive behaviors (problems). The next step is to individualize the key elements in the formulation to describe the particular case at hand. In other words, a formulation for a particular patient based on Beck's model will identify *which* early events (origins) caused *which* schemas that are now being triggered by *which* precipitants to give rise to *which* automatic thoughts, emotions, and maladaptive behaviors (problems).

Then the therapist extrapolates to account for all of the patient's problems. To do this, the therapist starts by identifying the problems on the Problem List that can be accounted for by the anchoring disorder itself and then builds the simplest story possible to account for the other problems.

An example is the case of Maria, a 35-year-old married graduate student who sought treatment for the following Problem List: depression, emotional reactivity, marital distress, chaotic interpersonal relationships, and difficulty settling on a career. She was studying for a PhD in biology but was considering dropping out of graduate school to pursue an acting career. Many of her problems were long-standing but they had flared up as Maria approached her comprehensive exams and confronted her career dilemma and as her husband became increasingly unhappy with her emotional instability.

Maria met criteria for MDD and personality disorder NOS. She had several symptoms of borderline personality disorder but did not meet full criteria for the disorder. I adopted borderline personality disorder as my anchoring diagnosis because it accounted for most of the problems on her list. I chose to adapt the formulation underpinning Linehan's (1993a, 1993b) DBT to Maria's case. Linehan conceptualizes the symptoms of borderline personality disorder as resulting from deficits in both the core emotional system (high emotional sensitivity to environmental stimuli, intense emotions, and a slow return to baseline after emotions are triggered) and the control system (a failure to learn and use good strategies to regulate emotion). Using this nomothetic formulation as a template led to the following formulation of Maria's case. The elements of the formulation are indicated in CAPITAL LETTERS.

> Maria grew up in an abusive home in which she was punished or ignored when she expressed distress in a reasonable way and only received attention when she dramatically and intensely communicated distress (e.g., by punching a wall). Her father appeared to have untreated bipolar disorder and her parents "fought like cats and dogs." They modeled maladaptive emotion regulation strategies and did not teach or model adaptive ones, and Maria may have inherited a biological predisposition to bipolar disorder (ORIGINS). As a result, Maria had high emotional sensitivity

and used maladaptive emotion regulation strategies. Maria tended to invalidate, minimize, ignore, and suppress her emotional reactions until they were so extreme that she lost control of her behavior (MECHANISM). For example, she ignored disrespectful or mean behavior from her friends until she became overwhelmed with rage and broke off the relationship. She experienced emotional reactivity (PROBLEM), especially outbursts of rage and anger (PROBLEM), and had chaotic intense relationships with all of the important people in her life (PROBLEM), including her husband, girlfriends, and dissertation chairperson. Her tendency to invalidate and ignore her emotional experiences also blocked her from getting the information she needed to identify her career interests and goals. She felt truly lost about whether to pursue a career as a biologist or an actress (PROBLEM). These mechanisms were chronically present but had been triggered more intensely by her upcoming comprehensive exams and by her husband's increasing unhappiness with her emotionality (PRECIPITANTS). Both of these events tended to push Maria to try even harder to suppress her feelings, which had led to increased volatility. She felt out of control. The accumulation of all these problems and her failed efforts to solve them made her miserable and depressed (PROBLEM).

This formulation individualizes and expands the DBT conceptualization of borderline personality disorder (Linehan, 1993a) to accommodate the details of Maria's case. The formulation will also help the therapist plan and guide treatment for Maria. The main treatment targets identified by the DBT conceptualization are the emotional sensitivity, the maladaptive emotion regulation strategies (avoidance, escape, and other poor strategies), and the absence of adaptive emotion regulation strategies. Maria's therapist would target those phenomena in her treatment and would likely add some interventions, perhaps couples therapy, to address Maria's marital problems.

Using Cognitive, Learning, and Emotion Theories

An alternative to the anchoring diagnosis strategy that was just presented is what I call the basic theory strategy, that is, using one of the basic cognitive, learning, and emotion theories described in Chapters 2, 3, and 4 as the foundation for a case formulation. Examples of this strategy include the use of learning theory to formulate the case of the young man who had a problem of psychogenic vomiting (see Chapter 3) or the use of approach and withdrawal theory to conceptualize the case of Susan (see Chapter 4). As already noted, a strength of the anchoring diagnosis strategy is that it is tightly tied to ESTs. However, the basic theory strategy, which I describe here, has its own advantages. One is that it is more directly tied to the phenomena (symptoms, behaviors, cognitions, and emotions) that are the treatment targets of CBT (Persons, 1986a). As a result, the basic theory approach to conceptualization can make it easier for the therapist to do theory-driven hypothesis testing and decision making. In addition, this strategy allows the therapist to develop conceptualizations of disorders and problems for which no EST-based formulation is available. The basic theory strategy is also useful when a single model underpins ESTs for two or more of a patient's disorders. Evidence-based formulations of many symptoms and disorders based on Beck's cognitive model and learning theory models have been developed and therefore those two approaches are particularly suitable for formulating multiple-problem cases.

There are three steps to developing a mechanism hypothesis based on basic cognitive, learning, and/or emotion theory. First, the clinician selects a symptom (as in the vomiting case presented in Chapter 3 on learning theory) or a group of symptoms (as in Susan's case in Chapter 4 on emotion theory) as a focus. Second, the clinician chooses a basic theory that can account for the symptom or symptoms. The third step is to individualize and extrapolate from the basic theory.

How does the therapist decide which theory or model to use? Again, the guiding principle here is treatment utility: which model is most likely to produce a formulation that leads to a treatment plan that will help the patient accomplish his or her goals? Helpful grounds for choosing include the strength of the evidence base, the model that seems to best fit the case (Haynes et al., 1999), the one that provides the most parsimonious account of the patient's problems, the one that is most likely to be acceptable to the patient, and the one with which the therapist is most familiar.

After a therapist selects a model, he or she must flesh out the idiographic details of the proposed mechanisms and extrapolate the formulation to describe how these mechanisms cause all of the patient's symptoms, disorders, and problems. Here I discuss strategies for doing this for Beck's cognitive model, learning models, and emotion theory.

BECK'S COGNITIVE THEORY

As described in Chapter 2, Beck's cognitive theory views symptoms as consisting of linked automatic thoughts, behaviors, and emotions that result from the activation of schemas by stressful life events. Thus, in Beck's model the schemas and the linked automatic thoughts, behaviors, and emotions are the mechanisms causing the patient's problems. To individualize a case-level formulation based on Beck's model, the clinician needs to identify the likely *origins* of the patient's schemas, the particular *schemas* themselves, the particular *precipitants* that are activating them, and the resulting *symptoms and problems,* perhaps identifying some of the typical automatic thoughts, behaviors, and emotions that make up those problems. Here I use Beck's model to formulate the case of Sharon, and I illustrate some of the strategies described in Chapter 2 for collecting the information to develop the formulation.

Sharon was a 52-year-old Caucasian housewife who lived with her husband, a mail carrier, and her mother, who was partially disabled by a recent stroke. Sharon sought treatment when she found herself increasingly overwhelmed by caring for her mother after the stroke.

Sharon and I worked together to develop the following Problem List for her case. I identified typical behaviors, emotions, and cognitions for each problem to aid in the process of developing a mechanism hypothesis for Sharon's case.

1. Depressive symptoms (BDI = 25). Behaviorally she was inactive and withdrawn. Emotions included sadness, guilt, and irritability. Cognitions included "I'm not as good as other people," "I'm not doing a good job with my mother," and "I'm selfish and self-indulgent."

2. Anxiety symptoms (Burns AI = 20) were also a problem, especially social anxiety in many situations. She tended to have cognitions of "I'm boring and uninteresting,"

"No one wants to spend time with me," and "I can't handle social situations." She was quite avoidant and socially isolated.

3. Worry was a major problem. Sharon worried constantly about social interactions ("I said the wrong thing") and other potential negative events. For example, if her husband arrived home late from work she worried that "Something bad has happened to him" and she called him to check on him. The most frightening worries were about her mother. Sharon had about 10 fearful thoughts/images about her mother daily, fearing she would fall and break her hip or experience some other medical catastrophe. A theme of these worries was "I have to be sure nothing bad happens because if something did I would not be able to cope with it." Emotions included anxiety, tension, and irritability.

4. Anger/irritability was a problem in its own right. Sharon was very upset by it ("I should be able to control myself!"). Especially troublesome to her was her tendency to lose her temper with her mother when she felt overwhelmed and frustrated by her mother's fears, helplessness, and constant requests for reassurance. "She shouldn't be so helpless and passive!" "I should be more patient and generous."

5. Sharon's marriage was distressed. She described her husband as a workaholic and said she had made repeated requests to him to change without results and had decided to accept the situation. "He's married to his job and there's nothing I can do about it." Emotions included helplessness and hopelessness.

6. No enjoyable work. Sharon was not employed or doing any volunteer work or activity that was gratifying and meaningful to her. "I can't handle a full-time job and I don't enjoy anything." She had previously worked as a teacher and had left her job some years ago when her mother began to have medical problems and came to live with the couple.

Sharon met criteria for MDD, dysthymia, generalized social phobia, generalized anxiety disorder, and avoidant personality disorder. Many of her problems were long-standing but the main precipitant of Sharon's acute distress was her mother's stroke about 6 months earlier.

I selected Beck's theory as the basis for a mechanism hypothesis of Sharon's case because its application to the symptoms of anxiety and depression that Sharon suffered had been elaborated in many places in the literature and had a good evidence base. Using Beck's model as a template (see Figure 2.4), I developed the formulation of Sharon's case that is presented in Figure 6.1. To obtain the schema (mechanism) hypotheses described in Figure 6.1, I used several strategies.

First, Beck's writings helped generate some schema hypotheses. Beck et al. (A. T. Beck et al., 1985) propose that anxious individuals have schemas of themselves as weak, fragile, and helpless and of the world as dangerous and threatening. And Beck's (A. T. Beck et al., 1979) conceptualization of depression suggested self-schemas that fit with other information I obtained about Sharon's case, namely that she viewed herself as inadequate, unimportant, and uninteresting.

Second, I looked for common elements that cut across the problems on Sharon's Problem List. I identified several automatic thoughts of this sort, including "I'm fragile/vulnerable," "I'm inadequate/not good enough," and "The world is dangerous and threatening." These thoughts suggested schema hypotheses that were consistent with

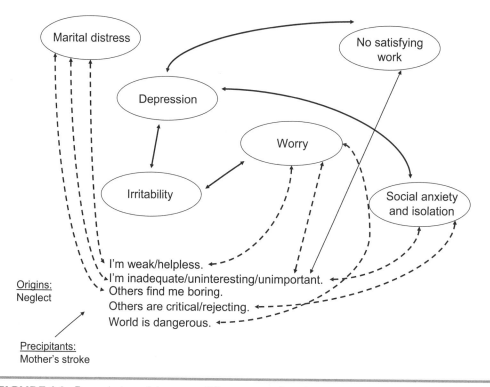

FIGURE 6.1. Formulation of the case of Sharon using Beck's theory.

the above ideas I already had. Behaviors that cut across her problems included withdrawal and avoidance.

Third, I used a Thought Record to dissect a recent problem situation Sharon had experienced. This helped to identify some of her automatic thoughts, behaviors, and emotions and to learn more about what situations triggered distress for her. The situation in question was "thinking about asking a neighbor to meet for coffee." This situation triggered a stream of automatic thoughts, including "She won't want to do it," "She thinks I'm boring," "She won't return my call," and "She'll think I'm lame for asking," and "I'll do it later." Emotions in this situation were anxiety and embarrassment. Sharon's behavioral response in this situation was to postpone making the call. Sharon's automatic thoughts in this situation supported the schema hypotheses I had already generated. Of course, my schema hypotheses based on a single Thought Record must be preliminary and the schemas that appear to generate distress in this situation may not be active in other situations. Nevertheless, the data from the Thought Record provide an excellent starting point for a mechanism hypothesis of the case. Finally, when I learned about Sharon's upbringing, I got information that was consistent with and thus supported my schema hypotheses. (I say more about origins later in the chapter.) Sharon was the middle of six children and she had had a younger sister who was severely retarded and required a huge amount of attention from their parents. As a result, Sharon always felt "invisible" in her family. Sharon's experiences of neglect helped me understand how she might have come to view herself as uninteresting and unimportant and others as not interested in her.

LEARNING THEORY

Learning models view target behaviors (Bs) as controlled by antecedents (As) and consequences (Cs). In these models the mechanisms causing and maintaining patient problems are described by the learning theories detailed in Chapter 3. Respondent theories explain behaviors as controlled primarily by antecedents, and operant theories explain behaviors as controlled primarily by their consequences.

To develop a case formulation based on learning models, the therapist first identifies a target behavior and then collects information about the antecedents and consequences of the behavior. Strategies for doing this were briefly described in Chapter 3 and include obtaining a timeline of the events leading up to the patient's symptoms and problems, asking the patient to self-monitor to track As, Bs, and Cs, and conducting a behavioral chain analysis to flesh out the As and Cs associated with a particular instance of B. Clinical interviews and reports from significant others about the As and Cs of problem behaviors can also be useful. I illustrate using some of these strategies to develop a learning theory hypothesis of Angela's case later in this chapter.

EMOTION THEORY

As described in Chapter 4, several models of basic emotion can be used to conceptualize and treat psychopathology. I illustrate here the use of Peter Lang's bioinformational theory and the model of emotional processing based on it that was developed by Foa and Kozak (1986) to conceptualize the case of Zoe.

Zoe was a 50-year-old divorced woman who worked as a project manager for a software development firm. She sought treatment for what she called "my fears of leaving home." Zoe met criteria for panic disorder and agoraphobia (PDA). She was experiencing few symptoms of anxiety and panic because she was assiduously avoiding situations that had triggered anxiety and panic in the past. However, her life was increasingly constrained by her inability to travel via bridges, crowded freeways, public transportation, airplanes, and elevators. Zoe also reported a history of trauma; she had been raped one day when she was working late alone in a client's office. She did not meet full criteria for PTSD because she reported only avoidance symptoms but no reexperiencing or arousal symptoms. She admitted to avoiding situations that reminded her of the rape (large open places at night and men wearing certain types of custodial uniforms), but she insisted that this avoidance behavior was rarely needed and that the past rape was not currently troubling her.

I used the methods described in Chapter 5 to develop a Problem List for Zoe. She had PDA and subsyndromal symptoms of PTSD. She was having some difficulty at work because she had been turning down projects that involved travel. Another problem was her relationship with her ex-husband. About 2 years earlier Zoe had finally gotten up the courage to leave her husband, whose verbal abuse and alcoholism had destroyed their relationship. However, she still needed to deal with him because they shared custody for their son.

My task was to develop a formulation of Zoe's case that helped me understand her PDA and PTSD symptoms, her work and family problems, and the relationships among them. Although Zoe was clear that she wanted to address her PDA symptoms and she stated that her rape and marital history were not problems for her, I had some concern that these problems were linked and that treatment of the PDA symptoms might trigger some PTSD symptoms. For that reason, instead of using a formulation based on the PDA diagnosis, I chose a more general model that made it easier to tie together Zoe's various anxiety and avoidance symptoms. I chose Peter Lang's model, which conceptualizes pathological fear as represented in memory by linked propositions that describe the stimulus, response, and meaning elements of a fear network. These are conceptualized as linked to a defensive motivational system in the lower brain.

To use this model to formulate Zoe's case, I needed to collect information about the stimulus, response, and meaning elements of her fears. To do this, I used information I obtained from the Adult Intake Questionnaire, from my clinical interview, and from some self-report scales. I used the Mobility Inventory (Chambless et al., 1985) to identify the situations Zoe avoided, the Body Sensation Questionnaire (Chambless et al., 1984) to identify the sensations she feared, and the Agoraphobic Cognitions Questionnaire (Chambless et al., 1984) to get some initial information about meaning elements of her fears. Stimulus elements she feared were large open spaces, bridges, crowded freeways, airplanes, public transportation, and elevators; she felt particularly frightened when she was alone in those places and when it was dark. Zoe's main response element to these situations was escape and avoidance. Later I worked through the interoceptive exposure exercises in Zuercher-White (1995) to get more details about the response elements of Zoe's anxiety, which included palpitations, sweating, and lightheadedness. The main meaning element of her fears was "I am going to go crazy." What's especially interesting here is the overlap of the cognitive network elements of Zoe's PDA and subsyndromal PTSD symptoms. Stimulus elements of large open spaces, being alone, and darkness, and response elements of escape and avoidance were common to both networks.

Now I confronted the challenge of considering whether Zoe's family issues could be tied to this formulation of her anxiety symptoms. Zoe and I speculated that for many years she had responded to the stimulus situations of her husband's drinking and abusive behavior by avoiding noticing them. She had learned to do this as a child by watching her mother's passive helpless responses to her father's alcoholism and violence. However, she had begun gradually to shift over time as she noted the effects of her husband's behavior on their child, and she eventually divorced. Her hypothesis that she had learned on her own to incorporate new response elements to stimulus situations in her marriage (and did not need more help there) was consistent with the observation that as she got up the courage to leave her marriage, her anxiety symptoms had improved. Following her success confronting the problems in her marriage, Zoe was ready to confront her PDA.

This conceptualization made some sense to me, and certainly Zoe was very clear that she wanted to focus her therapy on her PDA symptoms. Therefore, I developed a formulation of her case that emphasized the PDA symptoms and the view of them proposed by the Lang et al. model. I developed a formulation of her PDA that was similar to the formulation diagrammed in Figure 4.1 except that it also included stimulus and response elements related to her PTSD symptoms. And I pointed out to Zoe the overlap of the stimulus and response elements of her PDA and PTSD-related fears, and warned her that treatment of the PDA might activate some PTSD fears and that we would watch for these carefully as we proceeded.

As mentioned above, the treatment targets described by the Lang model are the stimulus, response, and meaning elements of the fears. The mechanism change goals of Zoe's treatment entailed activation of her fear network in a way that would allow her to obtain new response and meaning elements to the stimulus elements of the fear. We negotiated an agreement to focus our therapy on achieving goals of overcoming her PDA so she could travel freely in the Bay Area and could fly to Europe.

Zoe and I carried out *in vivo* and imaginal exposures to her feared situations and worked to handle them without escaping or using safety behaviors (e.g., clutching a bottle of water). Given our formulation, we made a point of carrying out some of the exposures at night and when she was alone. Not surprisingly, during those exposures, some memories and emotions tied to the rape emerged. However, because they were mild and/or because we were prepared for them, Zoe easily moved on through these and mastered them. In conjunction with exposures, I did some cognitive restructuring to help Zoe consolidate the new response and meaning information she obtained from the exposures. Zoe worked hard in treatment and quickly accomplished her goals. She reported, when I quizzed her about it, that she felt she was interacting more effectively with her ex-husband as a result of her newfound confidence.

Using More Than One Mechanism Hypothesis

In the above descriptions, the therapist relied on a single mechanism hypothesis as the basis for the case formulation. However, the therapist might elect to rely on more than one mechanism hypothesis to account for a single disorder or set of symptoms. For example, the therapist treating a patient with depression might simultaneously hold a formulation of the depressive symptoms (based on Beck's model) as resulting from schema activation and (based on Lewinsohn's model) as resulting from a dearth of positive reinforcers. These models do not conflict. Both might be simultaneously true. The therapist might use interventions from both models in treatment.

Or the therapist might use two models to account for different symptoms in a single case formulation. For example, the therapist might use Beck's theory to account for a patient's anxiety as caused by activation of schemas (e.g., of the self as weak and vulnerable and world as dangerous and threatening) and operant conditioning theory to account for the patient's excessive use of alcohol as negatively reinforced because it allows the individual to escape from anxiety. In fact, this approach is consistent with the approach used by some nomothetic formulations underpinning ESTs. For example, DBT draws on conditioning theory, emotion theory, and cognitive theory (and other sources, including zen philosophy!) to conceptualize symptoms and generate interventions.

The therapist might also use different mechanism hypotheses at different points in treatment. For a person who meets criteria for borderline personality disorder and PTSD, the DBT formulation is useful early in treatment when the main target behaviors are the impulsive suicidal and self-harming behaviors of borderline personality disorder. When those behaviors are under control, the treatment focuses on PTSD symptoms and one of the mechanism hypotheses underpinning one (or more!) of the ESTs for PTSD might be more useful.

As noted in Chapter 1, using more than one mechanism hypothesis as the basis for a case formulation can lead to muddled thinking or the use of conflicting models and interventions. However, relying on multiple mechanism hypotheses also has advantages. One is flexibility (the ability to shift to a different model to align with the patient's views or to generate new interventions when treatment based on the first model fails). Another is the potential for increased power arising from the use of multiple interventions flowing from more than one model. The final arbiter of the wisdom of this approach is treatment utility. That is, does the use of multiple mechanism hypotheses lead to an effective intervention plan for this patient? To answer this question, the therapist relies on a hypothesis-testing approach to treatment that is guided by careful process and outcome monitoring, as described in Chapter 9.

Information about precipitants, discussed next, often contributes to generating and testing mechanism hypotheses and developing a coherent formulation.

Identifying Precipitants of the Problems

Most cognitive-behavior formulations have a diathesis–stress format. The *mechanisms* piece of the formulation is the diathesis, and the *precipitants* piece, discussed here, describes the stressor that activates the diathesis. Precipitants can be internal (onset of diabetes), external (earthquake), biological (AIDS), psychological (guilt about father's illness), or all of the above.

Precipitants and problems frequently overlap. For example, Angela's marital problems were both a *consequence* of one of her other problems (e.g., her depression and irritability, which caused her husband to distance himself) and a factor that *precipitated or exacerbated* her symptoms. In a formulation of Angela's case based on Beck's model, for example, her husband's distance and disengagement activated her belief that no one cared and that she had to solve everything herself, causing her to feel sad, overwhelmed, and isolated. The term *vulnerability factor* can also be used to describe chronic stressors, like Angela's marital distress, that contribute to onset of a disorder or symptoms.

Information about precipitants is useful in many ways. First, information about precipitants helps the therapist generate mechanism hypotheses. For example, A. T. Beck (1983) proposes that events involving interpersonal loss and rejection would be expected to precipitate depression in patients who have schemas of themselves as unlovable and of others as rejecting/abandoning, whereas failure experiences would be expected to precipitate depression in patients who hold schemas of themselves as inadequate and defective. Thus, if the patient got depressed following his wife's decision to divorce him, this information about precipitants might contribute to the therapist's speculation that the patient has a core schema of himself as unlovable and of others as rejecting and abandoning. Information about precipitants can also be used to check the therapist's initial schema hypotheses. If the schemas do not "match" the precipitants, some adjustment in the schema hypotheses or the understanding of the precipitants or both may be needed.

Information about precipitants can also point to treatment targets. For example, if a patient's symptoms were precipitated by a harsh performance evaluation from an unstable and unreasonable boss, the patient may want to consider changing jobs.

Sometimes a clear precipitant is evident, as in the case of a woman who becomes depressed following a layoff from her job. However, even in a case like this, assessment is needed to identify exactly what aspect of the layoff is triggering the woman's depressive symptoms. Is it the loss of structure to her day? Is it the loss of social support? Is it the loss of reinforcement she received from doing work she enjoyed?

Frequently the precipitant is not immediately evident. Sometimes multiple precipitants cumulate over weeks or months or even years to trigger an illness episode. To obtain information about precipitants, the therapist can begin by asking the patient for her ideas about what external events might have triggered her current problems. However, often patients are poor reporters of this type of information. Working with the patient to construct a detailed timeline of events leading up to the development of symptoms is often useful in identifying precipitants. Often the best way to develop this timeline is to start by asking when the patient first noticed symptoms and asking "what happened around that time in your life?" This question is usually more productive than the question "what events caused those symptoms to develop?" because often patients (and all of us) are not very good at noting causes of symptoms. Patients often do not identify the links between events and symptoms until a detailed timeline is constructed. This task is a really interesting overlap of assessment and intervention, as patients often are not aware of relationships between events and symptoms and find it extremely helpful to learn them. Another valuable resource is family members, who sometimes are far enough removed from events to give useful information about precipitating circumstances.

When the patient has multiple problems and disorders, it can be cumbersome to assess the precipitants of every problem. Instead, the therapist can focus on identifying precipitants of the primary DSM disorder, the major symptoms, or the patient's decision to seek treatment. For example, a teacher who had long-standing symptoms of depression, OCD, generalized anxiety disorder (GAD), and social phobia sought treatment after she accepted an administrative job that required extensive public speaking that was quite anxiety-provoking for her.

Identifying Origins of the Mechanisms

The *origins* part of the formulation offers a hypothesis about how the patient learned or acquired the mechanisms that are causing his or her symptoms. Origins differ from precipitants in that origins are distal (distant in time) and precipitants are proximal (near in time). Origins can be external environmental events or experiences (e.g., the death of a parent or early abuse or neglect), cultural factors (Hays & Iwamasa, 2006), biological factors (e.g., an unusually short stature that might elicit teasing from peers), and genetics.

So, for example, if Beck's theory is used, the origins part of the formulation speculates about how the patient learned the schemas that are causing his or her symptoms. If a learning theory is used to conceptualize anxiety symptoms, origins describes any initial conditioning event, such as a trauma or panic attack that may have led to conditioned emotional responses. Origins of skill deficits can include models of maladaptive skills (e.g., parents who resolve disagreements through physical violence), the failure to be exposed to models of adaptive skills, or both. If an emotion theory is used, the formulation can describe, for example, how patients learned the maladaptive or inadequate emotion regulation strategies that contribute to their current symptoms.

CBT tends to focus on the present. Then why does the therapist, in the case conceptualization, seek information about origins? First, origins are a source of mechanism hypotheses. Certain types of origins are linked to certain mechanisms, as in the link between early abuse and emotion dysregulation (Deblinger, Thakkar-Kolar, & Ryan, 2006). Second, information about origins serves as a test of the mechanism or other elements of the formulation. If the origins don't match up well with the other elements of the formulation, the formulation is not cohesive and may need revision. Third, an understanding of origins can be helpful in treatment. Certainly the treatment of PTSD, which often involves exposure to memories of the trauma and stimuli that were present during the trauma, is an example. Sometimes the patient's understanding of the origins of his or her difficulties has powerful therapeutic effects. An example is the case of a suicidal young mother. Awareness that many of her difficulties originated in her mother's abandonment of her became a powerful motivator to not kill herself (so that her child would not experience the abandonment she had suffered).

Information about origins can be obtained from several sources. One is the patient's report of early upbringing, especially relationships with parents and other caretakers, and other significant childhood events, especially traumas, neglect, and abuse. Information about psychiatric illness in biological relatives can shed light on both biological and psychosocial origins. A discussion of racial or ethnic factors that may contribute to the patient's difficulties can also be illuminating.

Attention to the empirical literature can guide the assessment of origins. For example, Barlow and Chorpita (1998) reviewed findings showing that anxiety is related to perceptions of helplessness and that two parenting styles appear to contribute to a child's perceptions of helplessness: lack of responsiveness and overcontrol. For example, even a small child can signal nonverbally (by turning his head or crying) that he is overwhelmed by an overstimulating environment. The unresponsive parent who does not respond to these cues teaches the child that he is helpless and has no control over the situation. The overcontrolling parent blocks her child from exploring new and challenging situations and learning the skills to manage them and thereby promotes the child's perception of himself as unable to handle difficult situations. Thus, when seeking origins of anxiety, the clinician might profitably assess for parental lack of responsiveness and overcontrol.

Tying the Elements of the Formulation Together

As the therapist collects information about each element of the case formulation, he or she checks to see whether the elements seem to fit together. For example, Sharon's self-schema of "I'm unimportant" makes logical sense given the neglect she experienced as a child. This process of checking the elements of the formulation to see if they are consistent with one another tests the therapist's formulation hypotheses (Turkat & Maisto, 1985) and improves the overall coherence of the formulation.

One of the main ways the case-level formulation is useful is that it offers hypotheses about how the patient's various problems and disorders are related. Problems can be related in many ways. Multiple problems can result from the same mechanism. For example, a view of the self as vulnerable and helpless commonly leads to anxiety, avoidance behavior, and the failure to fulfill major life roles. The therapist tries to account for all of the problems using as few mechanisms as possible (Persons, 1989) so that the formulation is simple and easy to use to guide clinical decision making. Sometimes a single set of mechanisms, however, does not suffice. For example, it is possible to have both pneumonia and a broken leg, but these disorders are caused by very different mechanisms.

Some problems lead directly to others. For example, irritability leads to marital disruptions and binge eating leads to obesity. Often causal relationships go in both directions: anxiety leads to procrastination, which leads to more anxiety.

Some problems result from maladaptive coping with other problems. For example, the use of drugs and alcohol to cope with stressors can lead to addiction, poor health, or traffic accidents, and can fail to address or even worsen the problems these substances were intended to solve.

Although the formulation strives to tie all the problems and mechanisms together, efforts to do this exhaustively can lead to very long narratives and elaborate diagrams that are too complex to be clinically helpful. Strive for a simple formulation and add complexity only when a simple formulation fails to meet the clinical need.

The Process of Obtaining an Initial Case Formulation for Angela

At the end of my first session with Angela (as described in Chapter 5), I had obtained a Problem List, and some information about precipitants (the assault; see Figure 5.7). After the session, I had reviewed the Case Formulation Worksheet I had begun completing for Angela to see if I could flesh it out. As I reviewed in my mind what I had learned in the initial interview, I hypothesized that the assault had led to PTSD symptoms that Angela managed by avoiding and withdrawing, which led to a loss of reinforcers from usual sources of gratification (e.g., work) and thus to depressive symptoms. I planned to collect more information to test and evaluate this formulation hypothesis in the second pretreatment session.

I always begin the second session by reminding the patient that we are still in the pretreatment phase of assessing and making treatment recommendations. If I did not ask for feedback at the end of the initial session, I make sure to do this at the beginning of the second session. Then I set an agenda for the session. I typically propose that we do a brief check-in of developments since we met last and then return to data collection to help us understand the patient's situation in order to develop a treatment plan. Although I invite the patient to offer agenda items, in fact I am trying not to begin active treatment until the pretreatment tasks have been completed. This sometimes means I ask patients to postpone agenda items that involve active treatment until we have completed the pretreatment tasks.

At the end of the first session, I had let Angela know that she appeared to have some sort of mood disorder, probably MDD. However, in this session I needed to complete my diagnostic assessment. I also wanted to obtain some information about the origins of her difficulties and collect information to test and elaborate on my initial mechanism hypothesis. I wanted to follow up on her activity-scheduling homework, both as part of my efforts to inform her about what treatment would be like and to obtain more information about her behavior that would add to my diagnostic and formulation hypothesizing.

Angela reported that her week had been a bit better. She had gotten a lift from her initial session with me. Her report of feeling better, however, contrasted with her BDI score of 17, which was a bit higher than her initial score of 14. When I discussed this discrepancy with her, she let me know that in response to our discussion in the previous session she had "rescaled" her responses to the scale to override her tendency to minimize her symptoms. The fact that Angela had taken the initiative to do this indicated that she had already begun to engage in treatment—and to benefit. It also let me know that the minimization process we had identified in the first session was important (it had good treatment utility) and I would want to make sure to get it into the formulation somehow.

I wanted to test out my initial case formulation hypothesis, namely that the trauma had led to symptoms that she managed by avoidance (including experiential avoidance) and this had led to a loss of reinforcers that led to depression. This hypothesis depended heavily on the time sequence of events. To test it, I worked with Angela to make a timeline of the development of her symptoms.

I began by going forward from the trauma. She reported that after the trauma she had struggled to manage her symptoms while working and taking care of her responsibilities at home. However, she eventually felt so angry about how her superiors and colleagues responded to the trauma, panicky when she was at work, and overwhelmed at home that she asked for and obtained a temporary leave of absence from work. Although stopping work did reduce her anxiety, she noted that she had over time become increasingly withdrawn and depressed. This description of anxiety that she coped with by avoiding anxiety-evoking situations, which was followed by depression, was consistent with my initial mechanism hypothesis.

As another test of my mechanism hypothesis, I described the hypothesis to Angela and asked for her reaction to it. She reported that my formulation made sense to her. She agreed that the loss of her professional life had been a major blow to her, as she had been "at the top of her game," receiving lots of positive feedback from clients and colleagues, and lots of satisfaction from the work. She had expected to make partner and to have a long and successful career with the firm. All that seemed lost now.

This information was important because it was consistent with my mechanism hypothesis that depression was due to a loss of reinforcers that Angela had previously obtained at work. In addition, it disconfirmed a competing hypothesis I wanted to test, namely that receiving a disability income and having her treatment paid for by workers compensation might be reinforcing Angela's symptoms. Several other pieces of data also disconfirmed the hypothesis that the disability income was reinforcing. Angela reported that receiving disability payments caused her to feel bad about herself, the income she received was not sufficient to meet her family's needs, and she resented the hassles involved.

We also fleshed out a timeline going backward from the assault. As I questioned her in detail about her life before the assault, Angela realized that although she had not been aware of it, she had probably become depressed years earlier, when her husband began spending less time at home because of his long hours and commute. I suggested and she agreed that her depressed mood and low energy had promoted her use of avoidance to manage her distress following the assault.

As we discussed her depressive symptoms, I asked Angela's permission to fine-tune the diagnostic hypotheses I had developed in the first session. I used the ADIS (T. A. Brown et al., 1994) modules for MDD, dysthymia, and bipolar disorder to assess her symptoms. I determined and let Angela know that she appeared to have a "double depression," as she met criteria for both MDD and dysthymia, and that she did not appear to have a bipolar mood disorder. Because of the high rates of comorbidity among the anxiety disorders, I also used the other anxiety disorder modules in the ADIS to assess for other anxiety disorders. Angela met criteria for PTSD but not for any additional anxiety disorders.

Now I shifted the focus of the interview to obtain information about the origins of Angela's difficulties. I asked for more information about the intake questionnaire item in which she indicated she had been injured as a result of parental discipline.

Angela reported that she had thought of herself as having a happy childhood until some discussions with her brothers a few years previously had led to the realization that she and her siblings had been physically abused as children. Angela and her siblings had tiptoed around the house on eggshells because her father periodically lost his temper and lashed out at whichever of his children was nearest. Angela's brothers were the most common targets of their father's violence. However, on one occasion when Angela, at age 6, had ignored her father's request to turn off the TV, he struck her so hard that her eardrum ruptured. The family did not acknowledge the violence directly and in fact there was a running family joke that "regular beatings are part of life in a typical happy American family." We agreed that the chronic feeling of danger she had experienced as a child, the abuse she and her siblings experienced, and the family's minimizing of it were important contributors to the development of Angela's current symptoms. In fact, we tied Angela's underreporting of her symptoms on the BDI to her having learned at home to minimize the abuse she experienced and the distress it caused.

When we reviewed Angela's Activity Schedule, I learned that although she was mobilizing herself to get the kids to school in the morning and to pick them up from school in the afternoon, she was spending a lot of time in bed during the day. So the data from the Activity Schedule supported my initial mechanism hypothesis, which viewed inactivity as a key problem behavior.

Thus, the information I collected in the second session supported and elaborated on my initial mechanism hypothesis. Learning models seemed to provide the most elegant and simple account of all of Angela's symptoms and problems. Mowrer's two-factor theory accounted for her PTSD symptoms and Lewinsohn's operant theory accounted for her depressive symptoms and tied them to the PTSD symptoms. This thinking led to the following formulation of Angela's case. The elements of the case formulation are identified in CAPITAL LETTERS.

An assault by a client (PRECIPITANT) was a UCS that led to the development, through respondent conditioning, of PTSD symptoms (PROBLEM), including anger and irritability (PROBLEM) (which were CRs that were triggered by CSs in her environment), and, through operant conditioning, of escape and avoidance behaviors. Avoidance behaviors included stopping going to work (PROBLEM) and withdrawing from interactions with spouse and kids (PROBLEM). These escape and avoidance behaviors were negatively reinforced via their anxiety reduction effects (MECHANISMS). Depressive symptoms (PROBLEM) that preexisted the assault also promoted the use of avoidant coping with the assault and its sequelae. Angela's childhood experience of abuse and of learning to cope with it by avoiding and minimizing it likely facilitated these conditioning processes (ORIGINS). Avoidance led Angela to stop going to work (PROBLEM) and stop functioning at home (PROBLEM). This caused marital problems (PROBLEM) and a loss of positive reinforcers (MECHANISM), which led to depressive symptoms (PROBLEM). Avoiding work also led to financial problems (PROBLEM) and exacerbated marital problems (PROBLEM).

I added this formulation to the Case Formulation Worksheet for Angela (Figure 6.2).

Name <u>Angela</u>   Date _____

Problem List

1. Depressive symptoms (BDI = 14), symptoms of feeling discouraged about the future, not enjoying things she used to; feeling she may be punished, feeling disappointed in herself, crying more than usual, loss of interest in others, worry about looking old or unattractive, difficulty getting started doing things, early morning awakening, fatigue, and loss of libido. Denies suicidality. Cognitions include: "I don't know where to start to get my life back," "there's no use complaining," "no one will help me." Behaviors include excessive sleeping, not exercising, avoiding going to work or speaking to her employer. Emotions include irritability, anhedonia, sadness, and guilt.

2. PTSD symptoms. Intense fear reaction to physical assault by client followed by re-experiencing symptoms (panic and intense distress whenever she encounters work colleagues or other reminders of the event), avoidance (she is doing a lot of sleeping and has taken a leave of absence from work), and hyperarousal (irritability, insomnia). Cognitions include: "I can't cope," "My boss stabbed me in the back," behaviors include avoidance of work and sleeping, and emotions include panic and irritability.

3. Anger and irritability. Angry and resentful about being blamed by colleagues and supervisors for an act of violence against her. Has difficulty disciplining her kids without losing her temper. Resentful with husband, who is "never at home." She blows up at her kids about 3 times/week, at her husband about twice weekly.

4. Work problems. Recently took leave of absence b/c was having so many re-experiencing symptoms and resentment at work that she felt unable to function. Very distressed at loss of a previously rewarding professional life. She states, "I do not have any confidence that I will ever have energy and enthusiasm for my job again."

5. Marital problems. The marriage is "strained." Problems are chronic but exacerbated by her recent difficulties. Husband has a long commute and high pressure at work in a startup. Does not earn much money. "He's a good man but he's never at home and when he is he yells a lot."

6. Difficulty coping at home. Ongoing conflict with roof contractor, daughter with diabetes. "It's too much. I can't do it all." Coping style is do "do the minimum needed to get by."

7. Financial stresses due to loss of income from Angela's leaving work and husband's low-paying job.

Mechanisms

Assault → PTSD symptoms → avoidance → loss of reinforcers → depression

Precipitants of the problems

Assault at work

Origins of the mechanisms

Abuse by father/denial of abuse by family

The case formulation (origins, mechanisms, precipitants, problems):

An assault by a client (PRECIPITANT) was a UCS that led to the development, through respondent conditioning, of PTSD symptoms, including anger and irritability (which were CRs that were triggered by CSs in her environment), and, through operant conditioning, of escape and avoidance behaviors (including stopping going to work and withdrawal from interactions with spouse and kids) that were negatively reinforced via their anxiety reduction effects (MECHANISMS). Depressive symptoms that preexisted the assault also promoted the use of avoidant coping with the assault and its sequelae. Angela's childhood experience of abuse and of learning to cope with it by avoiding and minimizing it likely facilitated these conditioning processes (ORIGINS). Avoidance led Angela to stop going to work and stop functioning at home. This caused marital problems and a loss of positive reinforcers (MECHANISM), which led to depressive symptoms. Avoiding work also led to financial problems and exacerbated marital problems.

FIGURE 6.2. Completed Case Formulation Worksheet for Angela.

Writing the Case Formulation in the Clinical Record

The case formulation can be written in the clinical record in a paragraph, like the text above, or as a diagram, such as in Figure 6.1. Writing out a detailed case formulation in a paragraph or diagram is time-consuming. A shorthand strategy is to simply identify the nomothetic formulation(s) the therapist is using to conceptualize the case without writing down the details that are involved in individualizing it (Zayfert & Becker, 2007). The therapist using this strategy to formulate Angela's case could simply list Mowrer's two-factor theory and Lewinsohn's conditioning model of depression.

Which strategy is best? Unfortunately, no data are available to answer this question. I recommend the therapist choose the strategy that is clinically most helpful. Using this principle, the therapist might elect to use the shorthand strategy for simpler cases and to take the time to write out a detailed case formulation for complex cases (Haynes et al., 1997) or in a training situation.

SETTING TREATMENT GOALS

Although this chapter discusses developing a formulation before it discusses setting treatment goals, these tasks happen in tandem. In fact, the patient and therapist will likely set treatment goals even before completing a case formulation. In part, this is because the goals of treatment contribute to the formulation. That is, in a patient who has bipolar disorder under good control and panic disorder for which she seeks treatment, the formulation can be developed to emphasize the panic symptoms as a guide to treatment planning. In addition, the process of setting treatment goals helps patient and therapist decide if they are a good match for working together and if they are able to agree on a collaborative treatment plan. The therapist may, for example, ask the patient to commit to the goal of stopping suicidal behavior as a condition of treatment.

Treatment goals are the first element of a formal written treatment plan (see Figure 6.3). The other elements of the treatment plan are the treatment modality (e.g., individual or group), frequency, and adjuncts. In the next chapter, I describe using the formulation to guide decision making about those elements. I focus in this chapter on setting treatment goals.

Qualities of Good Treatment Goals

Good treatment goals are explicitly agreed upon by patient and therapist, focused on reducing symptoms and problems, focused on increasing desired behaviors or outcomes, emotionally compelling to the patient, realistic, measurable, and specific about when they have been met, and listed in priority order. It is not possible to meet all of these criteria for all goals. For example, goals that focus on reducing symptoms by definition do not focus on increasing desired behaviors or outcomes.

Agreed Upon by Patient and Therapist

Usually patients come to treatment because they have failed to reach important goals on their own. To have a fighting chance of achieving the goals in therapy, it is important that patient and therapist explicitly agree on them. Nevertheless, an initial failure to agree on

Name _____ Date _____

Goals

1.

2.

3.

4.

5.

6.

Modality

Frequency

Adjunct Treatment

FIGURE 6.3. Treatment Plan. Copyright 2008 by the San Francisco Bay Area Center for Cognitive Therapy. Reprinted by permission in Jacqueline B. Persons (2008). Permission to photocopy this figure is granted to purchasers of this book for personal use only (see copyright page for details).

goals or the priority order of goals is not uncommon. Common areas of disagreement include substance abuse, suicidality, and self-harm. Patients often consider these behaviors as solutions, whereas therapists tend to consider them as problems. Sometimes a compromise can be reached. For example, a patient who would not agree to a goal of stopping self-harming behavior did agree to log self-harming behaviors and to set a goal of learning alternative methods of reducing emotional distress that did not entail self-harm. The motivational interviewing and other strategies described in the next chapter can be useful in obtaining patients' agreement to goals they are not initially inclined to endorse.

Focused on Reducing Symptoms and Problems

Treatment goals are often the mirror image of the items on the Problem List (e.g., the problem is depressive symptoms and the goal is to reduce depressive symptoms). Thus, typical goals are to reduce symptoms of depression and anxiety, eliminate binge-eating episodes, reduce arguments with the spouse, or ease the distress caused by auditory hallucinations. However, usually it is unrealistic to try solving all of the patient's problems. And most patients don't wish to solve all of the problems on their Problem List (usually they want to tackle one or two). As a result, the list of treatment goals is usually shorter than the Problem List.

Focused on Increasing Desired Behaviors or Outcomes

As numerous behavior therapists (Kazdin, 2001; Watson & Tharp, 2002) have observed, it is more productive to focus on increasing a desired behavior (e.g., writing dissertation pages) than to focus on decreasing an undesirable behavior (e.g., watching TV). This dictum makes sense for the obvious reason that even if the goal of decreasing undesirable behavior is met (e.g., the person spends less time watching TV), desired behavior may not increase (the person may not replace TV watching with writing dissertation pages or any other desirable behavior). Goals involving increasing desired behaviors include such goals as increasing pleasure and enjoyment, getting to work on time, and spending more time with friends.

Emotionally Compelling to the Patient

In this aspect of goal setting, the therapist capitalizes on what emotion theory tells us about how emotions capture attention and provide motivation. So, for example, a teacher stated that her goal was to begin dating and establish a long-term relationship with a man. Upon assessing her, the therapist determined that the teacher met criteria for social phobia and that her avoidance of dating was in fact a symptom of social phobia. This diagnosis and formulation suggest the goal of overcoming symptoms of social phobia. However, the goal of dating to meet a husband is more emotionally compelling to the patient than the goal of overcoming social phobia and thus, at least in that respect, is a better goal.

Realistic

Curing schizophrenia or bipolar disorder is not a realistic goal. More realistic are goals to eliminate or reduce distress caused by certain symptoms (e.g., hallucinations, anhedonia) or to improve functioning (e.g., get a full-time job and function well at it or prevent another psychiatric hospitalization). Similarly, a person with dysthymia cannot realistically set a goal of eliminating depressed mood. More realistic are goals to reduce the severity and frequency of depressed moods and to increase positive mood and enjoyment.

Measurable

Good treatment goals are specified in measurable terms. Examples include goals to reduce depressive symptoms to the normal range (BDI < 10), eliminate panic attacks, and maintain abstinence from cocaine. Examples of good role functioning goals include goals to pay all bills on time, arrive on time for appointments and classes, and spend more time doing fun things with one's husband. To tighten up a vague goal, the therapist can ask the patient, "If you accomplished this goal, how would your behavior be different?"

Specific about When the Goal Has Been Met

Good treatment goals clearly specify when they have been met (Mash & Hunsley, 1993). That is, instead of stating the goal as "Eliminate suicidality," the goal is better stated as "Reduce suicidality to one fleeting thought weekly." The process of identifying what it means to accomplish a particular goal can be itself therapeutic for patients, who may not have thought this through for themselves.

Listed in Priority Order

To prioritize goals, the therapist refers to the priority list of problems on the Problem List described in Chapter 5. It is not necessary to assign a priority order to each and every goal but it is essential to be clear and to agree on the one or two or three highest-priority goals. Determining priority order of the treatment goals is not a one-time activity. In some sense, the therapist must examine priorities at every therapy session (during the agenda-setting process, see Chapter 10). However, the treatment-planning process presents an important opportunity to think through this issue carefully and discuss it with the patient.

The Process of Setting Treatment Goals

To begin the process of setting treatment goals, it is useful, as noted in Chapter 5, to ask patients at the end of the first or second pretreatment session to do a homework assignment of sitting down for 15 minutes to make a list of their goals for treatment that they can bring to the next session. Another option is to set goals with the patient in the therapy session.

Angela and I worked together in the second pretreatment session to develop the list of goals presented in Figure 6.4. Angela thought about her goals in very behavioral terms and it was easy to work with her to obtain a list of goals that described measurable, specific behaviors. In my paper-and-pencil clinical record (I am hoping to graduate soon to an online medical record), I place a colored paper clip on the Treatment Plan form, which includes the goals, so it is easy to locate in the chart and I can refer it frequently.

Name <u>Angela</u>   Date _____

Goals

· 1.   Reduce depressive symptoms to BDI score less than 10.

2.   Get back to work full time and enjoy it.

3.   Encounter "problem people" at work without a lot of distress, chest pain, shortness of breath.

4.   Welcome my husband home from work with a kiss and a hug.

5.   Have and enjoy sex 1.5 times/week.

6.   Be able to discipline my kids without yelling.

Modality

Frequency

Adjunct Treatment

FIGURE 6.4. Treatment Plan for Angela, with completed "Goals" section.

Angela and I had already begun weekly monitoring (she completed a BDI weekly before every session) to track progress on the first goal. A bit later, after we made a formal agreement to work together, I would work with her to set up a Daily Log to track progress on some of the other goals (e.g., yelling at the kids when disciplining them).

Typically the treatment goals flow directly out of the Problem List in the case formulation. In some cases, however, the mechanism hypothesis helps the patient and therapist select good treatment goals. The case of Elena illustrates this point.

Elena was 39 years old. Her biological clock was ticking. She had married Jim 2 years earlier. However, soon after she and Jim began talking about having a baby, she became consumed with fear that having a baby with Jim might be a terrible mistake. Elena admitted there were no big-ticket red flags. Jim was not an alcoholic or abuser, and he was eager to be a father. But Elena was tortured with doubt and indecision. She was spending at least an hour or two a day agonizing about her dilemma and monitoring Jim's behavior, her feelings, and their interactions, asking herself, "Will he make a good father? If I have a child with him, I'll be trapped in the marriage; I won't be able to just pack up and leave. Can I be happy with him over the long haul? Will this behavior of his make me miserable? Can I stand that one? Will we be a happy family?" And whenever Jim did something that triggered her fears (e.g., came home from work a few minutes later than he had said he would), Elena initiated a discussion of it with him. This happened two or three times a week and took up quite a bit of their time together. Elena also spent hours on the telephone talking with her girlfriends about her concerns and worries.

Although Elena did not meet criteria for GAD because she had only one worry and it had not been present for 6 months, Elena's therapist used the formulation of worry as avoidance behavior (Borkovec, Alcaine, & Behar, 2004; Orsillo & Roemer, 2005; Roemer & Orsillo, 2002) to conceptualize Elena's difficulties. The formulation proposed that Elena's worrying and her discussions with her husband and girlfriends about her doubts served the function of allowing her to escape and avoid her emotional experience of being in the relationship with her husband. The formulation proposed that paradoxically, the strategy (worry) that Elena adopted to prevent future misery was the main cause of her present-day misery. She was living "life in the future versus life in the present." (Borkovec, 2002).

The treatment targets identified by the formulation were Elena's worry behavior, the discussions of her doubts with her husband and girlfriends, and her disengagement from her relationship with her husband. The mechanism change goals identified by the formulation were to help Elena suspend the worry behaviors and discussions of her doubts and engage herself more fully in the present and in her marriage.

Elena's treatment (described in a moment) was quite successful. The decision about what treatment goal to set contributed in an important way to that success. The therapist, using the formulation just described, guided Elena to set the outcome goal of reducing her worry, the fruitless discussions of her doubts with her husband and friends, and the distress she was experiencing. If Elena had insisted in setting the goal of making the "correct" decision, this could have made the therapy more difficult. In fact it could have promoted worry behavior as Elena tried to figure out the "correct" answer to her question. Instead, the formulation cued the therapist to encourage Elena to set a goal of reducing the time she spent worrying. Efforts to achieve this goal helped Elena make the mechanism changes needed to accomplish it.

Elena agreed to the goal and to the interventions the therapist proposed. She agreed to stop discussing her worries with her husband and friends and to stop going over them in her mind and instead to disengage from the worries and engage herself fully in the relationship and her life with her husband and to accept and embrace whatever feelings this led to. These tasks, of course, were quite difficult. Nevertheless, Elena worked hard at them and was largely successful. Within about 8 weeks, Elena's worry was considerably reduced and she found that she felt comfortable with her husband and their life together and more connected to him than she had previously. In fact, engaging more fully in her relationship with her husband allowed Elena to collect the information she needed to make a decision about whether to start a family.

Elena decided to start a family and quickly conceived. She responded to her pregnancy with a flare-up of worry that she managed by recommitting herself to the strategies of curtailing worry behaviors and focusing on present-moment emotional experiencing.

Complications in Goal Setting

Sometimes the very problems for which a person seeks help interfere with the process of setting treatment goals. When this happens, the therapist can use the nascent case formulation to conceptualize the problem at hand and guide his or her response to it. For example, some individuals experience the process of identifying problems (a first step to setting goals) as stressful. They become defensive and antagonistic and avoid the task. In this particular case, the formulation might propose that a focus on problems triggers the person's schemas about being defective and likely to be rejected, and this triggers fear, shame, and anger. Using this formulation as a guide, the therapist can do two things. First, the therapist can focus on carrying out the task of developing a Problem List in a way that communicates acceptance and caring, using a warm tone, proceeding slowly, offering lots of support, highlighting the patient's strengths frequently, and stating (if it is true) that she expects she and the patient will be able to come to an agreement to work together and that she would like to work with him. In addition the therapist might be able to address the patient's emotions in the session and use them as an opportunity to teach the cognitive-behavior model, inform the patient about treatment, and address a therapy-interfering behavioral pattern. To do this, when the patient becomes emotional, the therapist can pause and highlight the patient's emotional reaction and ask to focus on it, saying, for example, "You know, what is happening right now is really a fabulous opportunity for us to work together and for me to teach you about how CBT would approach your situation. Could we work on the feelings that are coming up for you right now?"

Another complication can arise because most ESTs for a particular disorder are designed to accomplish the goal of treating that DSM disorder to remission. However, often patients do not have that goal. An example is Don, who had OCD and who sought treatment that would address some—but not all—of his fears and rituals. Don had contamination fears and rituals both at home and in his office. His goal was to address the issue at home so he could feel more comfortable and eliminate time-consuming cleaning rituals there. However, he did not want to tackle the fears and rituals at work. There he had a strategy of using certain avoidance behaviors and rituals that allowed him to get through the day without too much strain and he didn't want to upset the careful equilibrium he had achieved.

To address this (common) type of situation, the steps involved in deciding whether a non-optimal treatment plan is reasonable and obtaining the patient's informed consent to treatment provide good guidance. These are discussed in some detail in the next chapter. In Don's case, I spent some time explaining to him that if we treated his OCD symptoms at home but not at work he would be vulnerable to relapse because the fears and rituals in the two locations were so similar and many of the mechanisms underpinning them would remain intact and available to fuel a relapse (Foa, Steketee, Turner, & Fischer, 1980). We discussed advantages and disadvantages of his proposal. Don did not change his mind. I reluctantly agreed to his plan to tackle the fears at home but not at work. We did that and Don was successful in accomplishing his goal. Five years later he experienced a partial relapse and returned for further treatment. Even then he was not unhappy about his choice—and in fact made the same choice again.

* * *

At this point in the pretreatment process, the therapist has worked collaboratively with the patient to develop a Problem List, a diagnosis, an initial case formulation, and a list of treatment goals. It is now the second or third session and there is increasing pressure to begin intervening. However, two pretreatment tasks remain: completing the Treatment Plan and obtaining the patient's informed consent to proceed. Those tasks are described in the next chapter.

SEVEN

Using the Formulation to Develop a Treatment Plan and Obtain the Patient's Consent to It

To complete pretreatment, the therapist must develop an initial treatment plan and obtain the patient's agreement to it. This chapter describes how the case formulation, discussed in the previous chapter, helps guide these steps.

DEVELOPING A TREATMENT PLAN

The ESTs are valuable sources of treatment planning information. They serve as default treatment plan options. However, data from the randomized controlled trials offer useful information about the most effective treatment for the *average patient who participated in the randomized trial*. They do not provide information about the best treatment for the *patient who is in the therapist's office at that moment* (Howard, Moras, Brill, Martinovich, & Lutz, 1996). The individualized case formulation helps guide treatment planning for the individual patient.

The mechanism hypothesis of the case formulation helps the therapist identify the *mechanism change goals* and *compensatory strategies goals* of therapy. Information about these process goals helps the therapist select interventions, decide where to start when treating multiple problems, anticipate obstacles to success, and make decisions about the elements of the treatment plan, such as the modality, frequency of sessions, and adjunctive treatments.

The *mechanism change goals* of therapy are the psychological processes the therapy is attempting to change. For example, the *mechanism change goals* of treatment guided by a conceptualization based on Beck's cognitive model are to change the patient's schemas and modify the maladaptive behaviors and automatic thoughts that are elements of the patient's problems.

The *compensatory skills goals* of therapy are goals to teach the patient strategies that can reduce symptoms and suffering but that do not change the central mechanisms that cause the symptoms. In the case of a therapy based on Beck's cognitive model, compensatory strategies goals might include teaching the patient to avoid situations that are likely to activate his or her schemas.

The term *process goal* is used to describe both mechanism change goals and goals to teach compensatory strategies. *Process* goals are distinct from what might be called *outcome* goals, that is, the treatment goals that the patient and therapist set together and wrote on the Treatment Plan (Figure 6.3).

What I am calling *outcome goals* are what Mash and Hunsley (1993) and Haynes and O'Brien (2000) call *ultimate outcomes*. What I am calling *process goals* include what these writers call *intermediate outcomes*. I prefer the term *process goal* because it clearly refers to changes in psychological mechanisms and processes. However, the term *intermediate goals* captures the notion that the process goals are intermediate, or on the way to the outcome goals of the therapy.

However, it is important to remember that the formulation guiding treatment planning at this pretreatment point is only a rough formulation. So the treatment plan developed at this point is also provisional. After treatment begins, patient and therapist use the strategies described in Chapter 9 to collect data to monitor the process and outcome of therapy and make any revisions that are needed.

Using the Formulation to Identify the Therapy's Process Goals

There are two types of process goals: *mechanism change goals* and *goals to teach compensatory strategies.*

Identifying Mechanism Change Goals

Mechanism change goals are goals to change certain psychological mechanisms. The mechanism change goals of therapy flow directly out of the formulation and help the therapist make treatment planning decisions. For example, the case of Marge, who had anxiety about excessive blushing, could be formulated in two different ways. Each formulation led to a different treatment plan with a different mechanism change goal.

One formulation was that Marge's problem was due to faulty beliefs ("I'm red as a beet; my date will notice this and reject me for being strange"), an excessive focus on images of how she believes she appears, and safety behaviors (such as wearing a turtleneck sweater to hide flushing). This formulation points to a cognitive-behavior treatment plan that strives to accomplish the *mechanism change goals* of changing Marge's dysfunctional beliefs, shifting the focus of her attention from her internal image to the external situation, and dropping her safety behaviors (Clark, 2001).

A second formulation proposed that Marge's problem was due to a defect in vascular functioning (Malmivaara, Kuukasjaarvi, Autti-Ramo, Kovanen, & Makela, 2007). This formulation points to a surgical treatment plan that strives to accomplish the mechanism change goal of correcting the vascular defect.

A treatment plan usually entails more than one mechanism change goal. This was the case for Angela. The formulation of her case based on conditioning theory led to three mechanism change goals: to extinguish conditioned fear responses, eliminate avoidance behaviors, and regain old and acquire new positive reinforcers.

Identifying Goals to Teach Compensatory Strategies

Not all therapies achieve mechanism change, or intend to. In fact, a lively debate exists about whether Beck's cognitive therapy for depression accomplishes the mechanism change it seeks (that is, to change the schemas and automatic thoughts and maladaptive behaviors that drive symptoms) (Barber & DeRubeis, 1989; Brewin, 1989). An alternative view is that cognitive therapy teaches patients skills (e.g., cognitive restructuring, activity scheduling) they can use to manage the painful emotions they experience when their schemas are activated. Stimulus control interventions can be seen as teaching compensatory strategies. Stimulus control interventions change the problem behavior, B, by removing the antecedent As that trigger it. I stop my behavior of eating potato chips (B) by stopping the A of buying potato chips and leaving them on my kitchen counter. This intervention does not change the links between A and B, which remain intact (as I discover when I go to a picnic where potato chips are served). But the intervention does (mostly) help me accomplish my outcome goal of not eating potato chips.

Harm reduction strategies are a type of compensatory strategy. For example, supplying addicts with clean needles helps accomplish the ultimate goal of reducing the number of new cases of AIDS. It does not, however, lead to any change in the mechanisms that cause intravenous drug use and that link intravenous drug use to HIV and AIDS.

The distinction between changing mechanisms and teaching compensatory strategies is blurry. One could argue that the change in my potato chip–buying behavior may have resulted from some mechanism change. The repeated use of compensatory strategies might lead to mechanism change. Thus, the woman who learns to use distraction (a compensatory strategy) to tolerate panic symptoms may thereby experience some change in the mechanisms that drive those symptoms, which may include beliefs like "If I don't take immediate action to stop panic symptoms, I will go crazy."

Treatment plans that emphasize teaching compensatory strategies can be useful when we don't have the technology to change the mechanisms that cause symptoms or the patient is unwilling or unable to change the mechanisms. The case of Marla illustrates this point.

Marla was an elderly woman who was spending long hours at the hospital where her husband was hospitalized for a life-threatening illness. She sought help for her intense discomfort using public bathrooms. She feared that others would hear the noises and smell the odors she emitted and that she would feel embarrassed and humiliated as a result. Marla met criteria for social phobia. However, she had no desire to overcome her social phobia. She just wanted to get some relief of distress during her husband's hospital stay, which was expected to last for several more weeks. To address her goals, I designed a treatment that emphasized teaching compensatory strategies.

After some brainstorming, we determined that Marla would feel less uncomfortable about using the bathroom if it was one that was far from her husband's unit because this would reduce her chance of encountering someone on the unit who had been in the bathroom when she was there. She also developed a plan to simply stay in the stall until others left the bathroom if her embarrassment was high. She found that bringing a radio into the bathroom that would cover up some of the noises she made. Distracting herself by talking on her cell phone while using the bathroom also provided some relief of her discomfort. These avoidance and safety behaviors were not expected to alleviate Marla's social phobia (and might even make it worse, as I explained to her). However, they did help her achieve her goal of feeling more comfortable using the public bathrooms in the hospital.

Identifying Treatment Targets

Treatment targets are the phenomena the treatment focuses on. The formulation identifies the treatment targets. For example, in Marge's case the cognitive-behavior treatment targets were the beliefs about blushing, the focus of attention, and the safety behaviors.

Some therapies have the same treatment targets but different mechanism change goals. For example, Beck's cognitive therapy and mindfulness-based cognitive therapy both target distorted cognitions. But Beck's cognitive therapy has the mechanism change goal of changing the content of the cognitions, whereas mindfulness-based cognitive therapy has the mechanism change goal of reducing the patient's degree of engagement with the cognitions.

Using the Formulation to Guide Treatment Planning

Using Process Goals to Select Interventions

Information about the therapy's process goal helps the therapist select interventions. The case of Marla illustrates this point. Because the therapy's process goal was to teach compensatory strategies, I used interventions quite different from those I would have used in a therapy that sought to change the mechanisms causing Marla's distress. To give another example, if the mechanism change goal is habituation or extinction, interventions will include exposure. If the mechanism change goal is to reduce the patient's degree of engagement with negative thoughts, interventions may include teaching mindfulness skills.

However, there is not a one-to-one relationship between process goals and interventions. The *process goals* are like destinations that can be reached by a variety of routes (interventions). Many different interventions may accomplish the same process goal. For example, cognitive restructuring, behavioral experiments, and exposure can be used to accomplish a mechanism change goal of changing beliefs. The process goal helps the therapist generate new intervention ideas if the first ones fail or are not acceptable to the patient. The therapist can borrow interventions from multiple ESTs and other sources in order to promote the process goals of the therapy. Thus, case formulation-driven CBT involves "interventional eclecticism." What holds the treatment together and gives it coherence are the process goals, especially the mechanism change goals, which flow directly out of the mechanism hypothesis of the case formulation.

Using the Formulation to Anticipate Obstacles

The therapist who is aware of potential obstacles may be able to make a treatment plan that sidesteps them or, at worst, to use monitoring (described in Chapter 9) to identify and address obstacles promptly if they appear. Attention to the mechanisms hypotheses of the case formulation and the Problem List can be useful in identifying potential obstacles.

For example, I've learned from experience (and from Jeffrey Young, 1999) that sometimes patients who have "subjugation" schemas encounter several obstacles to making good use of therapy. One is that they don't view their needs as important (they subjugate their needs to those of others), and so they don't seek treatment until they are in a crisis. Then they often set up a relationship with the therapist in which they subjugate their needs and wishes to those of the therapist. As a result, they can become quite resentful at the therapist, feeling they are doing what the therapist wants but not getting their own needs met. They are also vulnerable to premature termination because they drop out of therapy as soon as their pain is less excruciating but before they have learned the skills needed to make any fundamental changes. They do not place sufficient value on their emotional health or comfort to remain in therapy as long as would be helpful. The therapist who can use the case formulation to anticipate these obstacles can take steps to prevent them (e.g., by discussing the potential for premature termination with the patient at the beginning of therapy or as soon as an early sign of it appears). The therapist can also monitor evidence of subjugation, including excessive deference to the therapist and resentment, to identify them early and address them promptly.

Sometimes items on the Problem List, such as financial problems, major interpersonal conflicts, or difficulty working collaboratively with others, can alert the therapist to potential obstacles. For example, a young adult's financial dependence on parents can become an obstacle if a goal of the therapy is to help the patient assert himself with parents. The patient and therapist need to be aware that the patient's assertiveness might jeopardize the parents' willingness to pay for the treatment! Or if the patient has a history of getting fired, the therapist would do well to think ahead a bit and perhaps even discuss with the patient what steps she will take (see the patient for free? reduce the fee? refer her out?) if the patient gets fired again and can't afford therapy.

Deciding Where to Start When Treating Multiple Problems

When there are multiple problems, the therapist must decide which to tackle first. The priority order of the Problem List (discussed in Chapter 5) is helpful when making the decision of what to treat first. The highest-priority problems are those that are life threatening. Next highest in priority are those that jeopardize the therapy itself, and third priority are "quality-of-life-interfering problems" (e.g., homelessness or severe substance abuse) that will interfere with solving other problems. The therapist need not treat *only* these problems when they are present, but it is risky not to prioritize them. In particular, when patients have chaotic out-of-control behaviors, it is a good idea to get those behaviors under control first before attacking other problems. This is especially true when treatment of some of the patient's other problems can be stressful. For these reasons, Linehan (1993a) proposes treating individuals who meet criteria for borderline personality disorder in stages. The first stage of treatment is devoted to teaching skills to manage emotion dysregulation and impulsive behaviors and later stages are devoted to exposure and other treatments for PTSD.

After the therapist attends to these three highest-priority behaviors, other factors guide the decision about what problem to address first. One consideration is whether treatment of a particular problem is likely to have positive effects on other problems (Haynes, 1992). I used this notion to guide my decision about where to begin my treatment of Angela. Because inactivity was a behavioral pattern that was common to nearly all of the problems on Angela's Problem List, I targeted it for change first, with the rationale that increased engagement would have positive effects in many areas of her life.

This focus on attacking behavioral inactivity first also appears in Beck's protocol for cognitive therapy for depression (A. T. Beck et al., 1979). The protocol targets the depressed patient's behavioral inactivity before it targets the distorted cognitions. This order seems to make good clinical sense, as I have found that individuals who are immobilized do not appear to be able to take in and make good use of cognitive restructuring interventions.

Similarly, it can be useful to spend some time increasing the positives and strengthening the patient's social and environmental support and comfort before undertaking a therapy (e.g., an exposure-based therapy) that may increase the patient's distress on the way to helping him or her (Kimble et al., 1998).

Often the patient does not have high-risk behaviors, and no obvious starting point presents itself. In these cases, the therapist can work collaboratively with the patient to make a decision about where to start and carefully monitor process and outcome to guide decision making about where to go from there.

Using Idiographic Details of the Case

The discussion so far has described how the formulation helps the therapist identify the process goals of the therapy, select interventions, anticipate obstacles, and decide where to start when treating multiple problems. The formulation also provides idiographic details of the case that aid the treatment planning process. Information about the patient's previous efforts to solve the problems, strengths and assets, and values and preferences can all be helpful.

THE PATIENT'S PREVIOUS EFFORTS TO SOLVE THE PROBLEM

When making treatment decisions, it is always useful to find out whether the patient has had this problem before and if so, what strategies were—or were not—helpful in solving it. A graduate student in history who sought help for social anxiety reported that a previous therapist had taught her to "focus on being in the present, not in my head" and to use calming self-statements that drew on her spirituality and reminded her of God's unconditional love for her. A treatment plan that helped her reestablish these strategies produced quick benefits.

Similarly, discussing with one of my patients how she had successfully stopped smoking helped her solve the time management problem she came to therapy to address. The key to solving both problems involved carefully examining the pros and cons to get *very* clear about why it was important to her values and life goals to solve the problem. Once she took this step, the patient was able, on her own, to implement several creative strategies to improve her time management. She set explicit deadlines and made public commitments to them, assertively declined to take on tasks that others wanted her to do but that she did not want to spend time on, and modified antecedents (e.g., scheduling meetings with subordinates immediately after the staff meeting so it was easier to arrive on time for them).

Details about failed problem-solving efforts can also guide treatment planning by helping prevent a repetition of previous failures. The Adult Intake Questionnaire (Figure 5.4) can help the therapist obtain basic facts about previous treatment. And sometimes family members or previous therapists are even better sources of this information than the patient.

STRENGTHS AND ASSETS

Effective interventions capitalize on the patient's strengths and assets. Thus, treatment for a patient with OCD whose wife is eager to participate and understands exposure and response prevention will look different than treatment for an unmarried person or one whose spouse is unable or unwilling to participate in the treatment.

VALUES AND PREFERENCES

Sackett, Haynes, Guyatt, and Tugwell (1991) point to the importance of considering the patients' values and preferences in treatment planning. Thus, for example, many patients have a strong preference for psychotherapy versus pharmacological solutions to their problems, for gradual over intense exposure-based intervention, or for cognitive therapy over exposure-based treatment for anxiety disorders. Cultural values can play a key role here as well. Interventions to help a Japanese American college student make direct assertive requests to her parents to modify their behavior run so directly against the grain of her culture that they are not likely to be acceptable or helpful and may even lead the patient to prematurely terminate treatment.

Using the Formulation to Guide Decision Making about the Elements of the Treatment Plan

In Chapter 6 I discussed how the formulation guides the setting of goals. The formulation also helps the therapist make decisions about the other elements of the treatment plan, that is, the, modality, frequency, and adjunct therapies.

Modality

In the pretreatment phase, the therapist needs to make a decision about modality. That is, can the patient benefit from individual therapy or is another modality, such as hospitalization or couple, group, or family therapy, needed? The case formulation can help the therapist make these decisions. For example, I evaluated a woman who sought treatment for her feelings of anxiety, depression, and constant worry relating to her efforts to care for her disabled child. She also had a marital problem. She felt resentful toward her husband, who was not providing her with any support in managing her overwhelming difficulties and who appeared to manage his distress about his home situation by gambling online and traveling on business as much as possible. The conceptualization suggested that a marital therapy would be more helpful than an individual therapy, as it could address all of her problems simultaneously. She agreed with this formulation and intervention tactic. I worked with her for three sessions to help her present this idea effectively to her husband and make the transition to marital therapy.

When is hospitalization needed? Certainly when the patient is suicidal the therapist often has the urge to hospitalize the patient. And the patient and his or her family may want this too. Sometimes hospitalization is a good idea. However, attention to the case formulation can guide decision making about the use of hospitalization to treat suicidality. In fact, there is no evidence that hospitalization provides effective treatment for suicidality (Goldsmith, Pellmar, Kleinman, & Bunney, 2002). In fact, if suicidal behavior is a maladaptive strategy the patient uses to escape stressful life circumstances, hospitalization can be countertherapeutic because it can reinforce the patient's maladaptive urges to escape and impede learning of more adaptive strategies for managing stressors (Chiles & Strosahl, 1995).

Frequency

Outpatient therapy is usually held weekly. Exceptions include the protocols for the first few weeks of Beck's cognitive therapy for depression (sessions are held twice weekly) and exposure and response prevention (ERP) for OCD (sessions occur three to five times weekly). Information about the details of the case at hand (e.g., the presence of a family member to help the patient practice ERP outside the session) and the mechanism change goals of the therapy (habituation that requires repeated prolonged exposures) can help the therapist make decisions about the frequency of therapy sessions.

Adjunct Therapies

Common adjuncts to individual CBT include pharmacotherapy, couple therapy, group therapy, and 12-step or other self-help programs. Information from published efficacy studies and from the case formulation helps the therapist make decisions about adjunct therapies. For example, psychotherapy plus pharmacotherapy is the treatment of choice for bipolar I disorder. However, the idiographic details of the case at hand can guide the therapist to a different treatment plan. For example, the therapist who is treating a person who meets criteria for bipolar I disorder might agree to a trial of psychotherapy alone if the patient wants it very much, has a good support network, has failed multiple pharmacotherapy trials, agrees to work hard in therapy to learn alternative strategies to manage his or her symptoms, agrees to monitor outcome carefully, and has agreed to a backup treatment plan if this one fails.

An example of an adjunct decision guided by the case formulation is a young woman whose symptoms of bipolar disorder were frequently triggered by criticisms from family members. This formulation hypothesis led to my recommendation that family therapy be added to her treatment plan.

After settling on an initial treatment plan, the therapist must, before moving forward to implement it, obtain the patient's informed consent.

OBTAINING INFORMED CONSENT TO TREATMENT

Imagine that you have a serious, even life-threatening, medical problem. What information would you want before you make the decision to begin a regimen of treatment? I recommend that mental health professionals consider this question when they work to obtain informed consent for treatment from their patients. In a formal informed consent process, the therapist:

- Provides an assessment, including a diagnosis and formulation, of the patient's condition.
- Recommends a treatment, describes it, and provides a rationale for the recommendation.

- Describes available treatment options.
- Obtains the patient's agreement to proceed with the recommended treatment plan or a compromise treatment plan.

The first three items listed here are things the therapist provides to the patient and the final item is something the patient gives to the therapist.

Providing Information about Diagnosis and Formulation

The patient is entitled to information about diagnosis and formulation. Sharing a formulation with the patient is particularly important. When the therapist and patient have a shared formulation and the patient feels the therapist "really gets it," he or she is more likely to accept and comply with the treatment plan the therapist proposes (Addis & Carpenter, 2000).

As was already described in Chapters 5 and 6, the best way to present formulation information to patients is in a guided, gradual way, as part of a process of mutual discovery. Nevertheless, as part of the informed consent process, the therapist provides some sort of summary formulation. It is not usually very helpful to simply review the formulation (e.g., the paragraph summarizing the formulation of Angela's case that was provided in Chapter 6). This information is so dry and complex that, in my experience, patients don't usually want it or find it helpful. Instead, it is helpful to provide one or two of the key pieces of the formulation, especially those that provide a rationale for the treatment plan, which the therapist will propose next.

Thus, when I presented a formulation to Angela, I presented my hypotheses about the key mechanisms driving her symptoms. I explained that the assault she experienced was a trauma that had led to conditioned fear responses. I explained the concept of conditioned responses by reviewing the experiments in which Pavlov had trained a dog to salivate in response to a bell by repeatedly pairing the bell with food. I explained that the trauma experience was a conditioning experience for her and that following that event, many stimuli that were present at the time of the trauma or related to stimuli that were present at the time of the trauma now evoked conditioned fear and other emotional reactions. These stimuli included her office, her colleagues, her work, and emotional and somatic responses she had experienced during the trauma. I explained that because she had been using avoidance, including experiential avoidance (S. C. Hayes, Luoma, Bond, Masuda, & Lillis, 2006) of her fear and other conditioned sensations, she had lost activities and connections with others that had been quite rewarding to her and this had caused her to become depressed. In fact, because she had been somewhat depressed even before the trauma occurred, she had been particularly vulnerable to coping by withdrawing. She even withdrew experientially, avoiding attending to how bad she felt, as she had noticed when she began completing the BDI as part of our work together.

Recommending a Treatment Plan

The next step is to recommend a treatment plan to the patient. The treatment plan needs to be clearly linked to the formulation that was just presented. A good way to begin is to describe the mechanism change goals and interventions of the treatment. For example, "As we have discovered during our assessment, your depressed mood appears to be tied to a huge raft of negative, distorted thoughts you are having. In therapy I'll teach you to identify, get distance from, and modify those thoughts so they don't run you around so much and pull your mood down."

The therapist also describes the treatment's evidence base, its benefits and risks, what role the therapist will take, what will be expected of the patient, any adjunct treatments the therapist recommends, and the problems or symptoms the therapist recommends tackling first. Of course, if the therapist is recommending that the patient seek treatment elsewhere, the therapist cannot provide all of these details. However, he or she must provide enough information to convince the patient that the referral is appropriate.

I encourage therapists to begin by recommending a strong treatment plan that they feel confident will be helpful. They can then see how the patient responds and, if appropriate, begin the process of negotiation (described below) to arrive at a mutually agreeable plan. Often therapists recommend a weaker treatment plan (e.g., therapy twice a month) because they fear the patient will reject it or can't afford it. However, the weakness of this strategy is that if they begin by proposing a compromise treatment plan, they are depriving the patient of the full benefits of the consultation process. They are not giving the patient the full story about what they believe is in the patient's best interest. When making a treatment recommendation it can be helpful to ask yourself the question: If this patient were a member of my family, what treatment plan would I want another therapist to recommend?

The therapist informs the patient about the evidence base of the proposed formulation and proposed treatment and about any major modifications he or she proposes to the evidence-based therapies, by saying, for example, "In your case, I'm going to modify the therapies that have been shown to be effective in the research in order to treat your mood and substance disorders at the same time." If the therapist is offering a novel, experimental treatment for a problem for which no EST is available, the therapist must inform the patient about that. For example, the therapist might state, "To develop a treatment for your shoplifting behavior, I'm going to be drawing on interventions and therapies for related problems and disorders, including bipolar disorder and borderline personality disorder, because the field has not yet developed an empirically supported treatment for shoplifting. The main elements of the treatment plan will involve your collecting data to monitor the details of the behavior and my teaching you skills to anticipate and manage urges to steal. You will need to do homework outside the session to monitor your behavior and practice new skills. We'll set some clear treatment goals and monitor progress carefully to make sure that what we are doing is helpful to you. If we do not make progress, we'll try to figure out why and what changes are needed in the treatment plan to accomplish the goals we set."

Patients often want to know how long therapy will last. This question is difficult to answer. One approach to answering this question is to take as a starting point the duration of the treatment provided in the ESTs that the proposed treatment is based on. The therapist can make adjustments to that duration depending on the patient's treatment goals, the presence of comorbidities, and other factors that might be expected to shorten or lengthen the treatment. Another approach to answering the duration question is to focus on the issue of when improvement is expected to occur. Patients who respond to CBT for depression generally show significant change in the first 4 to 6 weeks of treatment (Ilardi & Craighead, 1994); similar findings have been reported for bulimia (Wilson, 1996b) and substance abuse (Breslin, Sobell, Sobell, Buchan, & Cunningham, 1997). The therapist can inform the patient about this and recommend a review of the treatment plan if the patient does not make gains within 4 to 6 or 8 weeks.

Describing Available Treatment Options

Clinicians have a responsibility to inform the patient about *all* of the available therapies for his or her condition, including pharmacotherapy, electroconvulsive therapy, and the full range of psychosocial treatments, even those they cannot provide, so the patient has the information needed to make an informed choice about what treatment to pursue. The cognitive-behavior therapist may not have the expertise to describe these therapies in detail. However, she does have a responsibility to let the patient know that they are available and to provide some information about whether they might be helpful to the patient. To do this, the therapist must keep up to date with the efficacy and effectiveness literature for the problems and disorders she usually evaluates.

Obtaining the Patient's Consent to Proceed

After the therapist has made a recommendation and provided all the information described above, he asks the patient for a decision. The therapist asks the questions, "How does all this sound to you? Does the treatment plan I'm proposing make sense? Do you have questions? Do you want to go forward with this plan?" At this point, a formal pause is helpful. I often encourage patients to leave the office, go home, think about the proposal, and discuss it with family members before making a decision. Otherwise they may agree to what I am proposing just because of the interpersonal and emotional pulls in the room rather than because of a reasoned decision-making process. Treatment does not go forward until the patient makes an explicit agreement to the proposed treatment plan.

Negotiating the patient's agreement to treatment involves trade-offs. If the therapist sets the bar low (offers a nondemanding treatment plan), he may be able to induce the patient to begin treatment, but the treatment plan may be too weak to be very helpful. If the therapist sets the bar high, insisting on everything he needs to maximize the success of treatment, the patient may not get over the bar. The Trevose behavior modification program is an example of a very high bar (see Figure 5.1). How high to set the bar is a complex decision that is based on evidence, the details of the case, and the therapist's and patient's willingness to tolerate failure or crisis situations.

Sometimes the patient is eager to begin the treatment the therapist has described. However, sometimes interventions are needed to obtain the patient's agreement to proceed. And sometimes the patient and therapist cannot reach an agreement about the treatment plan.

Interventions That Can Help Get Consent

Sometimes the problems for which the patient is seeking help interfere with his ability to agree to a good treatment plan. For example, manic symptoms can prevent patients from perceiving that they have serious problems—or any problems at all! In a situation like this, interventions are needed to help the patient agree to an adequate treatment plan. It can be helpful to have a session in which family members or spouse can inform the patient about the effects of his behavior. I once treated a husband who had been unwilling enter treatment for his OCD symptoms until his wife told him that if he did not, she would divorce him. She told me this on the telephone when she called to schedule a consultation session. Just before the consultation session, she gave him the ultimatum and they came in together for the consultation session. Once the husband understood how miserable his symptoms were making his wife and that she was serious about her ultimatum, he agreed to get treatment (and made a speedy recovery!).

When the patient is reluctant to accept the therapist's treatment recommendations, the therapist can initiate a collaborative discussion to identify the patient's reservations and attempt to address them. The case formulation can be helpful here because sometimes the obstacles to undertaking treatment are the same ones that cause the problems for which the patient seeks treatment, as in the case of the depressed patient who believes that the future is hopeless and no treatment can help. The therapist may be able to use a Thought Record or guided Socratic discovery to address this issue or even suggest a behavioral experiment to test the patient's belief. In this case, a brief time-limited treatment contract, even for as few as six sessions, can evaluate whether the treatment can be helpful or is (as the patient fears) a waste of time and money.

A common situation occurs when the therapist recommends a combined CBT-pharmacotherapy treatment plan, say for a severely depressed patient, but the patient refuses to accept the pharmacotherapy element of the treatment plan. Although the evidence (Friedman et al., 2004) indicates that combined treatment for severe depression is superior to either psychotherapy or pharmacotherapy alone, many patients do not want to take medication. In this situation I will sometimes agree to the patient's plan with the understanding that if after 6 to 8 weeks of treatment (a recommendation based loosely on the data presented by Ilardi and Craighead, 1994) the patient has not shown substantial improvement, we will reopen this question. I warn the patient at the onset of treatment that when we reach the 6 to 8 week point, I might not be willing to go forward without the addition of pharmacotherapy or some other important change to the treatment plan. One of the beauties of this arrangement is that it can motivate the patient to work hard in CBT in order to forestall the need to take medication.

Motivational interviewing was designed to help patients overcome ambivalence about changing (see W. R. Miller & Rollnick, 2002) and emphasizes using empathic listening to help patients think through their goals and values, understand how their problems impede them from achieving those goals, and how treatment might help. It also aims to enhance patients' confidence that they can successfully reach their goals. Motivational interviewing strategies can help the patient accept a challenging treatment plan.

The process of carrying out interventions and negotiations in order to induce the patient to accept a treatment plan raises ethical issues. The therapist is providing some treatment before obtaining the patient's informed consent to treatment. In addition, the therapist (at least the therapist in private practice) has something to gain (the fee) from obtaining the patient's consent to proceed (W. R. Miller & Rollnick, 2002). These facts highlight therapists' responsibility to think carefully about these issues to be sure they are acting in the patient's best interest. Consultation with colleagues can be helpful in these situations.

Compromise Treatment Plans

Not infrequently the patient asks for changes to the treatment plan the therapist recommends. The patient and therapist can then undertake a negotiation to arrive at a treatment plan that is mutually agreeable. It is defensible to offer a patient a treatment plan that is different from the one with the greatest empirical support in the literature for two reasons. One, as already mentioned above, is that data from randomized controlled trials do not provide unequivocal information about what treatment plan is best for any particular patient (Howard et al., 1996).

Second, the question of what treatment plan a patient will benefit from is ultimately an empirical one. This is why outcome monitoring (described in Chapter 9) is so important. For example, Martin sought treatment for depression. Assessment indicated that he had an MDD and was drinking a bottle of wine daily after work with his buddies and more on the weekend. I recommended that treatment focus both on his depression and his alcohol use. Martin insisted that the alcohol was not a problem for him and, indeed, he functioned every day at a challenging job. To resolve the impasse, I proposed that we treat his depression while monitoring his progress weekly using the BDI. If, after 10 weeks, we had not made any substantial progress on his depression as measured by the BDI, he would agree to work with me to reduce his alcohol intake or I would refer him to another provider. Martin agreed to this plan. At the end of 10 weeks we reviewed his plot of BDI scores, which showed that he had made no progress (except for one week when he stopped drinking because he had the flu and was much less depressed). Despite this evidence, Martin was unwilling to address his alcohol use and I reluctantly referred him to another clinician.

When is it reasonable to agree to a non-optimal or compromise treatment plan? A compromise treatment plan can be a reasonable option under the following conditions (Gruber & Persons, 2008). First, the patient is not in imminent danger of dying (e.g., by suicide) or suffering grave danger from his illness (e.g., by getting fired from his job and becoming homeless). Second, no danger is on the horizon. Third, the patient has been informed that the treatment is non-optimal and knows the risks. Fourth, a backup plan has been established and agreed to. That is, patient and therapist have agreed on what treatment plan will be instituted if the compromise plan fails. Fifth, the patient agrees that progress will be monitored carefully and if the treatment appears to be failing, the backup plan will be instituted. Sixth, the patient agrees that the therapist has the option at any time to institute the backup plan. Before embarking on a compromise treatment plan, the therapist will want to document the treatment he or she recommended, the patient's refusal to accept the recommendation, and the rationale for and conditions of the compromise plan.

Deciding Not to Proceed with Treatment

Sometimes patient and therapist simply cannot agree on a treatment plan. Sometimes the therapist fails to induce the patient to accept treatment adjuncts (e.g., pharmacotherapy) or goals (stop suicidal behavior) or targets (alcohol abuse) that the therapist considers essential to adequate treatment. Sometimes assessment reveals that the patient's major problem is one the therapist does not have the expertise to treat or that the patient's problems require more intensive treatment than the therapist can provide. For example, the patient may be acutely suicidal and the therapist already has more of these patients in her caseload than she can easily manage or she does not have the collegial support she needs to manage a risky case.

If the failure to agree on a treatment plan seems like something that might be resolvable with a bit more discussion, the therapist can consider extending the pretreatment phase for another session. Other options are to establish a *monitor-only* plan or to refer to another treatment provider.

One of my colleagues (Michael A. Tompkins) uses a *monitor-only* strategy to maintain contact with adolescents whose parents want them to be in treatment but who are not ready to agree to any kind of treatment plan. This notion can also be helpful in community mental health clinics or other settings where the clinician does not have the option to refuse to provide services. In the monitor-only plan, the patient and clinician meet periodically (e.g., monthly) for assessment and progress monitoring. The clinician can use the monitoring sessions to carry out some interventions to increase the patient's motivation to participate in active treatment, for example by highlighting to the patient some of the ways his untreated symptoms interfere with his ability to accomplish important personal goals. Of course, a monitor-only plan is risky. If the patient's situation deteriorates, the clinician must step forward to provide active treatment until the crisis is averted.

Referring a patient to another provider when the patient and clinician cannot agree on a treatment plan raises complex issues. One is the issue of abandonment. The clinician must not abandon the patient. Therefore, the clinician may need to spend several weeks working with the patient to successfully transfer her to another provider. Second, the clinician is not serving the patient well (or building good professional relationships) by simply handing the patient a list of telephone numbers that she can call to ask for an appointment with another provider who may simply repeat the process the patient and clinician have just gone through. Instead, the clinician must (and can do this without giving the patient's name) call potential treatment providers, describe the situation frankly, and ask if they would be willing to meet with the patient for a consultation to discuss the possibility of treatment. The clinician must continue this process until she locates a treatment provider who agrees to meet with the patient.

Jane sought treatment for severe symptoms of panic disorder and agoraphobia (PDA). Jane had other problems as well. She had $40,000 in credit card debt and she was living with and financially dependent on a man who was physically abusing her. Despite extensive discussion, Jane was unwilling to address her financial and relationship issues in therapy. We agreed that I would refer her to another therapist who could accept Jane's wish to focus only on her PDA symptoms. I made several calls and located a therapist who agreed to "accept the patient where she is."

Therapists often have difficulty refusing to treat a patient who will not accept an adequate treatment plan. For example, the clinician may elect to refuse to treat a patient who has severe bipolar disorder and refuses pharmacotherapy (pharmacotherapy is generally considered to be an essential element of evidence-based treatment for bipolar disorder). The clinician may elect to refer the patient to another provider. Is this a valid and reasonable tactic? The reader may ask, "If the client would not agree to a treatment plan with this therapist that did not include pharmacotherapy, why would she behave any differently with another clinician?"

There are four answers to this question. One, as described above (in the section on using interventions to obtain consent), is that the patient's willingness to agree to a particular treatment is a dynamic process (W. R. Miller & Rollnick, 2002). Another clinician may well be more successful than was the first clinician at inducing the patient to accept pharmacotherapy. Second, different clinicians have different degrees of tolerance for risk. Even if one clinician is unwilling to provide treatment without pharmacotherapy, not all clinicians will take this position. Three, the fact that the patient refuses to accept an adequate treatment plan does not mean that the clinician must step forward to provide an inadequate one. A helpful concept here is one well stated by Grosso (2002):

"Seeking substandard care is the client's choice. Providing substandard care is the clinician's choice."

Four, sometimes therapists are tempted to agree to a substandard treatment. For example, Howard is severely and chronically depressed. He will not agree to weekly therapy sessions; instead he wants to call and come in whenever he feels the need. The therapist might think, "If I refuse to treat Howard he will just find another therapist who will do it his way." This thought might well be true. An idea that helps me hold firm in these types of situations is the notion that it is quite possible that before Howard will agree to an adequate treatment plan, he will need to meet four or five or six therapists who describe what is needed and refuse to agree to his treatment plan. I can be the first of those therapists. If I agree to Howard's treatment plan, I may not only fail to help him, I may be *impeding* him from getting the treatment he needs to accomplish his goals.

The methods described here for obtaining the patient's informed consent best fit a situation in which the clinician can elect not to provide treatment. Many therapists work in agencies where they cannot refuse to provide treatment. Several options are available in this challenging situation. I've already mentioned a monitor-only intervention. Another is to offer a less desirable treatment (e.g., a group rather than individual therapy) to patients who refuse adequate treatment. Another option is to set minimal goals that are consistent with the minimal intervention the patient will accept (e.g., a goal of rapidly identifying and intervening to address psychotic symptom flare-ups rather than a goal of preventing the flare-ups).

Obtaining Angela's Informed Consent

I carried out the informed consent process with Angela at the end of our third session. I summarized the diagnostic information I had provided her in the second interview (PTSD, MDD, and dysthymia). As explained earlier in this chapter, I spent some time describing my conceptualization of her problems, especially the mechanism hypothesis that was at the heart of my formulation of her case. To recap, these mechanisms were her conditioned fear responses, her avoidant mode of coping with the fear, and the loss of positively reinforcing activities because of avoidance. Angela found the account of her problems to be soothing and validating and it made sense to her.

Flowing out of the conceptualization, I recommended a treatment plan that was designed to help Angela regain previously important sources of reinforcement and also to extinguish the fear reactions she had learned. The key thing we'd be doing in treatment was helping her reengage in her life. We would do that gradually and would use standard cognitive-behavior interventions of behavioral activity scheduling, learning to cope with distorted thoughts, and other tools, like breaking tasks into parts. We'd be working in a here-and-now, present-focused way to teach her ways to overcome her symptoms and accomplish the goals she had set.

Because behavioral inactivity was common to her PTSD and depressive symptoms and because my formulation viewed disengagement as a key mechanism, I recommended to Angela that we address it first. I warned her that as she became more active, especially in approaching some aspects of her work situation, she would likely experience some anxiety symptoms. When that happened I would teach her tools to manage them, but I told her that treatment would involve her willingness to learn to tolerate and manage those symptoms without retreating and becoming inactive again. Homework would be a key piece of the treatment and she'd practice skills and tools outside the session that she learned in therapy.

I did let Angela know that my treatment plan involved some modifications to the evidence-based therapies for MDD and PTSD and that I would be combining interventions from cognitive-behavior therapies for depression and PTSD to address the fact that she had both problems. We would monitor her progress carefully and if she did not make good progress we would review the treatment to make whatever adjustments were needed to overcome whatever was getting in the way.

I offered a rationale for my recommendations. I recommended CBT, I told her, because it was supported by controlled studies that showed it was effective for treating both PTSD and MDD, her referring psychiatrist had recommended it, she seemed to have a good response to *Feeling Good* (Burns, 1999), I was trained to do it, and we seemed to have a good connection and be off to a good start. I also described other options, pointing out that in the San Francisco Bay Area there was a wide range of psychotherapies available, especially insight-oriented and psychodynamic psychotherapy. These other psychotherapies might very well be helpful to her but were generally not supported by evidence from randomized controlled trials. However, if the approach I suggested did not make sense to her or seem like a good fit for her I would certainly be happy to refer her to another therapist who could take a different approach.

As I thought about treatment modality, the presence of marital problems on Angela's Problem List raised the question of whether she might benefit from couple therapy. When I discussed this issue with her, Angela agreed that couple therapy might be helpful later but felt that now she needed individual therapy to get her life back on track. This thinking made sense to me. We agreed to hold in reserve the notion of a couple session with me and/or couple therapy as an adjunct later. The severity of Angela's difficulties seemed manageable in a weekly treatment format and given Angela's report and that of her psychiatrist that she was benefiting from pharmacotherapy, I recommended that she continue it.

I asked Angela if she liked the treatment plan I proposed (see Figure 7.1) and wanted to do it. It's good to wait here to get a clear response from the patient. Don't assume the answer is yes! In fact, sometimes, especially if I sense the patient is ambivalent or not really thinking through what is involved, or would have trouble saying no, I ask the patient to go home, discuss the treatment plan with family members, and think carefully about whether he or she wants to go forward before making a decision.

In Angela's case, I did not detect any reservations or ambivalence. She stated that she liked the plan I proposed and was eager to get started. We made an agreement to meet weekly on Tuesdays at 2 P.M. Before she left, I gave her a homework assignment to continue logging her activities, reading *Feeling Good*, and completing the BDI and Burns AI in the waiting room before each therapy session.

CONCLUDING PRETREATMENT

When the patient and therapist agree on a treatment plan, the therapist completes the Case Formulation Worksheet and Treatment Plan forms, as illustrated for the case of Angela in Figures 6.2 and 7.1. I highlight the Case Formulation Worksheet and Treatment Plan in my paper-and-pencil clinical record (I hope to shift to an online record

Name <u>Angela</u>   Date _____

Goals

1. Reduce depressive symptoms to BDI score less than 10.

2. Get back to work full time and enjoy it.

3. Encounter "problem people" at work without a lot of distress, chest pain, shortness of breath.

4. Welcome my husband home from work with a kiss and a hug.

5. Have and enjoy sex 1.5 times/week.

6. Be able to discipline my kids without yelling.

Modality
Individual CBT
Behavioral activity scheduling and cognitive restructuring focused especially on increasing engagement and reducing avoidance

Frequency
Weekly

Adjunct Treatment
Pharmacotherapy
Consider couple therapy or session later

FIGURE 7.1. Completed Treatment Plan for Angela.

shortly!) with a colored paper clip that allows me to retrieve them easily and use them to guide my work with the patient. Of course, if the patient and therapist have agreed not to work together, the therapist documents the disposition that was made and rationale for it, such as a referral to another clinician who had the skills the patient needed that the consulting clinician did not have.

When the pretreatment tasks have been successfully negotiated, typically after two to four sessions, the patient and therapist have the beginnings of a working alliance. The therapist has developed a diagnosis, an initial case formulation and a treatment plan, and the patient and therapist have agreed on the treatment plan. Treatment now begins.

* * *

The next chapter describes the therapeutic relationship in the case formulation approach to CBT. The location of this chapter is apt, because, as Bordin (1979) points out, agreement on the goals and tasks of treatment (described in detail in these pretreatment chapters) is an essential component of a good therapeutic alliance.

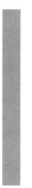

EIGHT

The Therapeutic Relationship

This chapter discusses the therapeutic relationship in case formulation-driven CBT. I describe the role of the relationship in therapy and offer strategies for using the relationship in therapy and working therapeutically with problems in the relationship.

THE ROLE OF THE THERAPEUTIC RELATIONSHIP IN CBT

The therapeutic relationship in case formulation-driven CBT is a synthesis of two views: the traditional view in CBT that the relationship is "necessary but not sufficient" to produce change and the newer (at least in CBT) view of the relationship itself as an assessment and intervention tool.

The Necessary-but-Not-Sufficient View

In the necessary-but-not-sufficient (NBNS) view, a good therapeutic relationship is necessary but not sufficient to achieve a good outcome (A. T. Beck et al., 1979). In this view, the main function of the patient–therapist relationship is to facilitate the technical interventions of the therapy. The technical interventions are seen as the key drivers of therapeutic change. The watchword of the NBNS view of the relationship is collaboration. The therapist's relationship task in this view is to build collaboration so that patient and therapist are working as an effective team to carry out the technical interventions of the therapy.

To unpack this notion a bit, the idea is that a warm, trusting, respectful, and collaborative relationship will help the patient accept the therapist's input, agree with the therapist on the goals and tasks of therapy, work hard to comply with the technical interventions of the treatment, and discuss with the therapist any problems that arise in the therapy. The NBNS view is consistent with the relationship as conceptualized by Bordin (1979). He proposed that the therapeutic alliance has three elements: bond (the liking, trust, and attachment between patient and therapist), agreement on the tasks of therapy (what interventions by therapist and activities by patient are needed), and agreement on the goals of therapy.

The therapist can use the case formulation to determine what type of relationship will be most helpful and comfortable for each patient (Turkat & Brantley, 1981). A. T. Beck (1983) discusses this issue for patients with depression. He describes depressed patients with core schemas of being unlovable (the dependent types) as wanting more interpersonal support and warmth from the therapist than patients with core schemas of being inadequate and bound to fail (the autonomous types). The autonomous types feel comfortable with a more distant relationship in which the therapist emphasizes the skills-teaching aspect of the therapy. Similarly, Karno and Longabaugh (2005) showed that reactant patients (those who perceive direct requests to change behavior as an infringement of their autonomy) who were being treated for alcohol abuse had better outcomes when therapists were less directive than when they were more directive.

The NBNS view predicts that good outcome results when the therapist and patient carry out the technical interventions of the therapy in the context of a good relationship. Studies of the NBNS view have produced mixed support for the model. In support of the NBNS view, Morris and Suckerman (1974) showed that systematic desensitization was more effective when carried out by a warm than by an aloof therapist and Rector, Zuroff, and Segal (1999) showed that changes in dysfunctional attitudes predicted outcome only in the presence of a strong therapeutic bond. Additional evidence supportive of the NBNS view was obtained by Castonguay, Goldfried, Wiser, Raue, and Hayes (1996), who showed that poor outcomes resulted when the therapist persisted in moving forward with the technical interventions of the therapy despite relationship glitches. Evidence disconfirming the NBNS view was reported by investigators Burns and Nolen-Hoeksema (1992); Persons and Burns (1985); and Santiago et al. (2005), who showed that technical interventions and the quality of the relationship each made independent contributions to outcome.

The NBNS view is clinically helpful. It reminds the therapist that when the relationship is not going well, taking the time to repair it before proceeding forward with the technical interventions can produce better outcome than simply plunging ahead (Huppert, Barlow, Gorman, Shear, & Woods, 2006). The NBNS view is especially helpful when patients have good interpersonal skills and the therapeutic relationship goes smoothly or is easily repaired. In this type of situation, the therapist can focus most of his or her energy on the technical interventions of the therapy.

However, the NBNS notion of the relationship is sometimes inadequate. This is the case when patients' problems—often the very ones for which they seek treatment—make it difficult for the therapist to establish a warm, trusting, collaborative therapeutic relationship. For example, Rector et al. (1999) showed that high levels of distorted thinking interfered with depressed patients' ability to form a strong bond with their cognitive therapist at the beginning of treatment. In these types of cases, the requirement that the therapist establish a positive collaborative working relationship in order to carry out the technical interventions of the therapy appears to place the therapist in a "Catch-22" dilemma in which he must cure the patient before he can carry out the treatment! The NBNS view comes up short in these cases. Another view is needed.

The Relationship-as-Treatment View

An alternative view is that the relationship itself is an assessment and intervention tool. This is the relationship-as-treatment view of the therapeutic relationship. The relationship-as-treatment view of CBT is based on the notion that the patient's behaviors in the session are samples of behaviors that also occur outside the session. As a result, the presence of these behaviors in the session provides opportunities for assessment, conceptualization and intervention. Moreover, in some therapies guided by this model (e.g., functional analytic psychotherapy [FAP; Kohlenberg & Tsai, 1991] and CBASP; McCullough, 2000), the therapist works actively to elicit patient problem behaviors that might not otherwise appear in the session. In a therapy based exclusively on this model, there are no technical interventions aside from those used to address the relationship transactions between patient and therapist.

The relationship-as-treatment view solves the Catch-22 dilemma mentioned above. Indeed, in the relationship-as-treatment view, problematic interpersonal patient–therapist interactions are not obstacles to the therapy (as in the NBNS view) but in fact are essential to the therapy because they provide opportunities to conceptualize and intervene with problem behaviors.

The view of the therapeutic relationship as an assessment and intervention tool has origins in psychodynamic theory, especially the proposal that successful therapy entails corrective experiences that occur in the context of the therapeutic relationship (Alexander & French, 1946). Many cognitive-behavior treatments capitalize on this notion. It is one of the ideas underpinning the "caring days" intervention (Stuart, 1980) that begins marital therapy, which is based on social learning principles. During "caring days," couples act "as if" they cared for each other in order to promote positive emotions that can serve as incentives to the couple to work on repairing the relationship. Similarly, Barkley and Benton's (1998) treatment for oppositional children counsels parents to begin intervening by praising and rewarding their child's the adaptive behaviors, no matter how small. By doing this, the parents become reinforcers for the child, which allows them to elicit behavior change from the child in the next parts of the treatment. Linehan's (1993a) DBT also uses similar notions. In Linehan's (1993a) words, "the therapist first develops a strong positive relationship and then uses it to 'blackmail' the patient into making targeted, but excruciatingly difficult, changes in her behavior" (p. 296).

Kohlenberg and Tsai's (1991) FAP relies on the relationship-as-treatment model. In FAP the therapist uses principles of operant conditioning to change the client's behavior in the session. The therapist works to increase the patient's adaptive behaviors by providing immediate and genuine interpersonal rewards for them (increased attention, for example) and to decrease maladaptive behaviors by extinguishing or punishing them, again with interpersonal consequences that are delivered in the session by the therapist. CBASP relies heavily on the therapist's in-session responses to the chronically depressed patient's maladaptive behavior (McCullough, 2006).

Empirical support for the curative effects of the relationship-as-treatment view is difficult to find. No outcome data for FAP are available. (Some outcome data are available for FAP-enhanced CBT for depression, which I describe a bit later.) Although efficacy data are available for CBASP (Keller et al., 2000) and DBT (reviewed by Scheel, 2000, and Koerner & Dimeff, 2000), the contribution of the therapeutic relationship to the effectiveness of these therapies is not yet known. Some support for the curative role of the therapeutic relationship can be seen in reviews by Lambert and Barley (2002) and Wampold (2001) showing that the alliance contributes more to therapy outcome than the technical interventions. However, most of these studies are of therapies that entail both technical and relationship interventions. One exception is the review by Elliott (2002) showing that the client-centered therapy developed by Carl Rogers, which consists mainly of the therapist's providing empathy to the patient in the session, is effective.

Although it has strengths (notably it solves the Catch-22 dilemma), the relationship-as-treatment view (at least the version of it described in FAP) also comes up short. If the patient's problem behaviors do not occur in the FAP session, the therapist cannot modify them. For example, if the patient's problem arises only in the context of relationships with subordinates or in a sexual relationship, it will not appear in the therapy session. Another problem is that behavior change accomplished in this way occurs slowly and does not readily generalize to situations outside of the therapeutic relationship.

A Synthesis of the Two Views

Case formulation-driven CBT relies on both the NBNS and the relationship-as-treatment views of the relationship. A synthesis of these views can capitalize on the strengths and compensate for the weaknesses of each. In the synthesized view, the therapist uses good interpersonal and other skills (e.g., motivational interviewing) to establish and maintain a strong relationship in order to facilitate the technical interventions of the therapy (NBNS).

The therapist also uses the patient–therapist interactions as opportunities for assessment, conceptualization, and intervention (relationship-as-treatment). Interventions include both therapist behaviors (e.g., the therapist leans in and is warm and supportive to reward the patient's improved behavior) and technical interventions (e.g., a Thought Record focused on interactions between the patient and therapist).

In one example, Alberto sought treatment for depression and problems at work. He had recently received a poor performance review from his supervisor, who pointed to Alberto's interpersonal clashes with his subordinates. Alberto was a manager and frequently found himself butting heads with his employees, who described him as insensitive, rigid, and unappreciative of their accomplishments and contributions. His work performance was extremely important to Alberto and his poor performance evaluation had precipitated symptoms of depression and feelings of worthlessness and inadequacy. In addition, he was baffled about what was going on, as he felt he worked hard to be fair and evenhanded with his subordinates.

I had begun assessing Alberto's depression and other problems. We seemed to have the start of a good working relationship. He was monitoring his activity and writing down some of his thoughts in upsetting situations. I did not yet understand what was happening at work and asked him to monitor some interactions there to give us more information. Here I'm using the NBNS view of the relationship.

I also observed Alberto's behavior when he interacted with me and my emotional reactions to his behavior. These observations contributed to my conceptualization of his case. Here I'm using the relationship-as-treatment view of the relationship. After an early session that I thought had gone very well, we set the next appointment. To do that, I had agreed (and let Alberto know I was doing it) to meet him at a time that was not very convenient for me but that worked well for him. The next day I got a brusque telephone message from Alberto in which he stated, "The appointment time we set yesterday doesn't work for me. Please call me to reschedule."

I noticed that my emotional reaction to Alberto's e-mail was to feel a bit discounted and annoyed. I reviewed the details of his message to see where my feelings arose. He did not apologize for inconveniencing me by asking me to reschedule, he did not acknowledge or thank me for initially offering him a time that was convenient for him but not for me, he did not offer me a reason for rescheduling that would make me feel better about it ("Oops, I forgot that I had a medical appointment scheduled that I made many months ago"), and his tone was cold and unfriendly.

These details of Alberto's behavior with me and my emotional reaction to it yielded some hypotheses about the causes of Alberto's work difficulties. I speculated that Alberto might have a sense of entitlement (if people are working for me they should do what I want and I shouldn't have to attend to their feelings), poor awareness of his own behavior (e.g., perhaps he was unaware his tone was cold), and/or poor awareness of how his behavior affects others. To collect information to determine which of these hypotheses was most accurate, I might use a role play or Thought Record to flesh out the details of the situation in which Alberto called me to reschedule his appointment. Thus, my conceptualization of Alberto's behavior in this situation relied on a view of the relationship that combined the NBNS and the relationship-as-treatment views.

The combined view of the relationship also aids in intervention. I made a plan to take up the telephone-scheduling exchange the next time I met with Alberto. I could use a Thought Record or an advantages and disadvantages exercise to address any entitlement beliefs that emerged or I could use role playing to help Alberto increase his awareness of his behavior and its effects on others if assessment indicated that this was part of the problem. I could use Socratic questioning to explore whether our appointment-scheduling interaction was related to some of his experiences at work.

I might also use my own behavior to intervene with Alberto's rescheduling request. I considered imposing a natural aversive consequence of his unskillful request by delaying returning his call, offering him only one or two appointment times even if I knew they would be hard for him, or being a bit cool. However, because it was early in therapy and I did not feel confident that Alberto was yet attached to me, I feared these behaviors on my part might prevent us from developing a trusting bond. So I decided, when I returned his call, to use a warm, pleasant tone that would promote a positive bond between us that would facilitate a productive discussion of the difficult rescheduling topic when we were sitting together in a therapy session. This tone would also provide a model of the tone he needed to use when telephoning me.

A practical and elegant way to think about the fact that the therapist can use both technical and *in vivo* interpersonal interactions to promote change is to focus on mechanisms of change (Goldfried & Davila, 2005). Thus, as Alberto's therapist, I was striving to teach him, by way of both technical interventions and interpersonal interactions, that his behavior and the beliefs underpinning it were causing him problems and that he might want to change them in order to have more successful relationships.

This combined NBNS and relationship-as-treatment view proposes that therapy happens on two channels: the technical interventions and the interpersonal interactions between patient and therapist. This notion opens up the possibility that an intervention might be therapeutic on one channel but not the other. For example, a therapist might teach problem-solving skills to a passive patient in an overly active way that reinforces the patient's passivity. Or I could teach Alberto social skills to improve his behavior at work and be endlessly warm and responsive to him even when his behavior with me was unskillful and would probably alienate others with whom he interacted. This strategy would likely be less effective and helpful to Alberto than if I strove to convey on both channels the same message about which of his behaviors were effective and which were not.

Thus, in the combined view of the relationship, the therapist uses the NBNS view of the relationship to build and maintain a strong relationship in order to support the technical interventions. The therapist also uses the relationship-as-treatment view of the relationship, viewing patient–therapist interactions in the therapy as samples of patient behavior. And the therapist strives to convey the same message on both channels.

Many patients have such excellent interpersonal and relationship skills that very little of the relationship-as-treatment part of the model is needed and the NBNS model goes a long way or even all the way to getting the treatment done. These are the easiest cases.

Angela's was one of these easy cases. Nevertheless, even in her case the combined view was helpful. One of the ways Angela's problems played themselves out in therapy was that her tendency to minimize her difficulties prevented her from seeking help with problems that needed attention. For example, on one occasion I learned only in passing about a meeting with her boss in which it was quite clear to me that he was not being supportive of her. However, she failed to notice this and assert herself to get the support she needed from him. And because she failed to notice his lack of support, she did not ask me for help with it either! Angela's initial (and fortunately short-lived) view of me as unlikely to be helpful to her is another example of the way her interpersonal difficulties (her schemas of others as unreliable and unhelpful) played out in her relationship with me. So even though the relationship-as-treatment view is less important in easier cases, it is always useful to keep it in mind.

The combined view is supported by findings from investigators (Burns & Nolen-Hoeksema, 1992; Persons & Burns, 1985; Santiago et al., 2005) who showed that technical interventions and the quality of the relationship each made independent contributions to the outcome of cognitive therapy for depression. Some empirical support for the utility of a therapeutic relationship that relies on both the NBNS view and the view of the relationship as assessment and intervention tool is provided by efficacy data supporting cognitive-behavior therapies that use this type of relationship (S. C. Hayes, Masuda, Bissett, Luoma, & Guerrero, 2004), including DBT (Linehan, 1993a), FAP-enhanced CBT (Kohlenberg, Kanter, Bolling, Parker, & Tsai, 2002), and CBASP (McCullough, 2000).

To summarize: in the combined view of the relationship, the therapist uses the NBNS to build and maintain a collaborative relationship in order to support the technical interventions of therapy. The individualized case formulation is helpful in this process. The therapist also views the patient's behavior with the therapist as samples of patient behavior that offer opportunities to assess, conceptualize, and intervene with those behaviors. The therapist uses both his or her own behaviors and technical interventions to assess and intervene. In the rest of the chapter, and, indeed, throughout this book, when I am discussing the therapeutic relationship I am referring to this combined view of the relationship.

USING THE RELATIONSHIP IN THERAPY

The therapeutic relationship aids in assessment and conceptualization and also in intervention. I discuss both here. I also discuss the potential for the relationship to cause harm.

To Aid Assessment and Conceptualization

Adele was not making progress in treatment. Losing her job had destabilized her and she had returned to her pattern of lurching from crisis to crisis. We had discussed her setback and agreed that she needed more intensive treatment. She had agreed to begin meeting twice weekly. One reason she needed so much treatment was that she had no support network.

Adele failed to follow through with our plan to meet more often. On the first week of the new plan, she called after the first session to cancel her second session of the week. When I called to urge her to reschedule, she agreed it was a good idea but said she felt so overwhelmed by her problems that she was having trouble scheduling the appointment. However, she agreed to try to sort out a time she could come and said she would call to let me know if she could meet. She did not.

I felt frustrated and let down. As I thought about the situation, I realized that Adele's behavior with me fit a pattern that occurred outside the therapy as well. Because she had grown up in an abusive environment, Adele had learned to say whatever was needed to placate powerful others on whom she depended when they wanted her to do things she didn't want to do or feel able to do. She had learned to give these people enough of what they wanted (I'll try to work it out) to placate them while simultaneously getting what she wanted. She had learned not to ask directly for what she wanted because when she did she was often attacked or abandoned or both. Thus, her behavior with me had been reinforced in the abusive environment in which she grew up. However, in her current environment, her behavior was maladaptive. In fact, it caused what she feared. That is, her behavior was alienating me even though I was one of the few supportive people in her life. In learning theory terms, Adele's behavior was extinguishing my efforts to help her.

Although my interaction with Adele was frustrating (the bad news), the good news is that it helped me flesh out my conceptualization of her case. In particular, it helped me understand why Adele had no support network! Also, conceptualizing her behavior as a consequence of her learning history and an example of her problems more generally, not just with me, reduced my frustration with it.

To Intervene

My conceptualization of Adele's behavior also guided my intervention. The conceptualization gave me some information about the ideas (distinction between abusive people and others) and skills (assertiveness and reinforcing those who offered help) I needed to teach Adele to help her build a support network. In addition to using those technical interventions, I could also use my interactions with her to intervene. One way of doing this is to verbalize the consequences of her behavior in the moment it occurs. I might say to her, "When you do this it really gives me a good feeling and I want to help you more" or "When you do that it demoralizes me and gives me less energy to help you."

Another client, Sandra, called to leave the message "I have to take my son Greg to San Francisco to a medical appointment at the time of our appointment. Could we meet on the phone? I could talk to you on my way over to the city." This behavior is an example of Sandra's problems. In fact, her chief complaint was "My life is not my own anymore. I'm living Greg's life, not mine." I considered pointing out to her in a light tone that her problem was currently present on the scene and demanding attention!

However, since she sounded rattled and stressed, I decided she was not likely to be able to receive that information without feeling unsupported by me.

So I decided to intervene via my own behavior to deliver some natural consequences. I called Sandra back and left her the message that I did not believe I could be helpful over the telephone. (This was true.) I recommended that we reschedule instead of meeting on the phone. This intervention provided a natural consequence (choosing to take Greg to his appointment caused Sandra to lose her therapy session that day). It also served as a model for Sandra of the type of assertiveness that she would need to begin practicing in order to achieve her treatment goals. Sandra responded! She called back to leave the message that she would handle the Greg situation in another way and would come to the session though she might be late. She arrived five minutes late and we had a very productive session in which I was able to get out on the table all of the ideas I presented here.

In Sandra's case I used my own behavior (refusing to agree to a telephone session) as an intervention to address both problems in our relationship and Sandra's problems in her life. Technical interventions can also be used in this type of situation. When one of my patients flew into a rage when I arrived 5 minutes late to the session, I responded first by apologizing and letting him know I would extend the session if he was able, to make up the time. Then I used a Thought Record to help him identify and address the automatic thoughts that drove his rage. He was quite willing to do this exercise with me and it proved very helpful.

The Potential for Harm

If the therapeutic relationship has the potential to be helpful, it must, logically, also have the potential to be harmful. The case of Alan illustrates the potential of well-meaning therapy for harm. Alan sought help overcoming his long-standing procrastination. My case formulation proposed that he had the central belief "If I make a decision and move forward to take action I'll do the wrong thing and bad things will happen that I won't be able to handle." Alan managed the fear and anxiety this belief produced by avoiding. Passivity, procrastination, and depression were his main problems. I was using activity scheduling, Thought Records, decision analyses (examining advantages and disadvantages), and the breaking down of tasks into parts to help him identify and address the causes of his passivity.

One in-session manifestation of Alan's passivity was his reluctance to set a therapy session agenda. When I asked him for agenda items, he tended to become passive and indecisive. However, I was so focused on the technical interventions of the therapy that for many weeks I failed to notice Alan's failure to contribute to the therapy session agenda. Instead, I sprang forward myself to set an agenda and make sure we had a "productive" session.

Fortunately, I eventually did notice Alan's failure to participate in setting the agenda. In fact I realized that his agenda-setting passivity was an example of his typical problem behavior of passivity and avoidance! At that point I stopped jumping in to make an agenda. Instead I used my own behavior (of waiting for him to take action) and some technical interventions. The latter included a Thought Record focused on the situation "Jackie just asked me to suggest agenda items for the therapy session."

My initial failure to identify Alan's avoidance of agenda setting meant that I missed a chance to help him learn to manage an important problem behavior. Even worse, I *reinforced* his problem behavior by stepping in actively to set the agenda for him. I fell into the trap of becoming too active when treating passivity, as McCullough (2000) describes so well. Thus, my therapy actually harmed Alan. McCullough (2006) used the word "lethal" to describe the effect of this type of error on chronically depressed patients.

Even a therapy that is not actively harmful can be inert. An ineffective psychotherapy harms the patient by costing him time and money that could otherwise be spent on another type of therapy that might be more helpful. Psychotherapists who have been in practice for any length of time can likely point to more than one patient who is unwilling to give up the relationship with the therapist despite failing to benefit from therapy. These cases are some of the most challenging for therapists. I offer some suggestions for managing them in my discussion of treatment failure in Chapter 11.

HANDLING PROBLEMS IN THE RELATIONSHIP THERAPEUTICALLY

Problems in the relationship include the patient's perception that the therapist is not competent or does not care about the patient, the patient's nonadherence to the treatment plan, failure to use the session productively, "yes-but" behavior, and the therapist's frustration or demoralization. I describe here how these problems in the relationship can be conceptualized and treated using the combined view of the relationship described above. In addition, I discuss nonadherence in detail in Chapter 11.

Problems in the therapeutic relationship are simultaneously a blessing and a curse. They are a curse because they interfere with the technical interventions that the therapist wants to carry out to help patients solve their problems and accomplish their goals. They are a blessing because, as discussed earlier, the presence of a problem behavior in the therapy session offers an invaluable intervention opportunity. The principles of operant learning theory tell us that reinforcers that are immediate and natural are most powerful. When the behavior is present in the office, the therapist can deliver an *immediate* reinforcer that is a *natural consequence* for an adaptive behavior (leaning forward in the chair and exhibiting warmth) or a punishment (e.g., leaning back in the chair and being a little cool) for a maladaptive one. Emotion theory also tells us that presence of the behavior in the session is an asset, because if the behavior is part of an emotional network as described by Lang and Foa and Kozak, then the network is likely activated. Activation is a necessary precondition of change (Foa & Kozak, 1986).

Identifying and Conceptualizing Problems in the Relationship

It can be difficult to identify that a problem behavior is on the scene. Instead, the therapist gets pulled into doing the dance with the patient and inadvertently colluding with the patient's maladaptive behaviors. Emotion theory tells us that this is easy to do. Emotional reactions in the patient evoke similar or complementary emotional reactions in the therapist (Keltner & Kring, 1998). This is part of what happened with Alan. I yielded to the pull to step in and set the agenda for him and I did this without at first being aware that I was doing it.

Thus, the first step in working therapeutically with relationship problems is to identify them. A useful general strategy is to match examples of patient problem behavior in the session to problem behaviors identified in the case formulation. Attention to the therapist's emotional reactions to the patient's behavior and to therapy-interfering behavior can also help identify problems in the relationship. I discuss all of these strategies here. Another clue to problems in the relationship and part of what tipped me off to the relationship problem in Alan's case is lack of progress, which I discuss in the last chapter of the book.

Identify Examples of Patient Problem Behavior in the Session

To identify problem behaviors in the session, the therapist can use the case formulation, especially the Problem List and the treatment targets identified by the case formulation. The therapist constantly watches the patient's behavior carefully to identify patient behaviors in the session that match the patient's problem behaviors outside the session. The therapist searches for examples of problems that are on the Problem List. For example, is the behavior the patient is exhibiting at this moment an example of the unassertiveness that is on his Problem List? The therapist also searches for mechanisms and treatment targets that are described in the mechanism part of the formulation. For example, is the behavior an example of the self-criticism or the distorted thinking that is a major cause of the patient's depression?

This strategy helped me identify the maladaptive aspects of Peter's behavior when he came to his session saying in a pleasant and easygoing way, "I didn't do my homework but it's OK because I did lots of other good stuff." His tone was so unconcerned and blasé that it pulled me into his point of view and I almost agreed with him! However, after a moment of confusion I was able to resist this urge because I recognized Peter's behavior in that moment as an example of problem behaviors that were identified in his case formulation. A major problem behavior for Peter was making a commitment to himself or another person and then failing to follow through. As a result, his life was stalled and he was not moving forward vocationally or personally. He was 37 and unemployed, supported by an inheritance. He was not dating despite his wish for a relationship. One of the mechanisms that drove Peter's failure-to-follow-through problem was his tendency to lapse into almost trance-like states of disengagement. He spent long hours sleeping or "zoned out" searching the Internet. Peter's statement to me was an example of his failure-to-keep-commitments problem. It was also an example of the "zoning out" mechanism. I could see by his bland tone that Peter had no awareness that a problem behavior was on the scene.

With this information at hand, I responded by saying, "I am glad to hear you got a lot of good things done. And you might be totally right that not doing the homework is OK. But I'm not sure about that. I'm wondering if this might be an example of the follow-through problem we were talking about last time. Would you be willing to think about this? If we look at it together, we can probably figure it out." Peter was quite receptive to my input and we had a good discussion that got out on the table that in fact it really was *not* OK that he had not done his homework. He also agreed that his zoned-out failure to recognize this was a key piece of the problem.

Attend to the Therapist's Emotional Reactions

The therapist's emotional reactions can signal the presence of a patient problem behavior. For example, Ruth, a data processor, tended to be excessively accommodating to others' needs, which caused her to become resentful and withdraw from people, leaving her isolated. To begin to address the isolation, she had agreed as a homework assignment to have lunch with her colleagues in the lunchroom instead of alone in her office. She came to the next session reporting that she had not done this homework assignment and stating categorically that her old pattern of behavior actually worked well for her. My emotional response was one of surprise, dismay, and a feeling of being pushed away. This emotional activation alerted me to the likelihood that a problem behavior was on the scene. After thinking about it for a moment, it was easy to tie my feeling pushed away to Ruth's problem of social isolation. That is, I recognized that Ruth's behavior with me was likely an example of the major problem behavior for which she sought treatment. I responded just as I had with Peter (described above), proposing that we stop and take a careful look at the interaction between us that was unfolding in that moment. I carefully used self-disclosure to give Ruth some information about my reaction to her pronouncement. This information was a surprise to her and led to a profitable discussion of how she likely inadvertently pushed others away as well.

Identify Therapy-Interfering Behavior

Violations of the typical structure of the CBT session can reveal maladaptive patient–therapist interpersonal interactions. Several of the examples already given, including Alan's failure to contribute to the therapy session agenda, Sandra's cancelling her therapy session, and Peter's and Ruth's homework noncompliance, illustrate this phenomenon. These problems are like the white towel my hairdresser holds up behind my dark hair that reveals flaws in the haircut. Homework is a particularly powerful part of CBT because it entails a transaction between patient and therapist. Poor process or outcome there can signal that something is awry in the patient–therapist relationship.

The patient's lack of receptiveness to the therapist's intervention suggestions can also signal a problem in the relationship. A focus on that problem, guided by the case conceptualization, can provide important details about the problem and help repair it.

Helen sought help for hip pain that had not responded to any medical interventions. I suggested that relaxation exercises might alleviate the pain a bit. Helen snapped irritably at me: "I have pain! I don't need to relax!" Helen's irritation and resistance to my intervention were signals that we had a problem in our working relationship. I sought consultation. My consultant Gary Emery (thank you, Gary!) suggested that my conceptualization of Helen's case was missing a key element. As a result my interventions were off-base and this accounted for Helen's irritability. He suggested that Helen's main problem was not the pain. Instead, her main problems were her refusal to accept the pain, her anger about it, and her belief "I shouldn't have this pain." He suggested that I target Helen's anger about her pain, not the pain itself. He hypothesized that until she overcame her view that she "shouldn't have to deal with the pain," Helen would not be receptive to learning strategies to manage the pain and would view my efforts to provide them as evidence that I did not understand her plight.

When I adjusted my formulation along the lines Gary suggested and shifted my line of intervention to provide more empathy and validation for Helen's anger and suffering, she felt heard and our relationship improved. She was able to join with me in the view that her anger about her pain was a key problem and was receptive to learning tools reduce it. Several weeks later, Helen came to her session reporting that she had found, in a bookstore, a relaxation tape that was really helpful in reducing her pain. Helen's resistance to my interventions highlighted a problem in our relationship that resulted from a conceptualization error which, when repaired, improved our relationship and Helen's treatment outcome.

Overcoming Problems in the Relationship

Jeremy Safran (Safran, Muran, Samstag, & Stevens, 2002) has written in detail about the way overcoming alliance ruptures can contribute to a positive therapy outcome. Evidence supporting this proposal includes the study by Strauss et al. (2006) showing that rupture–repair episodes in cognitive therapy were associated with improvement in symptoms of depression and personality disorders. I next take up strategies for overcoming problems in the therapeutic relationship. Problems in the relationship can result from therapist errors. I describe how to intervene to address these problems using the same methods as for other problems. I also highlight the importance of giving priority to therapy-interfering behaviors.

Identify and Repair Therapist Errors

Problems in the relationship can arise from therapist errors. For example, a patient's homework noncompliance can be a direct result of the therapist's failure to work collaboratively with the patient to agree on a clear assignment (Tompkins, 2004). An excellent first step when a patient–therapist problem occurs is to look for a *therapist* error and to make any apology or repair that is needed.

Therapist errors can often lead to useful therapeutic interactions. One afternoon at 4:20 I suddenly realized I had lost track of time and that Janice, who had an appointment with me at 4 P.M., was in the waiting room. I flew into a panic, ran into the waiting room to get her—and was amazed to discover that she was unfazed and even pleased about my mistake. Why? My error felt to her as it if relieved her of the burden of being perfect in her interactions with me! It also provided powerful evidence that errors were not catastrophes or signals of worthlessness. Janice grew up in a family where she had learned that any error she made signaled that she was worthless and would be abandoned. When Janice made a mistake, her mother frequently withdrew from her for days.

Even when the patient is not pleased about the therapist's error, attention to the error can lead to useful therapy. Therapists are not perfect. Like others in the patient's life, they make mistakes. However, what the therapist can do that is different from some other individuals in the patient's life is to acknowledge and apologize for the errors and make repairs for them. The therapist and patient can also treat the errors as a learning exercise. The therapist can help patients understand that relationships are made up of errors and repairs and can teach patients to tolerate errors and to make and accept repairs.

Because of the dynamic nature of patient–therapist interactions, a therapist error may be a response to a maladaptive patient behavior. The therapist error can bring the patient's maladaptive behavior and the maladaptive interpersonal dynamic to the therapist's attention. For example, my excessive activity in setting the agenda with Alan was a response to his passivity. Noticing my error and working to understand it and address it helped me increase my awareness of Alan's passivity and improve my conceptualization of his case and the treatment I provided him.

The monitoring element of case formulation-driven CBT (discussed in detail in the next chapter) can help prevent therapist errors or identify them early so they can be corrected promptly. Collaboration and consultation with other therapists can also help in these tasks. In Linehan's (1993a) DBT and Henggeler's (Henggeler et al., 1998) multisystemic therapy, one role of the treatment team is to help the therapist identify and address errors.

Intervene as with Other Problem Behaviors

The therapist addresses patient–therapist relationship problems the same way he or she addresses other problems. The therapist works to obtain a conceptualization of the problem, doing this collaboratively with the patient if possible, and then uses technical interventions and the relationship itself to address them.

For example, Sheila sought treatment for anxiety, depression, constant stress, irritable bowel syndrome, business problems, and a general tendency to lurch from one crisis to another. My formulation of her case proposed that all of these problems resulted from her persistent tendency to ignore her own needs and respond to the needs and demands of others. We had been discussing this issue in detail when she arrived 30 minutes late to her therapy session because she had stepped in to provide soothing and comfort to one of her employees who was distressed about the breakup of her marriage. I used a light tone to point out, "Well, hey, the good news is that now we have an example of your problem behavior right here in front of us!" Then I moved into a detailed chain analysis and solution analysis to help her think through how she had mishandled this situation and what she would need to do differently to manage this type of situation more successfully in the future.

Sheila's behavior of arriving late to her session because she chose to accommodate another person in her life occurred repeatedly. I found I had to intervene repeatedly with her on this issue. I used both technical interventions and relationship interventions. Using my relationship, I pointed out in a nonjudgmental way my emotional reactions of disappointment and concern that I seemed to be more committed to her health than she was. I used a matter-of-fact, curious, and direct stance: "How it is that you decided to do something that would make you late to your session instead of figuring out how to be supportive of your employee without shortchanging yourself?" I also used technical interventions. I used behavioral chain analysis, as I described above, and I also worked through a Thought Record in which Sheila listed and examined the thoughts that had caused her to accommodate someone else even when doing so would undermine her own health and goals.

Very occasionally I meet a patient I don't like. When this happens, I work to identify what behaviors are putting me off and to understand the mechanisms causing those behaviors. Usually a good understanding of why the patient is behaving as he is helps me feel more accepting and like the patient more. In addition, if the behaviors are really off-putting, I try to begin working right away to get those behaviors to change so they don't undermine my willingness to work with the patient.

Give Priority to Therapy-Interfering and Therapy-Destroying Behavior

Serious patient–therapist interaction difficulties, such as Adele's behavior of cancelling her session repeatedly, can undermine or even destroy therapy. Other behaviors that interfere with and can destroy therapy include coming consistently late, not doing homework, blowing up at the therapist repeatedly, lying to the therapist, calling the therapist incessantly, and failing to take medications as prescribed. These behaviors interfere directly with patients' accomplishing their therapy goals. Some also contribute to problems outside the therapy (e.g., the patient who is late to all appointments, not just therapy sessions). Some behaviors interfere with therapy by causing the therapist to burn out, feel demoralized, or want to fire the patient. Linehan (1993a) argues that these problems must be a high priority for intervention because if they are not solved the therapy will fail and the patient will not get help with *any* of his or her problems. Therapists who target a therapy-destroying behavior may face punishment from the patient who does not want to focus on the issue. Thus it can be helpful to remember that the *therapist* must take responsibility for doing what is needed to protect the therapy relationship. The therapist cannot let the patient continue to do behaviors that will destroy the relationship. In treating these behaviors, the therapist can use the same model as for all patient problem behaviors: identify, conceptualize, and use the formulation to guide intervention.

June sought treatment for PTSD and bipolar disorder. She was quite attached to me and reported the therapy was quite helpful to her. At the same time, she was quite volatile and reactive. When I behaved in a way that caused her to feel discounted or rejected, June's anger and fear flared up, and she frequently responded by impulsively quitting therapy. Then a few hours to days later she panicked and called me for reassurance that I still cared about her and wanted to work with her, and we scheduled another appointment and resumed working together. A few weeks later we repeated the cycle. I noticed that I was beginning to be worn down by this cycle and June was too.

June's impulsively withdrawing from relationships was a high-priority treatment target both because it had the potential to destroy her therapy and because it led to chaos in all of her relationships, not just the one with me. Therefore I targeted this behavior for aggressive treatment.

I began with assessment. June was resistant to looking at this behavior but I insisted. It was my responsibility to protect our relationship and save it from ending, as I explained that to her repeatedly until she agreed to examine this issue. I insisted that we could not ignore this behavior. I was firmer with June on this than I had ever been with anyone in my life on any topic. To increase her motivation to examine the behavior, I explained how her behavior with me appeared to be related to the difficulties for which she sought treatment and thus how addressing this problem in her interaction with me could have a payoff in other areas as well. Finally she agreed to examine her behavior. The moment she did, I warmly let her know how much I appreciated her willingness to do that.

We carried out a detailed assessment of her cycle and learned that June tended to quit therapy when something in the therapy triggered high fear for her. She then slipped into a PTSD-related mode of perceiving that she was in great danger and must flee or she might die. She literally believed this idea at times. We agreed that June would begin monitoring these fear states and work with me to identify early signals that she was vulnerable so she could ask for help before the fear was activated. If this failed, she agreed to use mindfulness skills to notice and ask for help with this state rather than let it drive her behavior. She agreed that when she had an urge to quit therapy she would call me to discuss it and get help with it rather than just acting on it. And she agreed that if she truly decided to quit therapy she could, but that before she did so, she would sit down in my office and collaboratively discuss her decision with me.

These interventions did not immediately eliminate June's quitting behavior. However, they did lead to an immediate improvement and they also set the stage for ongoing work on the behavior that did eventually eliminate it altogether.

I remind myself of this difficult experience when I experience therapy-interfering behaviors with other patients. These behaviors are gold. They provide invaluable opportunities for conceptualization and intervention that can improve both the therapeutic relationship and the patient's life.

* * *

This chapter describes the therapeutic relationship in case formulation-driven CBT. As noted above, to maintain a good relationship, the therapist must pay constant and careful attention to patient and therapist behaviors inside and outside the session, to the therapist's emotional responses, and to the patient's compliance and progress. Thus, monitoring is essential to maintaining a good relationship. I describe strategies for monitoring the relationship and other aspects of the process as well as outcome of treatment in the next chapter.

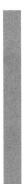

NINE

Monitoring Progress

Within moments of sitting down in my office, Janice was sobbing uncontrollably. "I'm out of control, my life is out of control, and this therapy is not helping." Janice's desperation sucked all the air out of the room and I began feeling panicky myself, thinking, "Maybe she really *is* out of control, and maybe I'm *not* helping her." I took a deep breath and began her session as I always did, by scoring the Beck Depression Inventory that Janice had just handed me and plotting the score (see Figure 9.1). The plot indicated that Janice was by no means well (she had a BDI score of 29 on that day (session 8 in the figure, indicating that she was severely depressed). It also showed that her BDI score tended to bounce up and down from one week

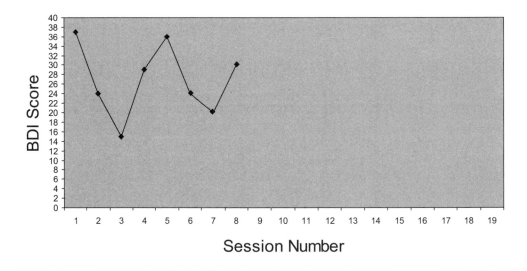

FIGURE 9.1. Using outcome monitoring to guide decision making in session 8 of Janice's therapy.

to another (no wonder she felt out of control). However, the plot also showed that the bounces were softening and smoothing out, and the peaks of the bounces were decreasing, indicating less severe symptoms at the worst points in the cycle. In fact, the plot showed that Janice *was* improving. This awareness helped me settle down, provide Janice with a calm presence, and focus on having a productive session (and series of sessions, with good results, as Figure 9.2 shows).

This vignette illustrates one of the many roles of monitoring in therapy. In this case, outcome monitoring helped me perceive that despite Janice's—and my own—panic in the room at that moment, Janice *was* improving.

Much monitoring that happens in therapy is informal and involves simple observation. In this chapter I describe the use of formal monitoring in therapy. Formal monitoring involves consistently tracking, over time, aspects of the process and outcome of therapy in writing or on the computer, using some sort of assessment tool. The tool can be a formal assessment instrument (such as the Quick Inventory of Depressive Symptoms) or an informal daily log or measure like a Thought Record or Activity Schedule. Formal monitoring is distinct from casual observation. It requires a commitment on the part of the therapist and the patient to think through what monitoring is needed and to consistently assess a variable or variables, collect the data, and use the data to inform the formulation and treatment plan.

This chapter begins with a discussion of *why* monitoring is so important in therapy and goes on to describe some of the details of *what, when,* and *how* to monitor. I end the chapter with a brief description of how to get the monitoring process started. For additional discussions of monitoring, see Bloom et al. (1995); Cone (2001); Haynes and O'Brien (2000); Ogles, Lambert, and Masters (1996); Sederer and Dickey (1996); and Woody, Detweiler-Bedell, Teachman, and O'Hearn (2003).

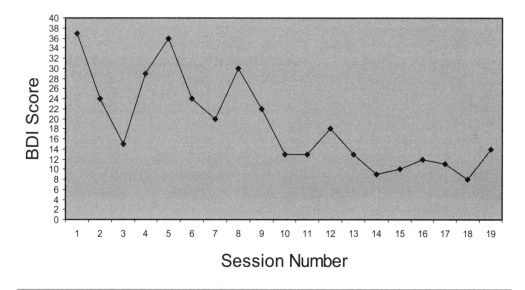

FIGURE 9.2. Weekly BDI scores for the entire course of Janice's therapy.

WHY MONITOR?

When psychotherapists collect data to monitor their patients' progress, patients have better outcomes. Michael Lambert and his colleagues (Lambert et al., 2005) have shown that patients who do not show a good response early in treatment have better outcomes when therapists receive feedback that the patient is doing poorly than when therapists do not receive this feedback.

Why and how does therapist monitoring improve outcomes? I offer here several clinical examples that illustrate numerous ways that monitoring aids clinical judgment and hypothesis testing.

Examples of Using Monitoring in Therapy

George, the Indecisive Actor

George was miserable. He had been coming to weekly sessions for nearly 3 months and was not feeling much better than when he started therapy. I had formulated his case using Beck's model and proposed that George had schemas of "I'm not good enough," "I'm fragile and I can't handle challenging situations," and "The world is threatening and dangerous." These schemas had been activated by his recent move and had given rise to anxiety, depression, and fearful ruminating about whether moving had been a good decision.

After many weeks of therapy it became clear that George was not improving. The plot of George's BDI scores (Figure 9.3) and his reports to me indicated as much. I began discussing George's lack of progress with him and consulted with a colleague. As a result of these discussions, I developed a new formulation, namely that George's negative thinking, which tended to be of a ruminative, obsessive sort, was a maladaptive problem-solving strategy (Borkovec, 1994; Borkovec et al., 2004; Orsillo & Roemer, 2005; Roemer & Orsillo, 2002) and in fact was avoidance behavior that prevented George from

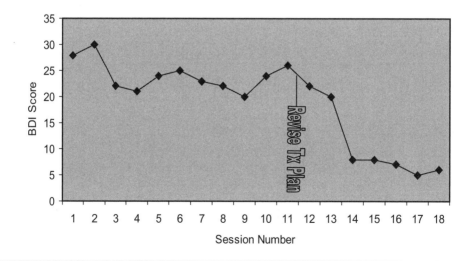

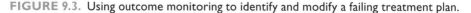

FIGURE 9.3. Using outcome monitoring to identify and modify a failing treatment plan.

engaging himself in his current life to test out his fear that he could not be happy in his new city. This formulation suggested a new line of intervention, namely that George work to distance from the worry thoughts, throw himself into his job, begin decorating his apartment, stop considering job opportunities in other cities, and in general participate in his current life. This would test out his fear that he could not be happy here. George was reluctant to try this approach; he feared he was "making a mistake." But he eventually agreed to try it for 6 weeks to see if it would help. As soon as George committed to the new plan and began working to implement it, he experienced an immediate and dramatic shift in his mood, as the plot in Figure 9.3 shows.

In George's case, monitoring helped both of us identify that he was failing to make progress initially, gave George a visual representation of his failure to progress that helped him muster the courage to try a new treatment plan, and helped us verify that the new treatment plan was more helpful than the original one.

Marie, Medication, and Depression

Marie was resistant to taking antidepressant medication. After considerable pressure from her therapist and her family, she had finally agreed to try them. Shortly after she began taking the medication, Marie proposed discontinuing it, saying it was not helping her. However, the weekly plot of Marie's BDI scores (see Figure 9.4) showed that 4 weeks after she began taking medication (as would be expected given the typical delay between taking medication and obtaining a response), her depressive symptoms showed a marked improvement. Although of course we can't be certain that the medication caused this change, these data did provide some evidence that, contrary to Marie's emotional impression, she was in fact benefiting from the medication. A review of the plot in the session helped her agree to continue to take them.

As in George's case, the plot of the monitoring data helped convince Marie to abandon the old treatment plan and try a new one. In addition, the evidence on the plot of its success helped her stick with the new treatment plan.

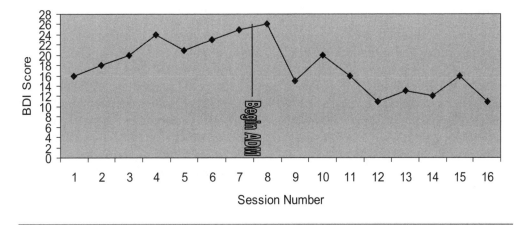

FIGURE 9.4. Using outcome monitoring to identify a response to antidepressant medication (ADM).

Stress, Headaches, and Insomnia

Jackie sought treatment for high levels of stress she experienced in taking care of her husband, who had Alzheimer's disease. She also reported experiencing frequent headaches and bouts of insomnia. As a first step to developing hypotheses about how these three things might be related, Jackie began logging them daily. She logged the severity of her stress (on a scale from 0 to 10), whether she had a headache and how severe it was, and several pieces of data about her sleep (time of sleep onset, time of waking up in the morning, and number of awakenings during the night).

Jackie brought her log to her therapy session every week and we reviewed it. Over the course of many weeks of keeping her log and discussing it with me, Jackie learned that increased stress led to increases in insomnia that night and headache and stress the next day. These observations led her to agree to a treatment goal of increasing her exercise. She hated exercise but had previously experienced good reductions in her stress level when she made herself take a long walk each day. She agreed to try this and to log its effects on her stress, insomnia, and headaches. When her monitoring data showed that the exercise helped her with all of those problems, her motivation to do it increased dramatically.

Monitoring data helped Jackie increase her awareness of the links between her stress, insomnia, and headaches. Awareness is a logical first step of the change process. Thus, many ESTs begin with a monitoring phase, including Beck's (A. T. Beck et al., 1979) cognitive therapy (patients complete an Activity Schedule after the first therapy session); CBT for bulimia (patients monitor eating, binges, and purges); DBT (patients complete a Diary Card that tracks key problem behaviors); and Barlow's (Barlow & Craske, 2000) protocol for treating worry (patients complete detailed logs of worry bouts). The monitoring data Jackie collected also gave her information that increased her readiness to change (cf. Prochaska & DiClemente, 1986), helped Jackie and I develop and test formulation hypotheses about the relationships among problems, and strengthened the therapeutic relationship by putting Jackie in the driver's seat of key treatment decisions.

Paul's Checking Behavior

Paul had OCD and he spent 30 minutes every night carefully and repeatedly checking all the doors and windows in his home before going to bed. He admitted that this ritual was time-consuming but insisted it was necessary because "If I don't check, I'll lie awake all night worrying." I suggested that he collect data to test his belief. He agreed to do this by abstaining from checking his doors and windows that very night and recording how long he lay awake worrying. Paul carried out the experiment and was amazed to report that he fell asleep after 30 minutes! Armed with this information, Paul immediately reduced his evening checking activities to a 5-minute routine.

Paul's case illustrates the use of monitoring data as a central element of an intervention, in this case, a behavioral experiment (see Bennett-Levy et al., 2004) that tested the dysfunctional belief underlying Paul's OCD rituals. Paul's case illustrates the point that monitoring is not just a procedure that is carried out to evaluate the effectiveness of therapy but can be a central ingredient of the therapy itself. Consistent with the view that monitoring has therapeutic effects, self-monitoring is associated with large reductions in binge eating (Latner & Wilson, 2002) and monitoring by parents of adolescents' behavior contributes to reductions in delinquency (Henggeler et al., 1998).

Andrew's Detachment

As I listened to Andrew, I noted that I felt a bit frustrated and thwarted. He was talking in a monotone, making poor eye contact, turning away from me in his chair, and seemed detached. Just as I began to notice these things, Andrew himself spoke up to say, "I'm talking to you but I'm not really in the room."

This observation helped me understand why I had felt thwarted and frustrated. Even better, I was able to identify Andrew's behavior in the session as an example of the avoidance behavior that was a major component of the difficulties that had led him to ask for help.

These observations prompted me to lean forward and thank Andrew for his observation. That is, I immediately used natural consequences (becoming more engaged myself and thanking him, which I judged he would find rewarding) to reward his shift from disengaged to engaged behavior. I also suggested that we take a closer look to try to figure out what was going on. Andrew explained that his halfhearted mode of interacting with me was his response to an agenda item he had taken up because I had proposed it even though he did not see it as relevant to his problems. He further revealed that he had agreed to this agenda topic in part because it helped him avoid a topic (the fact that he had not filed his tax return the previous month) that he knew he needed to tackle but was frightened to address. He stated that this pattern of behavior was common for him. He had a habit of avoiding scary problems, hoping they would go away, and of placating people rather than asserting himself to get his needs met. At this point, Andrew had shifted into an engaged mode and we had a good discussion of the various ways he avoided and disengaged. We were able to focus on the tax return issue and make some headway on it. Andrew left the office with a homework assignment to keep a log of instances of the behavior that he spontaneously labeled "pushing away," that is, avoiding something that he knew needed his attention.

This example illustrates monitoring of the patient–therapist interaction during the therapy session and monitoring that did not involve any objective measure. Instead, monitoring was done via the patient and therapist observations in the moment, including the therapist's observations of her emotional response. The example also illustrates the use of monitoring to flesh out the conceptualization of the case. I observed first-hand the details of at least one type of Andrew's disengaged behavior. Monitoring also guided my decision about what to focus on in the session and monitoring provided this information not just once, but at every moment in the session. Once we shifted to a focus on the avoidance and disengagement, Andrew shifted to an engaged mode of working, but I monitored this constantly and if he had shifted back to disengagement, I would have immediately highlighted it.

Reasons to Monitor

Lambert et al. (2003) showed that patients have better outcomes when therapists monitor outcome and process. This might be true for several reasons that are illustrated in the examples above.

Data from monitoring outcome helps:

- the therapist recognize stalled and failing treatments, prompting reformulation of the case and changing of the treatment plan (George)
- build patient motivation to change a failing treatment plan (George, Marie)
- the therapist recognize when treatment is helping despite the patient feeling no better or even worse (Janice and Marie)
- the patient build awareness of causes of symptoms, worsening, and improvement (Marie, George)
- patient and therapist test formulation hypotheses about relationships among problems (Jackie)

Data from monitoring process helps:

- the therapist identify therapy-interfering behaviors in session and move to treat them (Andrew)
- the patient test hypotheses about belief systems (Paul)
- therapist and patient track adherence and engagement (Andrew)

Finally, data collection helps the therapist build a sense of what works and what doesn't, specifically with each patient and more generally, which ultimately builds therapist expertise (Ericsson, 2006; Gawande, 2007; Thomas, 2008).

In addition to the data collected, the process of monitoring is a valuable skill to teach the patient. The process of monitoring can itself be an intervention, as the case of Paul in particular illustrates. Many of the new CBT interventions like dialectical behavior therapy, acceptance and commitment therapy, and mindfulness-based cognitive therapy emphasize mindfulness, which is another, more zen-like, term for monitoring. Monitoring provides patients with a way of approaching problems and collecting data that they will retain when treatment ends. It also encourages patients to take an active role in their treatment and can contribute in an important way to the building of a collaborative patient–therapist relationship.

Monitoring and Clinical Research

All of the clinical examples presented above, beginning with the opening example of Janice, illustrate how monitoring is used to develop and test clinical hypotheses in therapy. In addition, monitoring allows the therapist to accumulate data to test hypotheses that are important to the field. In fact, the questions clinicians want to answer are the same ones researchers want to answer: What therapies and interventions are effective? What mechanisms underpin effective treatments? As a result, clinicians can, without too much difficulty, collect data in the course of their daily work that can lead to a published paper that makes a contribution to the field (Persons, 2001, 2007).

However, joint clinical and research work requires care. When collecting data for joint clinical and research purposes, the therapist must attend carefully to ethical issues. Patients must give signed consent for this and the therapist may wish to locate an institutional review board to review the project.

WHAT TO MONITOR

In an ideal world, the psychotherapist monitors the *process* (what is going on?) of treatment and the *outcome* (is the patient getting better?). Monitoring *process* gives information about its three elements: *mechanisms of change, the therapeutic relationship,* and *adherence.* However, it is daunting to simultaneously monitor outcome, mechanisms of change, the relationship, and adherence. The therapist must make some choices. I offer several strategies for doing this.

First, if you can manage written monitoring of only one thing, focus on outcome. Monitor it at every session and track results on a plot or some other visual format that displays the patient's progress over time. Second, keep in mind that the function of monitoring is to guide clinical hypothesis testing. Monitor the phenomena that will facilitate the clinical hypothesis testing that is needed at that moment. For example, in Marie's case (the antidepressant medications) and George's case (the indecisive actor) we needed to monitor whether the change in the treatment plan led to better outcomes so we simply monitored outcome before and after the change in the treatment plan. In both cases I also monitored adherence (I did this informally through the patient's verbal report) because I was aware that if the patient was not adhering to the new treatment plan, the outcome data would not be very useful.

Third, often the phenomena you are trying to monitor overlap. Thus, activity level (measured with the Activity Schedule) is both a mechanism and a symptom of depression. In addition, the degree to which the patient completes the Activity Schedule and brings it to the session for review is an index of adherence.

Finally, quite a lot of monitoring requires little or no effort. Some is incidental; the therapist collects the data for other reasons. For example, the therapist notes the patient's attendance at the session in her progress notes and billing records. On an Activity Schedule, the therapist can note whether all the items on the log are written with the same pencil or pen. This low-effort measure can tell the therapist whether the patient completed the measure on a daily basis or recorded all the data in one sitting. The therapist can then institute high-effort monitoring of phenomena that are identified by low-effort monitoring as problematic. Andrew's case illustrates this point. Low-effort monitoring (via the therapist's emotional reactions and Andrew's verbal report) identified Andrew's disengagement behavior during the therapy session that led to higher-effort (via a written log) monitoring of his disengagement behavior.

WHEN AND *HOW* TO MONITOR

The therapist monitors outcome and process *at the beginning and end of each therapy session, during the session,* and *over the longer term.* At the beginning of *each therapy session,* the therapist collects data that guide the therapist's decisions about how to use that session. Data collected at the session's end guide subsequent sessions. *During the session,* the therapist collects data (usually simply by observing carefully) to evaluate the moment-by-moment progress of the session in order to guide decision making about the direction of the session. *Over the longer term,* the therapist obtains data after 1 to 3 to 6 months or at the end of treatment to determine whether the goals of therapy have been met and what processes have contributed to the progress or lack of it.

I describe next the *how* of monitoring, that is the tools the therapist uses to monitor outcome and process, at each of these times. Monitoring can be done in many ways, ranging from an objective scale the patient completes online to the therapist's observation of his or her own emotional response to the patient's behavior. I highlight tools and measures that are particularly useful to the outpatient therapist who is working with anxious depressed patients and the ones I and my colleagues use. Resources for other instruments are provided in Figure 5.5.

A key task is selecting the necessary monitoring tools. The therapist begins by using the patient's problem list and especially their treatment goals, to select one or two outcomes to monitor. The list of tools provided here can provide some suggestions for formal and informal ways to monitor outcomes. Then the therapist watches the outcome data and if outcome is poor, focuses on monitoring adherence of both the patient and therapist. If adherence is poor, the therapist continues monitoring while attempting to improve it. If adherence is good, a useful next step is for the therapist to evaluate the diagnosis and formulation to determine whether any revisions might be in order. If outcomes are good, the therapist can begin to track other aspects of the treatment to yield information about the causes (mechanisms) of the patient's symptoms and changes in the symptoms. In all these cases, monitoring helps keep treatment on the right path and helps the patient and therapist identify progress and lack of progress, as well as the aspects of treatment that are most helpful.

At Each Therapy Session

To make good decisions about how to use the session, the therapist needs information at the beginning of the session about *outcome* (that is, the patient's progress toward the treatment goals) and all aspects of *process* (mechanism, relationship, and adherence) that may be related to that *outcome*. I describe below several paper-and-pencil tools the therapist can use to track outcome and progress at every therapy session. An exciting development that is just around the corner is the creation of software and online tools that will allow the patient to track data on a handheld PDA or go online daily or before the therapy session to complete measures and transmit them to the therapist. The therapist will be able to access the patient's data, import them into the clinical record, and review a plot or other summary either before the patient arrives in his or her office or with the patient in the session.

All-Purpose Measures

The Daily Log (Figure 9.5) can be used to track any aspect of outcome or process at each session. It allows the patient to make a daily entry to assess any symptom, positive emotion, or aspect of functioning that the patient and therapist agree is important to monitor. This can include anxiety, self-harm behavior, suicidal thoughts, alcoholic drinks consumed, binges, assertiveness, trips to the gym, or social events with friends. The Daily Log can also be used to measure all aspects of process. It can track mechanism (e.g., use of mindfulness skills), the therapeutic relationship (e.g., feeling connected to the therapist), or compliance (e.g., urges to quit therapy). The patient can record a yes–no notation, a count, or a rating of intensity (e.g., on a scale of 0 to 10 or 0 to 100). Using the same tool to measure both outcome and process facilitates hypothesis testing about

Name _____ Date _____

Day	Date							
Mon								
Tues								
Wed								
Thurs								
Fri								
Sat								
Sun								
Mon								
Tues								
Wed								
Thurs								
Fri								
Sat								
Sun								

Notes

_____

_____

_____

_____

_____

_____

_____

_____

_____

_____

_____

_____

FIGURE 9.5. Daily Log. Copyright 2008 by the San Francisco Bay Area Center for Cognitive Therapy. Reprinted by permission in Jacqueline B. Persons (2008). Permission to photocopy this figure is granted to purchasers of this book for personal use only (see copyright page for details).

relationships between them. For example, a Daily Log showing that Sam's mood is less depressed on days he spends at his volunteer job supports the hypothesis that something about the volunteer job causes Sam's mood to improve. Some guidelines for using the Daily Log are provided in Figure 9.6.

Outcome Measures

The therapist selects outcome measures for each patient based on the patient's Treatment Goals, as discussed in Chapter 6. Goals generally involve *reducing symptoms* (e.g., depressed mood, panic attacks), *increasing positive emotions and behavior* (e.g., feelings of satisfaction, pleasant events), and *improving functioning* (e.g., work performance, interactions with spouse). Below, I describe measures of each type of outcome separately

1. Select a phenomenon to measure. This could be a behavior (using drugs), an urge (the urge to use drugs), a thought ("I want to die"), a group of thoughts (a clump of thoughts about how I'm failing at work), an emotional experience (a panic attack), a somatic experience (increased heart rate), or an external event (husband loses his temper). Use your case formulation (especially the Problem List and the mechanism hypotheses), the treatment plan (especially the treatment goals), and a collaborative discussion with the patient to decided what to measure. In general, it is useful to measure outcomes (that is, phenomena related to the treatment goals) and mechanisms (e.g., negative automatic thoughts, number of pleasant events). It is particularly useful to measure both outcomes and mechanisms simultaneously, so that relationships between them can be identified. Thus, for example, Cesar agreed to log intensity of urges to kill himself and intensity of self-critical and self-hating thoughts on his daily log, so we could track these to determine whether they were decreasing in response to treatment and to get more evidence about whether, as our behavioral chain analyses had indicated, they were related. It is useful to measure therapy-interfering behaviors (e.g., urges to quit therapy) when they are present.

2. Determine whether you wish to measure frequency, intensity, duration, or all of those.

3. To establish a scale for measuring intensity, use a 0 to 10 or 0 to 100 metric, whichever the patient prefers. Provide the patient with anchors for the lowest and highest scores, such as (in the case of anxiety) "Use 0 to mean 'totally relaxed, as relaxed as you have ever felt,'" and "Use 10 to imagine the most anxious you have ever felt or could imagine feeling." The details of these anchor points are not as important as the patient understanding the scale and using it in approximately the same way each time he or she completes it. Remember, you will not be comparing this patient's score to that of other patients; you will be comparing it to this same patient's scores at different time points. It may take a week or so of the patient's using the scale to settle into it.

FIGURE 9.6. How to measure anything. From Jacqueline B. Persons (2008). Copyright by The Guilford Press. Permission to photocopy this figure is granted to purchasers of this book for personal use only (see copyright page for details).

(symptoms, positive emotions and behavior, and functioning), and I also describe a handful of measures that address all three.

SYMPTOMS

When I am using a paper-and-pencil format, I assess symptoms of depression and anxiety at intake using the BDI or the Quick Inventory of Depressive Symptomatology (QIDS) and the Burns Anxiety Inventory (Burns AI) or Yale–Brown Obsessive Compulsive Scale (Y-BOCS) (described in Figure 5.3). Of course, many measures are available for this purpose. When patients have elevated scores on any of these measures, I initiate a discussion to determine whether, in the patient's view, these elevated scores reflect symptoms that the patient wishes to reduce and, if so, whether using these scales would provide a good way to track progress toward those goals. If so, I ask the patient to complete the measures before each session.

Using a measure that is used by outcome researchers, like the QIDS, BDI, or Y-BOCS, allows the clinician to evaluate a patient's progress in relation to that of the patients treated in the ESTs that are in published controlled trials. Using one of these scales also aids in setting treatment goals, as the patient can set a goal to reach a score in the normal range for the measure (that is, under 10 on the BDI, under 6 on the QIDS, and under 16 on the Y-BOCS; Franklin et al., 2000). Extensive normative data are not available for the Burns AI but data collected from a sample of students at the University of California, Berkeley, showed that this sample had a mean score of 16.01 with a standard deviation of 14.14 (Persons et al., 2006). These measures also provide a total score that the therapist can plot to get a visual representation of the patient's progress over time.

The Mood Chart (Figure 4.3) assesses both depressed and elated mood in a way that provides a visual representation of the valence of mood over time, collects data daily (useful both for hypothesis testing and for increasing the patient's awareness and therefore control), uses a monthly format that gives a longer-term perspective, and has spaces for logging other phenomena (sleep, activity, medications, life events, menstrual cycle, etc.) in a way that can reveal relationships among these things and mood.

Other useful tools for tracking symptoms weekly can be accessed using the resources in Figure 5.5.

POSITIVE EMOTIONS AND BEHAVIORS

Typical treatment goals involving positive emotions and behaviors include enjoying work to a level of at least 7 on a 10-point scale daily, doing at least one pleasant activity daily, and exercising three times weekly. The Positive and Negative Affect Schedule (PANAS; Figure 4.4) can be used to track 10 positive (and 10 negative) emotions at each session. The Mood Chart (Figure 4.3) and Daily Log (Figure 9.5) that were described above and some other measures described earlier in the book, especially the Activity Schedule (Figure 2.2) and the Event Log (Figure 3.5), can also be used to track desired emotional states and behaviors, such as elevated mood, enjoyment, sense of well-being, pleasant activities, workouts at the gym, numbers of fruits and vegetables consumed, or phone calls or e-mails to initiate social activities with others.

FUNCTIONING

Typical functioning goals include getting to work on time every day, exercising three times weekly, and completing all progress notes before leaving the office each day. The Daily Log (Figure 9.5) is ideal for tracking these sorts of things daily. Other useful sources of this type of information include the patient's self-report and the therapist's observation (e.g., of the patient's hygiene, follow-through with tasks like therapy home-work, and on-time arrival to the therapy session).

MULTIPURPOSE MEASURES OF OUTCOME

Several multipurpose measures track symptoms, well-being, and interpersonal and role functioning. The three best-established of these are the Outcome Questionnaire-45 (OQ-45; Lambert et al., 1996), the Clinical Outcomes in Routine Evaluation Outcome Measure (CORE-OM; Barkham et al., 2001), and the Treatment Outcome Package (TOP; Kraus, Seligman, & Jordan, 2005). These measures assess the typical symptoms seen in most psychiatric patients, thus saving the clinician the burden of selecting and obtain-ing different measures for each patient. All three measures have benchmarking features that allow the clinician to compare a patient's trajectory of change with those of large samples of similar patients. Software packages that score and plot the measure and compare the progress of the patient at hand to benchmarking samples are available in the United States for the OQ-45 and TOP and in Britain for the CORE-OM. The OQ-45 is notable for its published validity data showing that its use improves outcomes of patients who begin treatment with a poor outcome (Lambert et al., 2003). The measure is available at *www.oqmeasures.com*. The CORE-OM is available free for download on the Internet (*www.coreims.co.uk*) and can be freely photocopied so long as no modifications are made. TOP is available at *www.bhealthlabs.com*.

IDIOGRAPHIC MEASURES OF OUTCOME

Sometimes it is useful to develop a measure that assesses symptoms or behaviors that are unique to a particular patient. For example, my patient Charise and I developed a list of symptoms that typically presaged an episode of full-blown mania for her. She wanted to identify early symptoms so she could address them promptly in an effort to avert another manic episode. Charise's scale including sending long e-mail messages; wondering if she might be hypomanic; beginning the day without a clear plan for how she would spend it; feeling so well that she wanted to stop taking her medications; and lying to me, her psychiatrist, or family members about her symptoms. She completed the scale each week before her session (scoring each item 0 or 1) and reviewed the score with me when we met.

COLLECTING AND REVIEWING OUTCOME DATA IN THE SESSION

At our Center we keep files holding the main outcome measures we use (the BDI, QIDS, Burns AI, Y-BOCS, Daily Log, and Mood Chart) in our waiting room. We ask patients to arrive 5 minutes prior to their session to complete the measures they and their therapist have agreed will be useful in tracking their progress. When my patients come into my office, they hand me the measures they have completed, I score them and plot the scores,

and we look at the plot together. These data are invaluable, as the clinical examples provided at the beginning of the chapter illustrate. However, the data from these scales
alone are not enough to give therapists the information they need, for several reasons.

Measures have the potential for bias. Longwell and Truax (2005) and Sharpe and
Gilbert (1998) showed that repeated administration of the BDI consistently resulted in
lower scores over time, even when subjects were not depressed and were not receiving treatment. Reasons for this likely include statistical factors like regression to the
mean and clinical factors like the patient's wish to please the therapist by appearing to
improve. Similarly, it is well established that self-monitoring often causes changes (usually small and short-lived ones) in the desired direction of the behavior being monitored
(Nelson & Hayes, 1981).

Responses to measures can also be biased by current mood state. If a person is
depressed when he completes a symptom scale, this can bias his recall of the symptoms
he experienced during the week in an upward (more symptoms) direction. An elated
mood or a numb or dissociated state can bias recall in a downward (less symptoms)
direction.

Distorted scores can also result from the fact that symptom scales like the QIDS,
BDI, or Burns AI are quite transparent and the patient may use them to communicate
with the therapist or others, such as insurance companies or disability examiners. For
example, the patient who learned from her upbringing that she would not get any attention unless she was seriously ill may report an unduly high score in an effort to get the
therapist's attention. Or the patient who fears that if she does not meet the needs of others they will reject or hurt her may report an unduly low score in an effort to avoid antic-
ipated rejection or punishment from the therapist. For example, Janie reported scores
on the BDI that were surprisingly high given her pleasant and cheerful facial expression
and demeanor. When I questioned her about this, I discovered that her appearance of
cheerfulness was in marked contrast to her internal emotional experience of intense sadness and misery. The discrepancy appeared to result from Janie's experience of growing
up in an abusive environment in which she was punished whenever she exhibited any
signs of distress.

Distortions can also result from imperfections in measures. Even the BDI, a strong
measure with good psychometric properties, has a 1-week test–retest reliability (in
patient samples) of only about .70 (A. T. Beck, Epstein, Brown, & Steer, 1988). Thus, it is
important not to overinterpret changes in scores on measures like the BDI. Thomas and
Persons (2008) recently showed that large reductions in BDI scores (even as large as 10
points) are consistent with normal fluctuations in a gradual change process.

For all these reasons, scores on one or two measures alone do not give the therapist all the information he or she needs. In fact, sometimes a plotted score or scores
give exactly the wrong impression. Patients can seem to be getting worse when they
are actually better (as in the case of a patient who is experiencing more symptoms of
anxiety because she is now approaching feared situations she previously avoided). Or
they can seem to be getting better when they are actually worse (the BDI score is lower
because the patient is dissociated or otherwise experientially avoiding). Therefore, after
plotting the scores, I usually review them with the patient, saying, for example, "I see
that your depression score is lower and your anxiety score is higher, suggesting you
are less depressed and more anxious. Does that seem right?" I might also ask whether

others in the patient's life have noticed any change, examine items on the scales that are particularly important for that patient, or check to see whether other assessments show similar or consistent changes.

Mechanisms

The discussion of the patient's outcome progress (or lack of it or setback) leads very naturally into a mechanism discussion. I will generally ask the patient for his or her hypothesis about the mechanisms of any change on the outcome measures, asking, for example, "Why do you think you are feeling more/less depressed today than last week?" If I get a useful answer (I'm premenstrual, I had my performance review at work, I was on vacation, It feels like the medications are kicking in), I may write that information on the plot at the time point of the event in question in order to make a record of the possible causes of the upward or downward shift in the score. Thus, the weekly outcome monitoring data promote a constant process of patient and therapist working together to determine what mechanisms push symptoms up and down.

In addition to asking for the patient's ideas about mechanism, the therapist can use some of the measures described in Chapters 2, 3, and 4, which described cognitive, learning, and emotion-focused theories, to assess mechanisms. These measures include the Thought Record (Figure 2.3), the Activity Schedule (Figure 2.2), the Event Log (Figure 3.5), and the Daily Log (Figure 9.5). Often patients complete these measures as homework and a review of them at the beginning of the session together with the outcome measure can contribute to process-outcome hypothesis testing. For example, Christine's Thought Records helped her see that her anxiety and depression were both higher that week because she had gotten pulled into seriously distorted thinking nearly daily that week.

Tallying both symptoms and interventions intended to reduce the symptoms can provide useful data to test mechanism hypotheses. For example, my conceptualization of Moira's case was that her failure to attend to her internal state and use skills (that were already in her repertoire) to manage anxiety before it escalated out of control was a key mechanism leading to her panic attacks. I taught Moira some mindfulness skills and asked her to report her use of those skills and her panic symptoms on a Daily Log. Moira did this daily and brought her log to the session weekly for review. The log showed that, as predicted, increased mindfulness was associated with decreased panic. Even better, keeping the Daily Log itself helped Moira stay mindful.

Another approach to assessing mechanism is to ask for the patient's feedback about the session at its end or at the beginning of the next one. The therapist wants to know whether the patient found the session helpful and if so, what was helpful about it. Of course, patients are not always very good at observing or reporting this information. In fact, sometimes these deficits are part of the problem and these discussions can help patients develop needed observation skills. Useful questions at the end of the session include: Are you feeling better or worse or the same? If you are feeling better or worse, can you identify what we did in the session that is helping you feel better or worse? For example, a patient recently told me, "What really helped me was when you explained how *you* coped when you felt extremely anxious by just repeatedly asking yourself, 'Can I get through the next five minutes?' Your telling me that reduced my shame about having such high anxiety and needing to work so hard to manage it." This feedback gave me useful information about the patient's problems (shame), mechanisms that caused problems (shame interfered with coping), and change mechanisms (normalizing the experience of high fear and the need to work hard to cope reduced shame).

The Therapeutic Relationship

To assess the therapeutic relationship at each session, Burns (1997) has developed a 20-item Evaluation of Therapy Session scale that allows the patient to report on the alliance and other aspects of a therapy session (helpfulness of the session and satisfaction with it). Although no psychometric data evaluating the reliability and validity of the measure are available, I have found it to be clinically useful and it is easily and inexpensively available from Dr. Burns as part of his *Therapist Toolkit* (Burns, 1997).

I review the patient's report on the Evaluation of Therapy Session measure at the beginning of the session to get feedback about the previous session that can guide the current one. Of course, this strategy depends on the patient's willingness to give the therapist direct negative feedback. To address this issue, Burns's measure includes several items designed to assess that (e. g., "It would be too upsetting for me to criticize my therapist").

Data about the alliance can also be collected verbally. To do this at each session, the therapist can ask the patient to give feedback on the alliance, asking questions such as "Are we working well together?" "Does it feel like we are on the same team?"

Adherence

To monitor *therapist* adherence at each session, therapists can assess their use of the elements of a structured therapy session (e.g., agenda setting, homework assignment and review) after each session using the Therapy Session Log provided in Davidson, Persons, and Tompkins (2000) and reproduced here (Figure 9.7). Similarly, they can rate themselves on the Competency Checklist for Cognitive Therapists that appears in the Appendix of A. T. Beck et al. (1979). These tasks are too demanding to do routinely but are useful when the therapist is striving to improve adherence in a certain area (e.g., homework review or assignment) or has a difficult case. The therapist can also monitor, formally or informally, her adherence to the treatment plan that was agreed on in pretreatment.

To monitor *patient* adherence at each session, the therapist often relies on the patient's self-report and written homework assignments, such as a Daily Log, which indicate whether the patient, for example, practiced relaxation or exercised each day. Adherence can also be assessed by direct observation (e.g., of the patient's punctual arrival to the session), reports from family members, or even assays like urinalysis. Some adherence monitoring is incidental because it is already being done for other-than-clinical purposes (e.g., the clinician monitors the patient's attendance at the therapy session for billing purposes).

The therapist will also want to monitor the patient's adherence with interventions (e.g., pharmacotherapy, bipolar group) provided by other therapists and can do this by asking the patient and/or the adjunct therapist about whether the patient is taking the medications as prescribed, meeting with the couple therapist, or attending 12-step meetings.

Instructions: Select one or two components of the therapy session (e.g., agenda setting, homework review) on which you would like to focus. Write them at the top of the blank columns on the form. Then, for each patient you see during a week, record the date in the **Date** column and the patient's initials in the **Initials** column. In the columns corresponding to the components of the therapy session on which you are working, record a score of 0/1 indicating whether you used the component or not. In the **Comments** column of the form, note things you did well or poorly or things you learned and would like to remember for the future.

Date	Initials	Components		Comments

FIGURE 9.7. Therapy Session Log. Copyright 1999 by the San Francisco Bay Area Center for Cognitive Therapy. Reprinted by permission in Jacqueline B. Persons (2008). Permission to photocopy this figure is granted to purchasers of this book for personal use only (see copyright page for details).

During the Therapy Session

The most common approach to monitoring outcome and process during the therapy session is to carefully observe the patient's and therapist's behaviors, cognitions, and emotions as they emerge in a dynamic interplay. These data are available in real time, which makes it possible to formulate and test hypotheses about relationships among stimuli, responses, and mechanisms of change in real time as the session unfolds. Thus, for example, one of my patients, Sam, is prone to dissociation. I've learned that when dissociation is impending, he shows a facial expression of high fear and his eyes begin to dart around the room. I watch for those behaviors. When they occur, I try to attend to what triggered them to add to my formulation of the antecedents of Sam's dissociation. And I shift immediately to using validating and soothing interventions while instructing Sam to make eye contact with me. I coach him to stay engaged in the therapy task at hand (e.g., a backward chain analysis of an incident of self-harm) while remaining calm and focused myself (not always so easy!). As I do this, I continuously monitor Sam's facial expression and engagement with me (or even collect a rating of 0 to 10 to indicate how present he is feeling at that moment) to assess whether we are succeeding at aborting the dissociation. If not, I shift to grounding strategies and Sam and I get up and walk over to the books on the shelf and begin naming their colors and touching their textures to help him get back into contact with the present environment. When my observations of his facial expression and behavior and his report indicate that he is sufficiently grounded, we return to the therapy task that was interrupted by the dissociation. Sometimes the therapist can use more systematic measures to monitor outcome and process during the session. For example, during exposure sessions the therapist can collect a verbal report from the patient every 5 to 10 minutes on a 0 to 10 or 0 to 100 scale of subjective units of distress (SUDS). Or when using a Thought Record (Figure 2.3) to carry out some cognitive restructuring, the therapist can ask the patient to rate his degree of belief in his automatic thoughts before and after the intervention, his degree of belief in the coping responses, and the intensity of distress before and after the intervention in order to monitor whether the cognitive restructuring intervention is helpful and if not to get some ideas about why not. For example, if the patient rates her degree of belief in the coping responses as low, it can be useful to search for some additional more powerful responses or take another intervention approach altogether.

Similarly, the therapist monitors the alliance in the moment by attending to his and the patient's behavior, facial expression, and emotions. If the therapist notices a glitch, he can pause to collect more detailed assessment data, saying, for example, "Could we stop for a moment and take a look at what's happening here right now? It seems like we were working well together until about 10 minutes ago, when we started to get into a sort of a tussle. Does that seem right to you? Can we identify the moment we got off track and figure out what happened?" (Assessment of the alliance in the therapy session is also discussed in Chapter 8.)

The therapist can use similar strategies to monitor adherence during the therapy session. If the patient responds to interventions by ignoring them or proffering a "yes-but," the therapist can, as in the example just given, invite the patient to pause and examine the details of what is going on in the moment. The therapist can also use the formulation to generate hypotheses about the patient's nonadherence. For example, the observation that the patient's response to a recommendation from the therapist is a "yes-but" might lead the therapist to hypothesize that the patient is highly sensitive to a loss of autonomy and might benefit more from less directive interventions (Karno & Longabaugh, 2005). The therapist can test this hypothesis by shifting to a nondirective intervention style and monitoring the patient's response to it.

Longer-Term Monitoring

Longer-term monitoring can be done at a point in time that patient and therapist set at the onset of treatment (e.g., after 12 sessions). It may also be done in response to data generated by the weekly monitoring (e.g., if patient and therapist notice that no progress is being made), or at the end of treatment. A periodic formal review of progress helps keep a long-term therapy on track. In the review the therapist works collaboratively with the patient to evaluate progress toward the treatment goals, the mechanisms of change (or not), the alliance, and adherence.

To initiate a progress review, the therapist can say, "I suggest that we sit down soon, next session if that seems OK with you, to evaluate how your therapy is going. Let's review progress toward the goals we set. If we're doing great, that is fabulous. If we are not doing as well as we would like, we can start talking about why not and what changes we might make to get better results." I typically give patients a copy of the treatment goals we agreed on during pretreatment to review before the next session and encourage them to think about what is going well and what is not going so well in their therapy.

It is important for the therapist to keep in mind the formulation of the case as he or she initiates and carries out this progress review. Patients who fear abandonment, criticism, and rejection, for example, are likely to get quite anxious about a progress review, fearing that the therapist is going to kick them out of treatment. The therapist will want to be aware of this and work to address patients' concerns so they do not interfere with a productive review process.

Progress reviews can be difficult for therapists too. I find it very easy to avoid them, especially if things are not going well. Nevertheless, it is when things are not going well that a progress review is especially important. To overcome my discomfort, I push myself to adopt a nondefensive and curious stance, focusing on the goal of learning as much as possible about what is going on in the therapy that can help improve it. This stance improves my alliance with the patient and facilitates collaborative problem solving that can turn the therapy around (more details on overcoming failure are provided in Chapter 11).

The progress review can proceed quickly if the therapy is going smoothly, perhaps requiring half a session. If the patient is not making good progress, it can take the whole session or even all or parts of many sessions as patient and therapist collect data to develop and test hypotheses about the causes of the poor progress.

Several strategies can be used to assess progress toward the goals. One easy approach is to undertake a cumulative review of data collected weekly, for example, the plot of BDI scores over time or the monthly Mood Charts or the Daily Logs. The therapist can also ask the patient to complete measures that were given at pretreatment and that are relevant for tracking progress toward the Treatment Goals but are not suitable for weekly use, such as the Penn State Worry Questionnaire (Meyer et al., 1990). It can also be useful to ask the patient to ask whether his partner or others who are close to him have noticed any changes and if so what they have noticed.

To assess progress on idiographic goals, the therapist and patient can examine each goal to determine if it was met. Sometimes this is easy. It is easy to determine, for example, if a goal to return to work full-time has been met. When it is not immediately clear whether the goal has been accomplished, the therapist can ask the patient to rate, on a scale of 0 to 100%, the degree to which he or she believes the goal has been accomplished. This process works best if, as described in Chapter 6, the patient and therapist clearly identified in pretreatment what it would mean to reach the goal.

Rerating of a fearful patient's scores on his fear hierarchy can also provide a quantitative assessment of progress. Or the therapist can repeat a behavioral approach test measuring how close the patient can approach a feared object. Other options for measuring progress include using the Global Assessment of Functioning (GAF) scale of Axis V of the DSM (American Psychiatric Association, 2000) to assess progress in functioning.

In conjunction with assessing progress toward the treatment goals, patient and therapist also discuss process. It is especially useful to try to determine what mechanism changes have occurred. That is, has the patient made any changes in his or her thinking, behavior, emotions, or other processes that our treatments try to change. No measures are available to assess mechanism over the long term, and this piece of the assessment is best accomplished by discussion and review of mechanism assessments that were collected at each session, as described above.

To assess the alliance over the longer term, a well-known and well-validated scale that measures the therapeutic relationship is the Revised Helping Alliance Questionnaire (HAq-II; Luborsky et al., 1996). It is available free over the Internet (*www.uphs.upenn.edu/psycther/HAQ2QUES.pdf*). The HAq-II is a 19-item self-report scale that measures the alliance between patient and therapist. It can measure the alliance from either the patient or the therapist point of view. The rating from the patient's point of view is likely most valuable clinically, as it is most tied to outcome (Horvath & Bedi, 2002). Internal consistency and test–retest reliability have been shown to be high (Luborsky et al., 1996). Whipple et al. (2003) showed that outcome of psychotherapy (as measured by the OQ-45) for patients who began treatment with a poor start improved when therapists collected data on the patient's perception of the alliance using the HAq-II.

Especially when progress is poor, it is useful to examine adherence in order to determine whether the planned treatment plan is actually being implemented. Sometimes the answer is no! Exposure and response prevention was planned but somehow patient (and sometimes therapist; see Becker, Zayfert, & Anderson, 2004) just don't get around to carrying it out. In this type of situation, efforts to determine the reasons for the nonadherence may contribute to overcoming it.

Although the long-term progress review, like all monitoring, is a collaborative process, it can be helpful for the therapist to spend some time outside of the session reviewing the patient's progress. I find that often when I do this I get a different view of the case than the one I get when I meet with the patient, perhaps as a result of the emotional pushes and pulls that occur when the patient is in the room.

* * *

Collecting data to monitor outcome, mechanisms of change, the patient–therapist relationship, and adherence is demanding. However, the therapist needs these data to guide clinical decision making, which is described in Chapters 10 and 12.

TEN

Decision Making in the Therapy Session

Carol arrived 10 minutes late for her therapy session, apologizing profusely and feeling exasperated and upset with herself. She reported that she had planned her time so poorly that she had needed an hour and a half to complete a handful of errands that she should have been able to handle in an hour and had arrived late for her appointment.

As Carol's therapist, my task in the above situation was to decide whether to intervene at that moment, and if so, how. Ought I to focus at all on Carol's exasperated outburst? I could ignore it or give her a bit of empathy and move on. If I elected to focus on it, which treatment target should I address? Is it better to help Carol improve her time management skills, reduce her self-criticism, or do something else? These sorts of decision-making tasks are the focus of this chapter.

THE FORMULATION PROCESS
AS A GUIDE TO DECISION MAKING IN THE SESSION

Decision making during the session is guided by the same model that guides therapy as a whole (see Figure 1.1). That is, the therapist begins by collecting assessment data. Then the therapist uses the assessment data (and other information, including the case formulation) to develop a hypothesis (formulation) that helps him or her identify treatment targets and generate hypotheses about some likely causes (mechanisms) of those targets. The therapist uses the formulation to generate intervention ideas, obtains the patient's permission to proceed with an intervention, carries out the intervention, and collects data to monitor the effects of the intervention.

These steps comprise a full-bore intervention and often the therapist carries them all out in this order. However, sometimes the therapist skips steps. Sometimes the case-level formulation and the work of previous sessions provide information about the treatment targets and mechanisms that the therapist can use to guide intervention in the session without conducting a detailed assessment. Sometimes the therapist elects to carry out a very brief intervention to simply highlight and reward the patient's report of good coping by saying, for example, "Oh, so you got pulled for a moment into that old behavior and then you recovered. That was good" (Koerner, 2005). Or the therapist might change the order of the steps, perhaps asking for the patient's permission to proceed at the beginning of the process rather than in the middle. The therapist may also repeat steps, for example when addressing more than one agenda item in a session. Nevertheless, the steps of this model provide a good template to guide conceptualization and intervention during the session, as I describe in detail below.

Prepare for the Session

Presession preparation gives the therapist some ideas about good agenda items and likely interventions. Before the patient arrives, the therapist takes a moment to review several aspects of the case. One is the content of the previous session. The therapist reminds herself of how the patient was doing at the time of the previous session, what happened in the session, and what homework assignment was given. It is also helpful to review the Problem List (especially the priority order of the problems) and the case formulation (especially the treatment targets and mechanism hypotheses) (see Chapter 6), as well as the treatment plan, especially the treatment goals (e.g., to reduce symptoms of depression) and any mechanism change goals the therapist may have identified (e.g., to reduce negative thinking) (see Chapter 7).

For example, I find it particularly helpful when I am working with a passive patient with depression to remind myself before the session that a major process goal of the therapy is to help the patient overcome the passivity. I can do this not by mindlessly stepping in to offer solutions to the patient's problems but instead by targeting the passivity itself for treatment.

In addition, the therapist reminds herself of the quality of the patient–therapist relationship (is the relationship in good shape or is repair work needed?) and of the stage of treatment (I discuss this issue more in the next chapter). The stage of treatment is important because, for example, early in treatment the therapist takes more responsibility for things like agenda setting, whereas later the patient is expected to step up to take more responsibility.

The therapist usually doesn't make any final decisions about the session until she collects assessment data about the patient's current status. The therapist going into the session is like the tennis player waiting for the serve. She is poised and alert, and has some initial hypotheses about where, given past experience, the ball may come in. But she keeps her eyes wide open to see where the ball actually arrives before she makes a decision about how to return it.

Carry Out a Brief Assessment

The therapist begins the session with a structured check-in (Davidson et al., 2000) in which he asks patients to give a brief overview of how they are doing and of any important events that have occurred since the last session. The information obtained in the check-in contributes items to the therapy session agenda.

The therapist attends particularly to the presence of any treatment targets (identified in the case formulation) that appear in the patient's report of events. (This is why a presession review of the case formulation before the session is important.) For example,

I learned in the check-in that my patient June had decided to quit her job. In fact, she did not consider this to be controversial and would not have told me about it unless I had asked for a review of events since the previous week. However, this event was a treatment target. June's tendency to impulsively "bail out," as she termed it, was a problem on her Problem List, and one of her treatment goals was to stop doing this.

The therapist also attends to treatment targets that make their appearance in the therapy session itself. The therapist carefully observes the patient's behavior, both verbal and nonverbal. For example, I found myself "pulling teeth" to get a check-in from my patient Amelia. She was closed down and not very forthcoming. At first I made the mistake of focusing on the content of the bits of information Amelia was giving me. Then I realized that her shutdown behavior itself was more important, both because it was therapy-interfering behavior and because it was a treatment target for her. Passivity was an element of nearly all of the problems on Amelia's Problem List. The formulation of her case proposed that she had an emotion regulation deficit that manifested in many ways, including in her tendency to respond to emotional distress with avoidance and passivity rather than active problem-solving and coping strategies.

As soon as I shifted my focus to Amelia's passivity, she opened up and we began having a much more productive interaction. She was able to tell me that her passivity resulted from her feeling angry about how unhelpful I had been when she called me in an emergency the previous week. We put this issue on the agenda for the therapy session.

The therapist also attends to her own emotional responses to the patient's behaviors. For example, in the case of Amelia, my awareness that I felt frustrated by her shutdown behavior was one of the cues to me that this behavior needed attention.

During the check-in the therapist also reviews the monitoring data the patient collected as homework, as discussed in Chapter 9. If I am reviewing a QIDS, a BDI, or Burns AI, I score the measure and plot the score at the beginning of the session and the patient and I review it together. This interaction often leads to a discussion about the mechanisms that might be causing an increase or decrease in the patient's symptoms, and can lead to an agenda item. For example, if the patient's BDI score is much higher or the Daily Log reveals an instance of self-harm, I would probably suggest that we place a discussion of the worsening depressive symptoms or the self-harm behavior on the therapy session agenda.

The check-in part of the session is also a good time to monitor the patient's adjunct treatment. Is the patient taking his or her medications? How is the couple therapy going? Any problems in this area are candidates for agenda items for the session.

Develop an Agenda for the Therapy Session

Good therapy session agenda items include a symptom or problem the patient wants to work on, such as insomnia, hopelessness, anger, or anxiety. This might be a large vague problem (e.g., my job) or a small specific one (e.g., I am having trouble making this particular phone call to my boss). A review of homework, if it is not done in the check-in, is always part of the agenda.

Agenda setting is often easy, especially when the patient and therapist have a good working relationship and work is proceeding productively on a clear intervention path (e.g., using exposure and response prevention to systematically work through items on the fear and ritual hierarchies of the patient who has OCD). In this type of situation, it is easy to focus the agenda on the next step in the hierarchy or any problems the patient experienced in carrying out the exposure homework.

However, sometimes agenda setting is challenging. Common difficulties include selecting agenda items and obtaining the patient's agreement to the agenda items.

Selecting Agenda Items

The therapist must guide the process of agenda setting and take ultimate responsibility for what topics are addressed in therapy. The patient contributes to agenda setting and when patients do not play their part in this process it is often a sign of a problem. The patient (with help from the therapist) has chosen the goals of treatment. It is the therapist's responsibility to let the patient know what must be done to achieve those goals. Effective agenda setting is a key task of therapy (Burns, 1989a).

CRITERIA FOR SELECTING AGENDA ITEMS

I offer the following list of criteria the therapist can use when selecting agenda items for the therapy session.

A good therapy session agenda item focuses on:

- An important treatment target or mechanism described in the case formulation.
- A treatment target that is currently present in the therapy session.
- A high-priority problem on the Problem List.
- A high-priority treatment goal.
- A concern that is currently emotionally activated for the patient.
- A problem the patient wants to take up.

Of course, no agenda item can meet all of these criteria simultaneously but it is useful to consider them all when selecting agenda items.

This chapter began with Carol arriving late for her session in a state of high exasperation. How was I to decide how to respond to her? My decision making was guided by the list of criteria I just provided, and in particular by Carol's case formulation and her treatment goals. My formulation of Carol's case hypothesized that she held the schema "I'm inept and inadequate," and "Others don't care/find me boring/are critical," and that these schemas led to problem behaviors that included relentless self-criticism. Reducing self-criticism was a treatment goal. Thus, based on her formulation and treatment goals, I elected to focus on Carol's exasperation about her time management rather than ignoring it or just giving a bit of sympathy

Let me say more about identifying treatment targets in the therapy session. Matching a particular unique behavior that the patient reports or the therapist observes to a treatment target is a match-to-sample task that can be surprisingly difficult. For example, it is not so simple in the moment to see Carol's exasperation about her poor time management as an instance of self-criticism—a treatment target. One reason for the difficulty is that the behaviors described in the case formulation and Problem List are usually described in more general terms than the unique behaviors that appear in the session or that the patient reports. Another is that the patient's emotions or perceptions often pull the therapist in the wrong direction. This was true for the situation with

Carol. I initially felt confused because I was emotionally drawn into Carol's view of herself as inadequate and her request for help with time management skills. My emotional response here can be seen as an example of how emotions provoke emotions in others as discussed in Chapter 4. Distracted by my sympathy with Carol, it took me a moment to realize that the behavior in front of me was an example of self-critical behavior. However, as soon as I realized that, I could see that her self-criticism was a good agenda item, both because it was a treatment target identified in the formulation and also because it was present in the session and emotionally charged for Carol.

Some situations make it difficult for the therapist to select good agenda items. These include working with the high-risk multiple-problem patient, the patient who wants to work on a different problem every week, and the patient in the grip of intense emotion.

THE HIGH-RISK MULTIPLE-PROBLEM PATIENT

The high-risk multiple-problem patient faces multiple difficulties, some of which may be life threatening, such as suicide or self-harm, or risky, such as spousal abuse or homelessness. These patients often have poor judgment about what items belong on the therapy session agenda. As a result, the therapist can't simply accept the patient's agenda items, but must be prepared to identify important items. The criteria described above can help the therapist do that, especially in highly emotionally charged situations that can make decision making challenging.

To identify useful items for the agenda, it is particularly important to attend to the priority order of the problems on the Problem List. As discussed in Chapter 5, suicidality and self-harm problems are top priority, followed by therapy-interfering problems and by problems that interfere significantly with the patient's quality of life. After this, problems that the patient wants to address and problems that, if solved, can help solve other problems, merit attention.

Sometimes the case-level formulation clearly identifies treatment targets. But sometimes the therapist feels confused, perhaps by the strong emotion in the room. This type of situation is particularly likely to occur when the patient has multiple problems, including high-risk ones. In this type of situation, it can be useful to work collaboratively with the patient to identify useful treatment targets and agenda items. For example, the therapist might say, "Now I hear you describing problems A, B, C, and D. Let's think through which ones are the most important that we need to take up today. A collaborative discussion can teach the patient some useful decision-making skills, strengthen the alliance, and generate a good therapy session agenda.

THE PATIENT WHO WANTS TO WORK ON A DIFFERENT PROBLEM EVERY WEEK

When the patient comes in every week asking to work on a different problem, the therapist must try to determine whether shifting from topic to topic is a good idea or whether this is avoidance (and a therapy-interfering behavior). The case formulation can help the therapist make this decision. Sometimes agenda items that appear on the surface to be quite different are all driven by a common mechanism. If so, the therapy can do a good job of targeting that mechanism even if it addresses a different topic every week.

For example, Angelo was depressed and his case formulation proposed that a core belief driving much of his behavior was "If I make a full commitment and really put a lot of energy into something, I'll fail and then I'll feel even worse." Driven by this and related beliefs, he had a pattern of making halfhearted commitments to things as diverse as his undergraduate major (he changed his major so often that he had been an undergraduate for 5 years), his girlfriend (he was involved with her for years before he would agree to live with her), and his apartment (he delayed unpacking his boxes for months after moving in). Therapy sessions tended to bounce back and forth among these various problems. However, because all of the problems were driven by the same core mechanisms, therapy sessions taking up each of these diverse topics addressed his core belief. These sessions helped Angelo make slow progress on his treatment goals of reducing his depression and anxiety, completing his BA degree, unpacking his boxes and moving into his apartment, and improving his relationship with his girlfriend.

In other cases, the patient's difficulty addressing the same topic consistently from one session to another is a problem behavior. The case formulation helps the therapist make this determination.

THE PATIENT IN THE GRIP OF INTENSE EMOTION

The therapist's efforts to prioritize problems in order to select agenda items are sometimes impeded by the presence of intense emotion. Amiko came to her therapy session extremely upset about her dog's illness and her "out of control" eating. This distress occurred in the context of our current treatment focus on her unemployment, which was a very scary topic for her and one she had been avoiding for years (she was supported by a trust fund). She begged the therapist to postpone working on the job issue and to put the dog and eating topics on the agenda for today's session.

Emotionally charged topics often make excellent agenda items. The emotional charge can indicate that a schema or other core pathological mechanism is activated and available for modification (Foa & Kozak, 1986). Intense emotion can focus the patient's attention on the issue and motivate him or her to address it in order to get some relief from the emotional arousal (Levenson, 1999). In addition, of course, reducing emotional distress is frequently a goal of treatment.

In Amiko's case, urges to modify previously made plans in response to high emotional activation were a treatment target. Amiko's case formulation proposed that high emotional activation tended to pull her away from tasks she had planned for accomplishing personal goals ranging from going to bed on time to applying for a job. The main mechanism change goal of her therapy was to teach Amiko skills for tolerating emotional distress so that she could consistently pursue plans rather than being constantly derailed. So when Amiko, pulled by her emotions, asked to postpone the plan to work on the job issue, I reminded her of the formulation and proposed that she take this opportunity to practice distress tolerance while throwing herself into the job agenda item. I pointed out that if she worked efficiently, there would likely be some time left at the end of the session to address one of the topics that was distressing her.

This tack was quite difficult for me, as Amiko's emotions were intense and exerted a substantial pull. The collaborative formulation and treatment plan helped me hold steady in the face of strong emotion. The same concept can guide the therapist to propose important agenda topics that the patient is not at all concerned about. The patient's lack of concern about important matters (e.g., his boss's threat to fire him) may be an avoidance behavior that is a treatment target. In Amiko's case, my firmness and clarity carried the day and she accepted my recommendation to focus on the work issue. What if she had not?

Obtaining Patient–Therapist Agreement on Agenda Items

Patient–therapist disagreement on agenda items is not uncommon. The therapist cannot resolve it by simply yielding to the patient's wishes. Nor can the therapist simply strong-arm the patient and force her to capitulate to his plan. Instead, the therapist must skillfully induce the patient to agree to a productive agenda. This is the task of obtaining the patient's informed consent to treatment (described in Chapter 7) translated to the level of the therapy session.

The strategies that were described in Chapter 7 to help obtain the patient's agreement to the treatment plan are also useful in handling agenda-setting disagreements. Motivational interviewing is an example. The therapist can ask the patient to flesh out the details of what will happen if he continues to avoid discussing the item he doesn't want to put on the agenda. This tactic can enhance discrepancy between the patient's current situation and the life he wants. Careful empathic listening can help the patient see that placing this item on the agenda is essential to accomplishing his goals. Using another motivational interviewing strategy, the therapist can work with the patient to examine the advantages and disadvantages of avoiding the topic the patient wants not to address and can use empathic listening to overcome the patient's ambivalence about tackling it, as in "OK, so I hear you say you are at risk of being fired but you don't want to talk about that issue today. You're saying that focusing on it just makes you feel worse and doesn't really change anything, is that right?" Other strategies described in Chapter 7 are also useful, including offering the patient options and negotiating to reach a compromise. It can also be useful to remind the patient of his previous agreement to the treatment plan. "OK, so you want to take up the problems with your boyfriend and we agreed [in pretreatment] that we will address suicidal behavior whenever it comes up. So since suicidality was up for you last week, let's be sure to take that up today too." A confident and matter-of-fact tone is helpful here. Although suicidality is the top-priority agenda item and must be addressed at some point during the session, it need not be addressed first.

If the patient is reluctant to place a high-priority item on the therapy session agenda, this is therapy-interfering behavior and the therapist can target that reluctance itself: "So you say you are on the verge of being fired but you don't want to take up this topic in the therapy session. Could we talk about that?" During this discussion it can sometimes be useful to ask whether the behavior of ignoring important situations—what one of my patients called "head-in-the-sand behavior"—is a pattern for the patient. If the patient sees the behavior as a pattern, he or she may be more willing to address it.

If the situation is extremely high priority, Linehan (1993a) uses the strategy of "talk it to death." Here the therapist simply refuses to go on to address any other agenda items until the urgent one is addressed in some way. This is essentially a contingency management strategy. The therapist can also explicitly spell out the contingencies: "If you are able to give me another no-harm agreement, we can move forward to take up this issue about your boyfriend but if you don't feel able to do that, let's talk more about the self-harm and what is getting in the way of your giving a no-harm agreement."

Frequent patient–therapist disagreements about the therapy session agenda may indicate a need to impose a pause in the treatment and renegotiate the treatment plan. I discuss this issue in more detail in the last chapter of the book.

Develop a Formulation of the Problem Being Addressed in the Session

The choice of agenda items is itself often a powerful intervention, as the decision to focus on some phenomena but not others has significant emotional and cognitive effects on the patient and the therapy. Nevertheless, agenda setting is only the first step. Once the agenda items have been set, the therapist must decide how to intervene with each. To make this determination, the therapist works with the patient to develop a collaborative formulation of the problem that is being discussed.

The first step to developing a formulation of the problem is to focus on a particular instance, not a generality. Why focus on the concrete specifics? Focusing on a concrete, specific event appears to facilitate activation of the emotions connected with the incident, and Foa and Kozak (1986) propose that activation is necessary if emotional processing is to occur. Activation (unless arousal is too high) also allows the patient to access more details of the problem because it allows the patient to reference his or her current sensations or memories. Thus, focusing on a particular emotionally charged incident (e.g., my boss frowned at me when I met him in the cafeteria) generally leads to more productive problem solving than does a focus on a general issue (I feel unappreciated at work), which tends to lead to sterile, overly intellectual, and unproductive discussions (Burns, 1989b).

To begin to develop a formulation of a particular instance of the symptom or problem, the therapist consults his case formulation. The case-level formulation can provide an initial hypothesis about the mechanisms underpinning the particular instance of the problem behavior at hand. For example, in another session when Carol came in feeling particularly depressed following a social interaction, even before I learned the details of the situation, I adopted the tentative hypothesis that her "I'm defective" schemas had been activated in that situation.

Previous symptom-level formulations of that same behavior for that patient can also lead to some initial formulation hypotheses. For example, in the case of Amelia, I knew from previous work on this symptom that her shutdown behavior typically was an escape response to high-intensity emotion, usually fear. The fear, in turn, was triggered by perceptions of abandonment by important others that she felt dependent on for survival. So I was not surprised when she told me her shutdown behavior was triggered by feeling that I was unresponsive to her when she called me for help.

Thus, the case-level formulation and previous symptom-level formulations provide initial hypotheses about the mechanisms driving a particular symptom or problem. The therapist can use those preexisting formulations as the basis for an intervention. However, it is nearly always a good idea to conduct a detailed assessment of this *particular instance* of the problem before moving forward to intervene.

The tools provided in Chapters 2, 3, and 4 can be used to develop a formulation of a particular instance of a symptom or problem behavior. Often this formulation is based on the same model that was used as the basis for the case formulation. For example, if Beck's theory was used for the case-level formulation, as in Carol's case, the therapist may use Beck's model to formulate Carol's exasperation and self-criticism. A Thought Record (Figure 2.3) can be used to do that.

Sometimes (as was discussed in Chapter 1) the therapist uses a model different from the one used for the case-level formulation to formulate the symptom or problem in the session. This was true for my work with Angela, which is described in more detail in the next chapter.

The therapist might even use more than one formulation simultaneously to guide intervention. For example, I worked recently with Andrea, who was struggling with hopelessness. We used cognitive restructuring interventions based on Beck's conceptualization of hopelessness as driven by cognitive distortions (Burns & Persons, 1982) to tackle some of the thoughts driving Andrea's hopelessness, such as "I will never have the life I want." We also used interventions based on a functional analysis of hopelessness as a behavior that allowed Andrea to escape intense emotions of fear and shame. Based on the functional analysis, we worked to develop alternatives to hopelessness that could help Andrea achieve some relief of those intense states; these included mindfulness, distraction, and compassionate mind training (Gilbert & Procter, 2006). Thus, interventions to address Andrea's hopelessness flowed out of the simultaneous use of two different conceptualizations. One rationale for this strategy is that it yields additional leverage that can help solve tough problems. Another, as already noted, is that both conceptualizations might be true. The conceptualizations and interventions underpinning the various cognitive-behavior ESTs are usually complementary rather than conflicting.

Similarly, cognitive restructuring and exposure and response prevention (ERP) can be used simultaneously to address the obsessions and compulsions of OCD (Rector et al., 2007; Wilhelm & Steketee, 2006).

Sometimes the therapist is confused about how to apply the case-level formulation to the current situation but must make an intervention decision nevertheless. When this happens, the therapist can simply develop a formulation of the symptom or situation at hand and collect data to monitor process and outcome as she goes, as in the case of Eileen, described next. Usually, this work clarifies the relationship between the patient's behaviors in the current problem situation and the case-level formulation.

Eileen and the Theoretical Math Course

Eileen, a PhD student, was anxious and depressed. My main formulation hypothesis was that she had a schema of herself as weak, helpless, incompetent, and needing help and support from others at every step in order to make her way in the world. One of the major problems on her Problem List was that work on her dissertation was proceeding at a snail's pace. One of her treatment goals was to finish the dissertation.

Eileen came to her therapy session agonizing about a theoretical physics course that she wanted to audit. She had evaluated the advantages and disadvantages of the plan as a homework assignment. She stated that intellectually she knew she shouldn't take the course because it was tangential to her work but emotionally she felt driven to register for the course and had done so. She asked for help managing her anxiety about the course, which was quite challenging.

As therapist, I felt torn. It seemed clear (even Eileen agreed) that taking this course was not in Eileen's best interest and did not promote her therapy goals. If I agreed to work with her to reduce her anxiety about the course, I feared that I was colluding in her maladaptive behavior. Nevertheless, it was clear that challenging Eileen to drop the course was not going to be productive. She was locked into taking it. So I discussed the situation with her. I explained my dilemma and concluded by saying that although I had some concern that I might be colluding, I would agree to her request to help her with the course with the proviso that we would monitor the process carefully to be sure it was helpful.

We began developing a detailed formulation of her anxiety about the course. We worked through a Thought Record that identified the thoughts she had about performing poorly. These included: "I won't be able to handle the work," "The professor will disapprove of me," and "I must get his approval in order to feel good about myself, feel competent, and be successful in the field." As soon as I saw this list of automatic thoughts, I felt much better about agreeing to work with Eileen on her anxiety about this course. I could see that these thoughts were directly tied to the schema hypotheses identified in the case formulation, which proposed that she viewed herself as not good enough and not able to succeed without intensive and constant support and approval from others. This congruence indicated that helping Eileen manage her anxiety while taking the course addressed the same schemas that drove her to take the course despite her better judgment.

We spent a session working through a Thought Record in which we identified and developed responses to her automatic thoughts about the course. At the end of the session, Eileen stated, "You know, if I solve this stuff, I won't have to take the course. I'm already thinking that maybe I won't go to class today!" Two weeks later she quit the course.

I have repeatedly found that helping a person manage the distress that arises when he is doing a behavior that is not in his best interest often involves work on the central psychological mechanism that drives the problem behavior. For example, work on the distress a woman feels when her married lover does not call her on her birthday (e.g., automatic thoughts of "This proves that I'm unlovable and no one could care about me") can address the central vulnerability (her self-schema that she is unlovable) that keeps her in the destructive relationship in the first place.

Use the Formulation to Generate Intervention Ideas

Obtaining a formulation of the patient's current problem or symptom is often a kind of intervention itself. Pointing out to Carol that her self-criticism was an example of her problem behavior is an example of this type of intervention.

However, formulation is not usually enough. Intervention is needed. After a formulation has been obtained, it is frequently helpful to ask the patient what strategies or tools, if any, he or she has found helping in previous efforts to address the problem. In addition, the therapist can use the formulation to generate interventions that address the mechanism described in the formulation. Carol's case formulation proposed that a mistake, criticism, or disapproval by another person activated her schemas ("I am inept and inadequate," "Others don't care/find me boring/are critical"). Her schema produced feelings of embarrassment and distress, and a barrage of self-critical automatic thoughts that she frequently did not identify as problematic. Instead, she accepted the content of the self-criticisms. This formulation suggested several interventions. I could ask Carol to monitor self-criticism with a counter to help her increase her awareness of it and disengage from it, teach her to use compassionate self-statements to counter self-criticisms, encourage her to examine advantages and disadvantages of self-criticism, help her develop behavioral experiments to test her view of herself as inadequate and boring to others, or use a Positive Data Log to tally evidence supporting an alternative schema of herself, perhaps that she is capable and interesting. Many other interventions could be suggested to address the deficits described by the formulation of Carol's case.

Obtain the Patient's Permission to Proceed

After offering some intervention ideas, the therapist asks for the patient's permission to proceed. A good way to get the patient's buy-in to an intervention is to first make sure he or she agrees with the formulation that underpins the intervention. For example: "OK, so now we're working on that situation last Saturday where you had a fight with your mother, got highly agitated, got in your car, and drove away really fast, half-hoping you might crash and kill yourself. Based on our discussion just now, it seems like you suck it up, suck it up, suck it up [the patient's words] and then you get overwhelmed and do something impulsive to escape how bad you are feeling. Does that sound right?"

A useful next step is to offer a choice of intervention strategies, asking the patient to select one. For example, in the above case the therapist might say, "I'm thinking of two possible things we could do here. We could develop a list of things you could do to calm yourself down when you get so upset you want to jump in the car and go speeding away. Or we could flesh out the chain of events leading to that intense emotional distress you experienced on Saturday and generate ideas for ways you might have been able to interrupt the chain at an earlier point and prevent the intense upset in the first place. Which seems most useful to you?"

Before carrying out the intervention, the therapist monitors the patient's receptiveness to it to determine if he or she is fully committed to trying it or exhibiting signs of reluctance. If the latter is true, the therapist would do well to work to reduce the patient's ambivalence before proceeding, perhaps by using empathic listening. Another option is to change the intervention tack to one that is more acceptable to the patient.

If patient and therapist are working well together, the therapist may elect to skip the step of asking for the patient's permission to carry out the intervention, especially if he or she has already asked for permission at earlier points, such as at the point of agenda-setting or formulation. It is simply too cumbersome to ask for permission at every step.

Intervene

Now the therapist moves forward to carry out the intervention. The therapist might help the patient work through a Thought Record to identify and respond to cognitive distortions, break an intimidating task down into parts, identify pleasant activities, list advantages and disadvantages of diverse courses of action, carry out a behavioral chain and solution analysis of a problem behavior, develop an exposure hierarchy and begin working through the items on it, or any other interventions in the cognitive-behavior therapist's armamentarium. The therapist might even develop and carry out a novel intervention that is not written in any paper or EST protocol. Most important is that interventions flow from the formulation and address the process goals of the therapy in one way or another.

Monitor the Effects of the Intervention

The therapist collects data to monitor both the outcome and process (mechanism, alliance, and adherence) of the interventions. As described in Chapter 9, most of the monitoring that occurs during the session involves the therapist's observations of the patient's emotions and behavior and the therapist's emotional response.

Because the therapist collects monitoring data at every step of the process and uses those data to guide the session, the content of the session can differ quite a bit from the ideal sequence described in this chapter (assess, formulate, select an intervention, obtain the patient's permission, intervene, and return to assessment). I find that, based on the monitoring data, I often begin and abort conceptualizations and interventions repeatedly. When the monitoring data indicate that the patient does not accept or benefit from my intervention efforts, I back up to collect more assessment data and try again. For example, the patient might agree to a formulation (e.g., "Let's take a look to see what thoughts you were having that caused you to get so angry at your husband") and to the intervention (cognitive restructuring) that flows out of that formulation. But then monitoring may show that this approach is not very helpful or that the patient doesn't accept it or like it. When this happens, I am likely to abort the intervention and go back to collect more assessment data before selecting another intervention or even focusing on a different agenda item. All these changes in direction are based on monitoring data I'm collecting in the moment. Thus, monitoring data provide an essential guide to the process of formulation and intervention in the therapy session.

OTHER CLINICAL DECISIONS

Clinicians make many decisions that are focused on administrative, scheduling, and billing issues. Many of the interactions between patient and therapist in these arenas are quite straightforward. However, some are not. To identify which are which, the therapist attends carefully as these interactions transpire to identify any instances of patient problem behaviors or treatment targets that appear in these interactions. When treatment targets are observed, the therapist can use the steps of clinical decision making described above to conceptualize and intervene in these situations. Many of these happen in the session but some happen outside the session, such as on the telephone.

Caroline called to ask to reschedule her therapy session. Principles of operant conditioning helped me decide how to handle her request. She and I had met several weeks previously and made an agreement that before the next session she would carry out a list of tasks for making progress on her dissertation, which she had been avoiding. We had agreed that one of the main ways she could use me was to hold her accountable for keeping her commitments. This strategy was effective because Caroline agreed it would be punishing for her to have to come to the session and tell me that she had not done what she had agreed to.

A week before her scheduled appointment, Caroline called to say that she had not had time to carry out all the tasks on her list and wanted to postpone her appointment for a week to give herself more time to get everything done. Caroline's request sounded reasonable at first. But a moment of clear thinking told me that if I agreed to Caroline's request, our contingency management system would fall apart. I called her back and explained this to her. She quickly understood it and agreed to keep the appointment she had originally scheduled and suffer the consequences of not keeping her commitments!

In another case, Jonas and his therapist were at the end of a session, scheduling the next one. The therapist consulted his calendar and offered Jonas a time: "How about next Wednesday at 1 P.M.?" Jonas's immediate response was "Sure, that's fine!" The therapist observed that Jonas had agreed to the therapist's suggestion without consulting his calendar. The therapist's formulation led him to hypothesize Jonas's behavior in this situation was probably a sample of unassertiveness driven by his belief that unless he met others' needs they would get angry and reject him. Jonas's therapist gently put this hypothesis out on the table for Jonas to consider. When Jonas agreed it had some validity, he and his therapist revised their plan for scheduling the next therapy session. Jonas would go home and review his calendar, which was posted on his refrigerator, and call the therapist to offer some appointment times that would work for him.

One of my patients, Jane, walked into my office and sat down. She began describing, in great detail, in an emotionally compelling way—which I found quite engaging—an exchange she had just had with the postman who was delivering mail to my office. As Jane's therapist, I faced a question: Was Jane's decision to begin the session with this vignette a pleasant ice-breaker or a problem behavior?

A review of the formulation of Jane's case helped me decide that her vignette telling was a problem behavior. My formulation was that Jane had significant deficits in emotion regulation. She repeatedly made plans for her day and found at the end of the day that she had not accomplished any of them. She had allowed herself to get drawn away from her plans by her emotions, which pulled her to spend hours every day doing things other than those she had planned. She typically spent long hours on the telephone chatting with her friends or getting their help with emotional distress. As I listened to Jane and saw how much time she spent on the vignette and how little work she was doing in the therapy session, it was easy to see that her vignette telling was an example of the emotion-driven avoidance behavior described in her case formulation. Moreover, a major goal of her treatment was to use her time more productively. We had agreed that in order to achieve this goal, she needed to learn to guide more of her behavior on the basis of her plans and less on the basis of her emotions. This was the mechanism change goal of the treatment. Thus, the formulation and mechanism change goals of Jane's treatment cued me to speak up to ask, "Could I interrupt you? Do you see what is happening here?"

These examples illustrate the point that although many decisions about scheduling and business matters are not controversial and many interactions are pleasant ice-breakers, a constant awareness of the case formulation and treatment plan helps the therapist notice when treatment targets appear on the scene and respond to them therapeutically.

* * *

To summarize, clinical decision making in the session proceeds through the same steps described in Chapter 1 for the therapy as a whole. That is, the therapist begins with assessment, then develops a formulation and uses it to guide agenda setting and select an intervention, obtains the patient's permission to proceed, intervenes, and monitors the process and outcome of the intervention. The next chapter discusses how to address obstacles and failures in therapy.

ELEVEN

Handling Nonadherence and Treatment Failure

Setbacks, obstacles, and failure occur frequently. One of the strengths of a case formulation-guided approach to psychotherapy is that it provides a systematic way to address these unwanted events. This chapter describes how to use that model, which is illustrated in Figure 1.1, to handle nonadherence and treatment failure.

NONADHERENCE

Nonadherence is the failure to carry out a behavior that has been agreed to or is expected, such as an intervention or a homework assignment. Nonadherence can occur on the part of the patient or the therapist. It can slow down therapy or cause it to fail.

Therapist Nonadherence

Examples of therapist nonadherence include not monitoring the progress of therapy, failing to obtain the patient's informed consent to the treatment plan, and not reviewing the patient's homework assignments.

CBT is a lot of work and adhering to its every element is not easy. The therapist can establish systems to promote adherence. For example, I typically keep a plot of the self-report scales the patient and I are using to monitor outcome at the front of the patient's chart so it is the first thing I notice when I open the chart. This prompts me to ask the patient for the scale at the beginning of the session.

Using monitoring tools to identify nonadherence is the first step to addressing it. The therapist can use the Daily Log (Figure 9.5) described in Chapter 9 to track his use of the components of the cognitive-behavior therapy session (e.g., homework review and assignment, agenda setting). It is impractical to track each component in every session but if the therapist knows or suspects he is having difficulty with one or another component, he can track that component. Other monitoring tactics that can identify therapist noncompliance include listening to tapes of therapy sessions alone or with a consultant and carrying out periodic progress reviews (described in Chapter 9) to evaluate compliance with the treatment plan. I recently reviewed each of my patients' charts for evidence that I was using a measure (of any sort) to monitor progress at every session. I was surprised and disconcerted to learn that I was doing written progress monitoring at every session for only 16 of 22 (73%) of my active cases!

When the therapist realizes he is not doing what he has agreed to do, he can work to obtain a conceptualization of his nonadherent behavior. The conceptualization can help him generate ideas for solving the problem. The therapist's willingness to notice and examine errors in a nondefensive way is essential to this process. To overcome my progress monitoring nonadherence, I will need to review each case where this occurred, obtain hypotheses about what is interfering, and do what I can to solve the problem.

The same assessment tools we use with our patients can help us carry out these tasks. The therapist can use a Thought Record or carry out a functional analysis to conceptualize her own behavior as a guide to changing it. A functional analysis might reveal that my failure to monitor progress with my patient Suzanne is being reinforced because Suzanne frowns and punishes me when I ask her why she has not completed her Daily Log. Therapist lack of accountability (contingencies) can contribute to nonadherence. For this reason, working as a team and consulting with colleagues can improve therapist adherence by imposing some accountability on the therapist.

Using Beck's cognitive model to conceptualize, the therapist may fail to adhere to the agreed-upon treatment plan (or even to propose an adequate treatment plan!) because she "buys in" to the patient's distorted beliefs. This might include the belief that the patient is fragile and can't carry out the interventions the therapist is recommending. This is probably one of the main causes of my failure in the case of Julie, whom I treated when I was an intern.

Julie was a fantastically bright and charming nursing student who had OCD. She feared contamination by household cleaning agents and spent hours washing every day. She refused my recommendation that we undertake ERP, insisting that it was too scary and she simply could not do it. I continued to see her weekly, doing what I could to help her and hoping that eventually she would agree to ERP.

As the school year came to an end, Julie was worse. She still had all of her OCD symptoms, and in addition she was depressed and hopeless, telling me desperately, "I might as well kill myself. I'll never get better. I've spent 9 months in therapy and I haven't made any progress!"

I was horrified. I realized that by agreeing to meet with Julie and not do ERP (which was scary to me too), I had provided her with evidence to support her belief that she was too fragile for ERP. Even worse, my therapy helped her develop an even more harmful belief—that therapy could not help her. I would have been more helpful to Julie if I had obtained consultation to address my own ambivalence about ERP and then held firm to my ERP recommendation. If Julie had refused to proceed with ERP, I could have invited her to call me when she was ready to do ERP and referred her to a therapist who could provide supportive psychotherapy in the interim (Caire, 1991).

Patient Nonadherence

Examples of patient nonadherence include not doing therapy homework, not attending regular sessions, not proposing agenda items for the therapy session, and not using therapy time productively.

Preventing Nonadherence

The pretreatment phase attempts to prevent nonadherence by obtaining the patient's full informed consent to the proposed treatment plan before beginning treatment. Other aspects of CBT, such as the therapist's structured approach (e.g., setting an agenda for the therapy session and following it) also help prevent nonadherence.

The case formulation can also be used to predict and prevent nonadherence. For example, Marcia's self-schema was that she was unimportant and her needs didn't count. Marcia had learned from her family (her parents were needy and alcoholic) that her relationships with others went most smoothly if she focused on their needs, not hers. However, her attempts to meet the many, often conflicting needs of her family members had led to quite a lot of anxiety that propelled Marcia, unwillingly, into treatment. I taught Marcia progressive muscle relaxation, which she reported was extremely helpful when we did it in the session. We agreed it would be useful for her to practice relaxation at home. However, the formulation of Marcia's case made it easy to predict that homework practice to take care of her own needs would be quite difficult for her.

To address this issue, I carried out a role play with her in the session to help Marcia overcome obstacles to practicing relaxation at home. I played the role of her husband. Just as Marcia was getting ready to do her relaxation exercise, I said to her, "Honey, this button is just about to fall off my jacket. Will you sew it on for me so I don't lose it?" Marcia practiced asking me to put my jacket aside so she could take care of it when she had finished her relaxation exercise.

Identifying Nonadherence

When nonadherence occurs, it can be surprisingly difficult to identify. The patient and therapist are enjoying working together, and the therapy *feels* comfortable and successful. And so I unmindfully stepped into the gap to set the session agenda for passive Alan (discussed in Chapter 8). He was so pleased that I did it that I failed to notice for many weeks that I, not he, was setting the agenda.

The therapist can establish some monitoring systems to help identify nonadherence. My progress note for a session always describes the homework assignment I made and I review the note before the next session. This system helps me identify homework nonadherence right away.

Assessing, Conceptualizing, and Intervening

When nonadherence occurs, the therapist moves into assessment and intervention to address it. Of course, the therapist can't address every single item of nonadherence he or she encounters. It is necessary to use clinical judgment and focus on nonadherence that is interfering with therapy or that exemplifies a typical patient problem behavior, especially one that is significantly interfering with functioning.

Nonadherence behaviors can be conceptualized and treated in the same way as other target behaviors, using the methods described in Chapter 10. It is important that the therapist take a nonjudgmental problem-solving approach, viewing nonadherence behavior the same way we view the patient's other behaviors. Remember, it is the therapist's job to figure out how to help the patient identify and change this behavior. It is not helpful to simply blame the patient for the behavior or to assume that he or she does not want to change it. Ambivalence about change can certainly contribute to nonadherence. However, if it does, it is the therapist's job to identify it and help the patient resolve it.

When seeking a conceptualization of patient nonadherence, be sure to consider that therapist nonadherence may be a cause of patient nonadherence (Tompkins, 2004). For example, the patient's failure to complete a homework assignment might be due to the therapist's failure to make a clear assignment. A patient's failure to arrive on time for the therapy session can result from the therapist's tendency to start the session late. Even worse, the therapist's tardiness undermines his or her ability to address the patient's tardiness.

To begin to conceptualize nonadherence, it can be useful to simply ask the patient, for example, "What do you think got in the way of doing the homework assignment?" Another useful question is "Did the thought of doing the homework pass through your mind?" If so, the therapist can exclaim, "Good! That is a good start. What happened next?" This situation can be a good one for a Thought Record, where the Situation column reads "I remembered the homework assignment," and the patient and therapist work to identify what thoughts came up in that situation that got in the way of doing the assignment. Typical thoughts in this situation include "It won't help," I'll do it later," or "I'm afraid of making a mistake." If the assignment did *not* enter the patient's mind, the therapist will want to try to find out why not. Useful questions to sort this out include: When the assignment was agreed on in the session was the patient committed to doing it? Did he schedule or plan a time to do it?

Corey did not follow through with her homework assignment to log episodes of binging and purging. When she and her therapist began discussing what got in the way, Corey described chaotic and disorganized behavior and revealed that 2 weeks earlier she had decided, against her psychiatrist's advice, to stop taking the lithium he prescribed to treat her bipolar disorder because she was so upset about the weight gain it caused. Thus, her homework noncompliance seemed to be at least in part a result of her disorganized and chaotic behavior, which itself was a result of her unilateral decision to stop her medication. This conceptualization suggests that in order to treat Corey's bulimia, it will be important to improve her ability to collaborate with her treatment team on effective treatment of her bipolar disorder.

When seeking a conceptualization of nonadherence behavior, it can be helpful to consider whether the behavior might be a typical problem behavior for the patient. If so, the mechanisms part of the case formulation might provide an initial hypothesis about the mechanisms driving the nonadherence behavior. Paulo was depressed, not dating despite his desire for a relationship, and unhappy at work. We hypothesized that a failure to value his needs and speak up assertively to get them met was a factor in all these problems. Following a session in which we tackled his work issues, Paulo did not carry out his homework assignment to ask his boss for a raise. When we explored this, I learned that Paulo had felt that speaking up to his boss was not likely to succeed and might make his boss angry. I also learned that Paulo had known when we discussed the assignment that he wasn't planning to do it but he had been reluctant to tell me this for fear I would get angry! This information led to an important discussion that improved our working alliance and, in the process, addressed Paulo's central fear that if he asserted himself by asking to get his needs met, others would refuse his requests and get angry at him.

Similarly, when Sharon and I investigated why she had not done her homework, she reported that she felt I wanted her to do it for my own reasons, not because it would be helpful to her. Sharon had grown up in an invalidating family in which, for example, her parents sent her to a school that specialized in music and the arts when she was a child, not because she wanted to go but because it met *their* needs to have an artistic child. This issue was a central one for Sharon and we had a very useful discussion of it in the context of working together to address her homework nonadherence.

Despite the importance of doing so, it can be difficult for the therapist to address nonadherence. I frequently have to override a desire to ignore nonadherence and hope it will go away. Sometimes I worry about annoying or alienating my patient by taking up a topic he doesn't want to discuss. This concern doesn't make sense, for several reasons. First, if the issue is handled skillfully, the patient is not usually upset. In fact often the work on nonadherence is powerful and important, and most patients perceive that and are appreciative. In addition, if the patient's nonadherence is interfering with treatment, I am not doing anybody a favor by ignoring it. In fact, if I don't point it out, the patient may not even be aware that his nonadherence is undermining his therapy. I am the therapist, and it is my responsibility to point out the elephant in the living room. If the patient becomes upset when I do so, this is important information that contributes to my formulation of the case. When the time is right, I can highlight and address that problem behavior as well.

To ease my way into discussing nonadherence, sometimes I start by pointing it out with a light touch, saying, for example, "Oh, it's too bad we are starting a bit late today." If the behavior does not change, I increase the intensity of my intervention in small steps. I might escalate next to a request to start on time, for example, saying warmly, "Listen, I'm really committed to doing my best for you, so if it is possible for you to get here so we can start on time that would be terrific." If all that fails, I will point to the recurrent problem and ask to put it on the therapy session agenda. As I move through all these steps, I take care to notice and reinforce improved behavior (e.g., "It is terrific we can start on time today!").

I can also impose natural consequences, ending on time even when we start late and pointing out that a consequence of starting late is that we are not going to be able to finish a piece of work we started today. Natural consequences are especially useful for handling homework nonadherence. The therapist can elect to start the session by completing the homework assignment that the patient didn't do before the session. I do this most commonly when the patient failed to complete the symptom scales or the Daily Log before the session. This tactic imposes immediate contingencies that are often quite effective, as most patients don't want to spend the first part of their session completing their self-report measures.

Although it is a problem, nonadherence is also an opportunity. Nonadherence often provides powerful *in vivo* opportunities to identify and address central issues in the patient's psychopathology. In fact, nonadherence can be good news, as it can bring the patient's problem behaviors into the therapy itself, where the details of the behavior are available for examination, the mechanism causing the behavior is activated and ripe for intervention (Foa & Kozak, 1986), and the results of the therapist's efforts to address it can be monitored in the moment.

Premature Termination

The patient's decision to terminate therapy prematurely is a type of nonadherence. I define premature termination as ending before the treatment goals are reached or patient and therapist agree they will not be reached. Premature termination deserves extra attention because it is common (Foulks, Persons, & Merkel, 1986; Persons et al., 1988) and because, by definition, it is therapy-destroying behavior.

The case formulation can help the therapist predict and prevent a premature termination. For example, patients like Marcia, who do not view their needs and comfort as important, are prone to terminating therapy when they are no longer excruciatingly miserable but before they are truly well. Similarly, sometimes patients who are highly emotionally reactive can fly into a rage and impulsively fire the therapist. Another predictor of premature termination is a treatment history that includes previous premature terminations. In all these cases, it can be useful to initiate a discussion of the patient's potential for premature termination to arrive at a collaborative conceptualization of it, a commitment from the patient not to end treatment without discussing it with the therapist, and a plan for handling urges to prematurely terminate therapy.

Sometimes it is difficult to determine whether the patient's decision to end therapy is reasonable behavior that the therapist should accede to or a problem behavior that the therapist should target and treat. To answer this question, it is helpful to consider whether the patient's urge to quit is an example of the problem behaviors for which the patient seeks treatment. A clear example of this phenomenon is the patient with bipolar disorder who, during a manic episode, decides to terminate her therapy because she feels she is doing so well that she doesn't need it.

In these cases, the therapist would do well to view the patient's quitting as an example of therapy-interfering behavior and intervene accordingly. One of my patients, Estelle, in the middle of a crisis, impulsively threatened to quit her therapy. I ignored this verbalization and kept working with Estelle to resolve the crisis. When the crisis was over, I initiated a discussion of Estelle's threat to quit her therapy. We had a good discussion and were able to conceptualize her behavior as an example of her typical escape behaviors when stressed. She made a commitment to stop threatening to quit therapy impulsively and instead to sit down calmly in the therapy session to discuss the issue if she had the urge to quit therapy.

Sometimes pointing out that the decision to quit is maladaptive is unavailing. The patient insists she is going to stop therapy. When that happens, I validate the patient's wish to quit (usually there are some valid reasons) and say in a calm way, "Of course it is your decision but I would not recommend that you stop your therapy now. I hope you will come to your session and I will keep the time for you and hope to see you then." If she does not come to the session, I will continue to reach out for as long as I feel comfortable keeping her chart open without seeing her, sending occasional messages attempting to reengage her in treatment.

TREATMENT FAILURE

Failure to respond to treatment is unfortunately common. Treatment can be inert, like the therapy illustrated in Figure 11.1. The meta-analysis by Westen and Morrison (2001) showed that 63% of patients with depression, 57% of those with generalized anxiety dis-

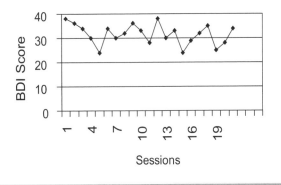

FIGURE 11.1. Plot of weekly BDI scores of a patient who is failing to benefit from treatment.

order (GAD), and 46% of those with panic disorder did not improve during treatment with an EST. These are substantial figures. Deterioration is less common but does occur. Ogles, Lambert, and Sawyer (1995) reported that 3 to 5% of the patients who completed treatment in the National Institute of Mental Health Treatment of Depression Collaborative Research Program (Elkin et al., 1989) got worse. These data remind us that having a well-meaning and caring therapist providing compassion, empathy, good-faith effort, and empirically supported treatment does not ensure that the patient will benefit.

Despite its frequency and importance, therapists do not appear to be very skilled at handling treatment failure. Kendall, Kipnis, and Otto-Salaj (1992) found, in a survey of Division 12 and AABT (Association for the Advancement of Behavior Therapy) therapists, that in 41% of cases that therapists identified as not responding to treatment, the therapist had not planned or initiated any change in the treatment plan. Instead, the therapist was planning to continue to provide a treatment that he or she knew was failing.

Therapists are in need of heuristics to guide clinical decision making when treatment fails. Case formulation-driven CBT offers a systematic way to think about preventing, identifying, and overcoming treatment failure (Persons & Mikami, 2002). I also describe the process of accepting failure and ending treatment when efforts to overcome failure are unavailing.

Preventing Failure

Elements of case formulation-driven CBT that help in the task of preventing failure include the use of pretreatment to obtain the patient's full informed consent to the treatment, reduce ambivalence about change, and establish a good therapeutic alliance before beginning treatment; the use of EST formulations and interventions as templates for the first-line idiographic formulation and treatment plan; efforts to set realistic and mutually agreed-on treatment goals; and strategies for managing problems with adherence and coordination of care by multiple providers described above.

Identifying Failure

A method to identify failure may seem to be unnecessary, but data suggest it is not. The findings by Lambert et al. (2005) described earlier tell us that when therapists are notified that their patient is showing an initial poor response to treatment and is at risk of failing, outcomes of those patients improve. The progress-monitoring piece of the model (described in Chapter 9) helps identify failure. A flatline plot of the patient's weekly scores on a key outcome measure, as illustrated in Figure 11.1, can provide both patient and therapist with a visual depiction of the cold hard fact that treatment is failing. However, monitoring data alone are not enough to conclude that treatment is failing.

The monitoring data are only part of the story and are subject to biases. When the patient is not improving, a useful first step is to discuss the issue with the patient. I initiated this discussion with my patient Larry when we observed that his BDI scores were not changing. Larry acknowledged that his scores were unchanged but pointed out many other positive shifts that I had not been aware of. In fact, Larry told me that he had been afraid to let me know he was improving for fear that I would refuse to continue seeing him. I (gently) explained to him that in fact the opposite was true: unless he benefited from treatment, I could not continue to provide it.

Overcoming Failure

The Therapist's Stance toward Failure

If treatment is failing, the clinician must try to determine why and get the patient's permission to make some change in the treatment plan that has a chance of turning the case around. In general, if efforts to remediate the situation fail, the therapist must refer the patient to another treatment setting.

These tasks are the most difficult ones a clinician faces. I find that I frequently need help from my colleagues as I move through these steps. Patients often are very comfortable with treatment as usual and don't want to make a change. In fact, if things aren't going well they may be especially reluctant to consider giving up the support and comfort of their therapist for something new. Therapists encounter inertia and obstacles here too. In fact, therapists in private practice are reinforced when patients continue therapy indefinitely without getting well enough or confident enough to discontinue it.

Despite these obstacles, aggressive action to address a failing treatment is needed for several reasons. First, it is not ethical to continue to provide a failing treatment (American Psychological Association, 1992). Second, the therapy may be iatrogenic—that is, harmful to the patient. For example, in the case of Julie, described above, the therapy I provided seemed to support and even strengthen Julie's belief that she couldn't handle ERP. Even when the patient does not get worse, therapy can be iatrogenic. For example, the patient may be using therapy as a way of obtaining a supportive social contact rather than learn skills to obtain this outside of therapy. Finally, continuing an ineffective treatment can be harmful by preventing the patient from obtaining another therapy that might be more helpful.

The reader may object that some patients who do not respond to the treatment they are receiving are not likely to respond to any treatment. Therefore, referral to another treatment setting, especially in the face of the patient's preference to remain with the current therapist, seems unnecessary or even cruel. That is, for example, some patients simply are unable to learn skills to obtain a supportive social network and it is reasonable for them to obtain social support through a relationship with a therapist. This argument has some validity. Certainly there is much we do not know about psychopathology and its treatment. There are many patients we can't help because treatments for their problems have not yet been developed.

How does the therapist decide whether "this is as good as it gets" or the patient could improve and the therapist should change or discontinue the treatment? It is frequently impossible to definitively answer this question. However, useful strategies for answering this question include using benchmarking data to compare outcomes of the case at hand with other similar cases; consulting with another clinician; asking the patient to obtain a consultation from another clinician; and discussing the options in detail with the patient and his or her family.

Strategies for Overcoming Failure

To attempt to overcome treatment failure, the therapist can evaluate the adequacy of the treatment plan, the formulation, and the diagnosis. Consultation with other clinicians can also be helpful.

EVALUATE THE TREATMENT PLAN

The therapist can ask several questions to evaluate the treatment plan.

- *Are we adhering to the agreed-upon treatment plan?* It is entirely possible for patient and therapist to agree to ERP for OCD but then somehow never to get around to it (Zayfert & Becker, 2007). This is not surprising in view of how unpleasant it is to carry out ERP. Efforts to identify and remove obstacles to adherence like ambivalence about change or a weak patient–therapist relationship can help resuscitate a failing treatment.

- *Are treatment goals realistic?* Sometimes treatment fails because its goals are unrealistic. The goal of overcoming bipolar disorder in six sessions is unrealistic but the goals of providing the patient with some psychoeducation about his disorder, helping him accept pharmacotherapy and get a referral to a good psychiatrist, and referring him to a support group for patients with bipolar disorder are not.

Sometimes the patient shows a partial response to treatment, and the patient and therapist can elect to view the treatment as a success by deciding that a partial response is adequate. Sometimes this decision results from a shift in view of the patient's problem from one of curable acute disorder to a chronic one unlikely to remit (Scott, 1998). The goal can be shifted from treating the problem to preventing it from worsening. Similarly, patient and therapist can agree to shift the treatment contract from active treatment to palliative care. That is, the goal can be shifted from the goal of treating psychopathology to the goal of reducing suffering.

I used the "partial success is good enough" strategy to continue caring for Jonas for over a dozen years. He had a chronic, unremitting depression and multiple medical problems. After my initial efforts to treat Jonas's depressive symptoms failed, I made multiple changes in the treatment plan in an effort to get a better result. I held conjoint sessions with his wife, I sent Jonas for a consultation with a geriatrician, and consulted with multiple clinicians myself. At about the 2-year point, I reluctantly gave Jonas an ultimatum, telling him that I would not continue to treat him unless he stopped drinking. He did, but his depression still did not remit. Jonas's psychiatrist tried numerous medications and a sequence of electroshock treatments. Jonas's depression continued. I repeatedly encouraged him to seek treatment from another provider and Jonas steadfastly refused to do so.

As our efforts to treat his depressive symptoms failed, I shifted my focus to Jonas's medical problems. He had early symptoms of diabetes but was not complying with his physician's recommendation that he monitor his blood sugar and use exercise and diet to manage it. Jonas complained that he didn't like his physician. I referred him to my own primary care physician, who he liked and who helped Jonas get on board with monitoring his blood sugar. Jonas and I shifted our goals to those of keeping his depressive symptoms from worsening and improving his management of his medical problems. We had enough success accomplishing those goals that I felt I could justify continuing to provide Jonas with treatment. I continued to care for him until he died at age 85.

• *Is the treatment plan adequate to meet the patient's needs?* To get at this issue, therapists can ask themselves: "If this patient was a member of my family and I wanted him to get top-notch treatment, what treatment plan would I recommend?" The exercise of thinking through the answer to this question can expose discrepancies between the treatment plan that is in place and the one the therapist truly believes the patient needs. Often therapists find themselves providing treatment they know is inadequate (e.g., meeting whenever the patient can get the funds to pay for a session even though more intensive treatment is needed) because of financial or geographical or other limitations. Efforts to address these limitations can rescue a failing treatment.

James did not follow through with his homework agreement to do exposures to the fear items on his OCD hierarchy. Careful questioning revealed that he was highly motivated but his fear was too high. He could only do the exposures in session with a lot of help. The therapist concluded that even twice-weekly outpatient therapy sessions were simply not enough for James. He needed more help doing exposures outside the session. This hypothesis was supported by evidence that James could do his exposures and made great progress when he received intensive treatment in a partial hospital setting.

When CBT alone fails, it can be helpful to ask whether adding pharmacotherapy to the psychotherapy might produce better results. For example, sometimes pharmacotherapy can alleviate anxiety enough to allow a phobic patient who cannot otherwise do it to tolerate exposure-based therapy.

• *Are therapist vulnerabilities getting in the way of treatment?* When Alisa called a few hours before her therapy session to leave a breezy message announcing that she was cancelling her session because she did not need to meet this week and would see me at the following week at the usual time, I felt devalued, irritated, and offended, and had maladaptive thoughts like "I shouldn't have to work so hard to get her in the office" and "She should treat me with more respect." I had the urge to not respond to her telephone message, feel superior and self-righteous, sulk, and passively–aggressively wait to see her at her regular session the following week.

All of these feelings and thoughts made it difficult for me to think clearly to conceptualize Alisa's therapy-interfering behavior and make a plan to manage it. When I was able to discipline myself to do that, I saw that her behavior was an example of the impulsive, mood-state-driven maladaptive behavior that was a key treatment target for Alisa and that we had discussed repeatedly. Based on that conceptualization, I decided that the most therapeutic way for me to handle Alisa's message was to call her (hoping I did not get her but could just leave a quick message) and pleasantly point out that I suspected that her cancelling her session was one of those problem behaviors we had been discussing and tell her that I would hold her regular appointment time for her and hope she decided to come for her session. I also reminded myself that when she came in (as she did), I needed to reward that behavior by being happy to see her (not miffed). I also needed to review with her the conceptualization of her urge to cancel and generate strategies for handling that urge differently the next time it arose. I was able to do all of these things, with excellent results.

In this example, I was able to identify and manage my vulnerability myself. Sometimes this is not possible and the therapist needs help from a treatment team, a consultant, or a therapist to manage feelings and behaviors that undermine effective work.

After evaluating the treatment plan, a review of the diagnosis is in order.

EVALUATE THE DIAGNOSIS

Diagnostic error can contribute to treatment failure. For example, if the treatment plan is founded on the notion that the patient has unipolar depression and GAD when she actually has bipolar disorder and a substance abuse disorder, the treatment plan is likely to be misguided and the outcome poor.

EVALUATE THE CASE FORMULATION

A change in the case formulation can sometimes suggest a new and more effective approach to intervention. I list here several questions therapists can ask themselves to evaluate the formulation and I provide examples of how revisions to the formulation can lead to new and more successful interventions.

• *Have I accurately identified the fearful patient's central fear?* Erin had PTSD following an incident in which she was knocked down and assaulted by a homeless person. She developed PTSD symptoms and began avoiding all public situations where she might encounter a homeless person. In treatment, she worked hard at practicing going to public places and approaching homeless people. Although she was able to handle those situations with more comfort, weekly progress monitoring showed that her symptoms did not change. A careful reassessment yielded (with difficulty, as Erin at first was not able to verbalize her fear) the information that Erin was not just afraid of being in a place where there might be a homeless person. She was afraid of being pushed and knocked over. After we got this new information, I shifted the focus of treatment and we practiced exposures in the office in which I pushed her and bumped against her. The first time we did this, after asking her permission to do so, I tapped her gently on the shoulder. She burst into tears! Once we had identified the details of her fear and designed exposures that activated the fear network, Erin made rapid progress overcoming her PTSD symptoms.

George's case illustrates the same point in a more complex situation. He sought treatment for hypochondriasis. My initial conceptualization was that he was afraid of dying of cancer and therefore I carried out *in vivo* and imaginal exposure to those fears, asking him to read newspaper and other articles about cancer and to carry out imaginal exposures to dying of cancer. George did not improve. Further assessment revealed that George also had social phobia, especially a fear of public speaking. As part of the process of assessing his hypochondriasis and social phobia, George and I completed the Thought Record illustrated in Figure 11.2. I learned from this Thought Record that a fear of humiliation underpinned both George's performance anxiety and his hypochondriasis. George, it turned out, feared cancer not because he feared death (as I had assumed) but because he feared he'd miss work, make a mistake, get fired, and be humiliated.

This new conceptualization suggested that treatment of George's fears of humiliation would cause both his performance anxiety and his hypochondriasis to remit. That proved to be the case. *In vivo* and imaginal exposures to fear of humiliation led to significant improvements both in his fear of public speaking and his hypochondriasis, as Figure 11.3 shows (this case is described in detail in Persons and Mikami, 2002).

• *Have I selected the wrong target behavior?* Sometimes treatment fails because the patient and therapist focus on a target behavior that does not help the patient reach his or her treatment goal (see Hawkins [1986] for an outstanding chapter on treatment target selection). For example, I first began working with a graduate student, Ann, whose treatment goal was to complete her dissertation, by helping her increase the amount of time she spent working on her dissertation. Ann was effective in doing this—but did not make much progress on her dissertation because she spent hours reading in the library but did little or no writing. When we changed the target behavior from "spending time on the dissertation" to "writing manuscript pages," Ann made much more progress.

• *Have I failed to identify all of the causes of a problem behavior?* Joseph, a depressed anxious elderly man, complained of severe fatigue. My initial formulation hypothesis was that the fatigue was a symptom of his depression, which I viewed as due to a loss of reinforcers he suffered when he retired. In line with this formulation, I used behavioral activity scheduling in an attempt to help him come in contact with reinforcers that would activate his behavior and reduce his depression and fatigue. Results were poor. His fatigue and depression were unabated.

I began collecting more data to determine if I had missed an important piece of the puzzle. I spoke to Joseph's daughter, a nurse, and she alerted me to her concern that Joseph was misusing his sleeping medications (I hadn't known that he was taking sleeping medications!). He tended to not take medications at bedtime, but did take them when he awoke at 4 in the morning. This dosing schedule led to fatigue and low energy that persisted throughout the day. This new hypothesis about the causes of Joseph's fatigue led to changes in the dosing of his insomnia medications that produced improvements in his insomnia, fatigue, and depression.

• *Might a different formulation lead to a more helpful intervention plan?* The cognitive theory described in Chapter 2, the conditioning theories described in Chapter 3, and the emotion theories described in Chapter 4 offer distinct conceptualizations of some of the same problem behaviors that lead to different interventions. For example, Beck's model conceptualizes depressed emotions and mood as due to distorted thoughts and treats them by intervening to change the content of the thoughts. In contrast, behavioral activation (BA) views depressed mood as due to disengagement from reinforcing activi-

DATE	SITUATION (event, memory, attempt to do something, etc.)	BEHAVIOR(S)	EMOTIONS	THOUGHTS	COPING RESPONSES
	Colleague says, "Oh you're sick again."			It could be cancer. → I'll miss work. → I'll drop a ball. → I'll lose my job. → I'll be humiliated.	

FIGURE 11.2. Thought Record leading to change in formulation and treatment of George's hypochondriasis.

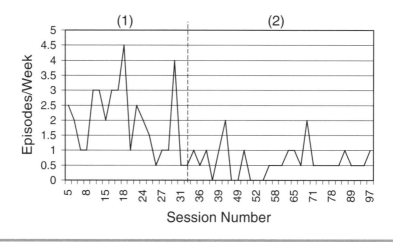

FIGURE 11.3. Hypochondriacal episodes during interventions focusing on hypochondriasis (1) and on public speaking (2).

ties and excessive focus on depressive ruminations, and treats it by helping individuals with depression reengage and actively participate in their lives and turn away from negative cognitions. To take another example, Beck's model conceptualizes suicidality as due to hopelessness and works to change that. In contrast, conditioning models view suicidal behavior as an operant that allows the individual to escape aversive situations and/or gain desired consequences (caring from others, a safe hospital bed) and works to change those contingencies.

The different conceptualizations lead to different interventions. This fact offers the therapist valuable flexibility. If a conceptualization of a behavior guided by one model does not lead to a helpful intervention, a reconceptualization guided by another model might yield a more helpful intervention strategy.

Serena's typical response to stressors was thoughts like "I can't do it," and behaviors of withdrawing and giving up. For example, she reported that when she was under a lot of pressure at work to meet a deadline, she repeatedly told herself, "I'm never going to make it." My initial efforts to help her drew on a structural (Beck's cognitive therapy) approach to this thought. I helped her develop responses to it, such as "I have done similar projects in the past," "I can get help if I need it," and "The world will not come to an end if I do not meet this deadline." I used these interventions repeatedly with Serena. She reported they were not helpful and she continued to pull back and collapse whenever she encountered stressors.

I consulted with a colleague (Kelly Koerner) and she helped me find another conceptualization of Serena's behavior that led to a much more helpful line of intervention. Kelly suggested a functional conceptualization of Serena's "I can't do it" thought, namely that the thought functioned to reduce the pressure Serena felt in the situation. When I proposed this hypothesis to Serena, she reported that it made sense to her. We worked together to identify some more adaptive thoughts and strategies that could serve the same function. She decided that when she felt pressured by an overwhelming task, she would break it into parts and focus on small goals like (in the case of the work deadline) completing the first part of the project. Serena reported that this strategy helped her complete a large work project on a tight deadline without melting down from the pressure.

Alice sought treatment for painful bouts of anxiety and worry that arose when she began graduate school. She spent hours worrying that she was not going to be happy in her new graduate program. She considered withdrawing, studying to improve her GRE scores, and applying again the next year to schools that she might like better. I first treated Alice's distress by using a structural model (Beck's cognitive therapy) to help her identify the thoughts that appeared to be causing her anxiety, pinpoint and respond to the distortions in those thoughts, and think through the advantages and disadvantages of her options. This line of intervention was not helpful. Alice got worse and in fact began having thoughts about suicide.

I stepped back and reviewed my formulation and intervention plan. A consultation with a colleague (Gary Emery) and a review of a Thought Record Alice had recently completed helped me reformulate Alice's case in functional terms that led to a new and more effective intervention plan. The Thought Record is presented in Figure 11.4. Alice completed it when she left a school event that was anxiety provoking for her and went home to complete a Thought Record to help her manage her anxiety. My operant formulation proposed that Alice's behavior of leaving a scary situation to go home to do a Thought Record was maladaptive avoidance behavior that was negatively reinforced because it alleviated the anxiety evoked by her central fear, which was that she had chosen the wrong graduate program and was doomed to unhappiness. In fact, my earlier efforts to help her identify cognitive distortions and think through the advantages and disadvantages of her options also promoted her avoidance behavior (Persons, 1990).

This operant formulation led to a new intervention plan that called for Alice to throw herself into her new graduate program, go to all her classes, complete all her homework, and attend social events and reach out to new friends. I asked her to view her worry thoughts as avoidance behavior and to use anxiety and worry as cues to reengage in the feared situation and wait for her anxiety to go down. Alice courageously and rigorously followed the new intervention plan and within 2 weeks she was feeling much better and functioning well as a first-year graduate student.

- *Are there any significant problems that I am not addressing?* Patients frequently seek treatment for some problems and want to ignore others. Common problems that patients want to "take off the table" include substance abuse, suicidality, self-harm, and marital problems. If treatment is failing, it can be useful to collect more assessment data to be certain that *all* of the patient's problems have been identified and that an unidentified or untreated problem is not undermining the therapy. I once participated in a panel discussion at an international conference in which I and some colleagues provided consultation to clinicians who asked for help with their tough cases. Over the course of an hour, the panel consulted on four cases of patients who were not making progress. Every one of these patients had a significant substance abuse problem that was not being addressed in treatment!

Accepting Failure and Ending Treatment

Failures are inevitable. Our field has not yet developed therapies that will help all of the patients we treat. Accepting failure and managing it effectively are some of the hardest parts of good clinical care. Therapists' unwillingness to accept treatment failure is likely one of the factors that contribute to our tendency to persist too long with failing treatment plans (Kendall et al., 1992).

DATE	SITUATION (event, memory, attempt to do something, etc.)	BEHAVIOR(S)	EMOTIONS	THOUGHTS	COPING RESPONSES
	At a party where I don't know anyone	Go home to do a Thought Record	Anxious	I don't fit in here. I can't stay here while I'm so anxious. Maybe I chose the wrong school.	I'll go home and do a Thought Record to feel better.

FIGURE 11.4. Thought Record leading to change in formulation and treatment of Alice's anxiety and worry.

If after repeated efforts to turn the therapy around, the patient is not responding, the therapist must refer the patient to another provider. It is not ethical to continue indefinitely to provide failing treatment (American Psychological Association, 1992). One exception is, as described above, when patient and therapist agree, ideally after some consultation from others, that the treatment being provided and the results that are being achieved are likely the best that can be obtained.

An important strength of a case formulation-driven approach to clinical work is that it sets the stage for ending a failing treatment even before the painful moment of truth arrives. The steps of setting treatment goals at the onset of therapy and monitoring progress and process at every session serve as constant reminders to the patient (and therapist) that if the treatment plan fails, a change will be needed or the treatment must be ended.

Nevertheless, ending a failing treatment can be difficult for both patient and therapist. Often the failing therapies are ones in which therapists and patients have invested significant amounts of time and energy. Patient and therapist are often quite attached to one another and it is painful to say good-bye. The patient may be happy with the therapy despite its failure. Therapists fear they are, or will be sued for, abandoning their patient. These situations are difficult and I typically need consultation and help from colleagues to address it.

Implementing a decision to end a treatment and refer the patient to another treatment setting can sometimes be accomplished in a session or two. However, if the therapy has been going on a long time, this process can require many weeks. During that time, the patient and therapist discuss treatment options, review the results of the patient's meeting with another therapist to aid the patient in making the transition, and bring the treatment to a good close. As I carried out these steps with one of my patients, she complained bitterly, "You are giving up on me!" In a certain sense she was right. I agreed that I had concluded I could not help her. At the same time, I pointed out, "Notice there is some sense in which I am *not* giving up on you. If I was giving up on you I would continue to see you every week even though you are not making any progress. I believe you can do better than you are doing now. However, you are not doing it here so I need to refer you to someone who has a chance of helping you more than I have." Obviously, the therapist cannot abandon the patient and must provide the patient with treatment alternatives that are feasible, affordable, and available, and take steps (e.g., telephoning the alternative providers) to help the patient make contact with those providers.

Failure—flat-out failure—that cannot be overcome, is tremendously disappointing for all involved. But it is inevitable, if only because our field has not yet developed adequate treatments for many of the disorders and problems we treat.

* * *

The next chapter describes decision making and intervention over the course of treatment when things go well, including the process of bringing therapy to a close.

TWELVE

Decision Making
over the Course of Therapy

This chapter describes decision making over the course of the therapy. I discuss treating multiple problems, coordinating the work of multiple providers, and stages of treatment, using illustrations from the case of Angela, who was described in Chapters 5, 6, and 7.

TREATING MULTIPLE PROBLEMS

When patients have multiple problems (most do), the clinician must decide whether to treat problems in sequence or address them all simultaneously. I use the word *problem* here to refer to symptoms, disorders, and psychosocial and environmental difficulties.

Treating Problems in Sequence

It is usually a good idea to treat problems in sequence, focusing first on one or two and putting others aside. Tackling several problems simultaneously can make it difficult for the patient to focus enough energy on any single problem to solve it.

However, the disadvantage of sequencing is that the multiple-problem patient must wait to work on some problems until others have been addressed. Linehan (personal communication, October 31, 2005) developed distress tolerance skills in part for this reason. Another (partial) solution to this dilemma is layering, described below. In layering, after work on one problem is under way (but not completed), work on others begins. Another solution is to tackle a problem that, when solved, will lead to improvements in other problems.

When Treating One Problem Resolves Other Problems

Often treatment for one disorder or problem leads to improvements in others even if those other problems are not addressed directly. Treating panic (Tsao, Mystkowski, Zucker, & Craske, 2002), OCD (Franklin et al., 2000), and bulimia nervosa (Fairburn,

Kirk, O'Connor, & Cooper, 1986; Garner et al., 1993) often leads to improvements in other problems and disorders.

Why does treating one problem sometimes lead to improvements in others? There are several possible answers to this question. One is that generalized gains can occur if, when the therapist treats one problem, he treats mechanisms that underpin other problems. The case of George, described in Chapter 11, illustrates this point. In George's case, interventions to reduce his fear of humiliation led to improvements in both hypochondriasis and social phobia because this core fear underpinned both disorders. Another example is the treatment of a young woman who had fears of death, fears of loss of control, and hypersensitivity to criticism (Persons, 1986b). Interventions to reduce her fear of death also reduced her fear of losing control, as was predicted by the formulation that the two fears shared stimulus elements in the young woman's fear network (Foa & Kozak, 1986).

Treatment of one problem can also lead to gains in other areas if the treatment teaches the patient skills (e.g., cognitive restructuring, mindfulness) he or she can use to manage other problems. This notion is different from the proposal made a moment ago that treatment of one problem leads to improvement in others by changing mechanisms underpinning all the problems. Instead, this notion is based on the idea that therapy teaches patients compensatory skills rather than changing dysfunctional mechanisms (Persons, 1993; Barber & DeRubeis, 1989).

Alternatively, treating one problem might lead to improvement in others because remission of some problems helps the patient solve others. For example, alleviating the low energy symptom of depression can give a person more energy to solve other problems. Similarly, alleviating the hopelessness symptom of depression can give a person optimism that can help him attack other difficulties.

Also, treating one problem can lead to improvements in other problems that were caused by the first problem. For example, treating depressive symptoms might lead to improvements in a depressed woman's marriage because when she is less depressed she has fewer irritable and more pleasant interactions with her husband. Or treating panic disorder and agoraphobia (PDA) allows a person to get a more satisfying job because she can now drive on the freeway to get to that better job.

As these examples illustrate, the therapist can use the case formulation, especially the formulation's proposal about how problems are related, to guide decisions about which problem or mechanism to target first in order to get "the biggest bang for the buck" (Haynes, 1992). Despite the help provided by the formulation, the way ahead is frequently unclear. Usually a trial and error process is needed to guide these types of decisions. I begin by collaborating with the patient to develop a hypothesis about the relationships between the patient's problems that helps us decide where to start and what interventions might be helpful. Then at every step I monitor the results of my interventions carefully (Are they helpful? Harmful? Useless? Do they produce narrow specific effects? Broad general effects?) in order to decide what to do next.

When Treating One Problem Exacerbates Other Problems

Sometimes treatment of one problem worsens other problems. Sometimes this is progress and the therapist and patient should hold the course. Sometimes it is a setback and evidence that a change in the treatment plan is needed. To determine whether the worsening is progress or a setback, the therapist can use the case formulation, careful monitoring, collaborative discussions with the patient, and, if needed, consultation.

How can symptom worsening be progress? A. M. Hayes, Laurenceau, Feldman, Strauss, and Cardaciotto (2007) offer some very interesting ideas about how therapeutic progress can entail a period of chaos and disorganization on the way to a new integration. Gary Emery (personal communication, 1985) aptly described this phenomenon as the difference between feeling better and getting better. For example, when Jason came to therapy and courageously agreed to stop using maladaptive strategies (self-harm, dissociation, and suicidality) to regulate his emotions, he began having frequent and extremely painful and frightening PTSD reexperiencing symptoms. He and I conceptualized this development as progress because even though he felt much more distressed than before, his behavior was now much less dangerous and more in line with his personal values. The next steps were to provide self-soothing and distress tolerance strategies to help him get through the distress, teach adaptive emotion regulation strategies, and treat the PTSD.

Layering

Layering (Zayfert & Becker, 2007) is a useful strategy when treatment of one problem makes others worse or leaves them unchanged or only partially remitted. In layering, the therapist begins by tackling one or two problems. When patients have learned a tool or two that they are using consistently to manage those problems, the therapist begins treating another problem while monitoring the patient's continued progress on the first ones. For example, I began working with Ariel, who had bipolar disorder and sought treatment when she was in the depths of a severe depressive episode, by teaching her to use activity scheduling to counter her passivity and depression. After she was regularly using activity scheduling to stay active and was feeling less depressed, I taught Ariel assertion skills to improve her relationships with friends and family who tended to take advantage of her.

Treating Multiple Problems Simultaneously

Sometimes it is quite effective to treat multiple problems simultaneously. This way of working is especially helpful if the various problems are all related to one disorder that manifests itself in multiple domains or if all the problems appear to be caused by one mechanism.

An example is the case of Mark, who was depressed and had interpersonal, work, and leisure problems. All these problems appeared to be driven in part by the core dysfunctional attitude, "If I compromise, I'm not being true to myself," and a behavioral pattern of disengaging when situations did not immediately meet his exacting standards. This belief and behavioral pattern appeared in his leisure time activities (if the weather was not perfect for skiing when he arrived in the mountains, he returned home and went to bed); at business meetings (if the discussion did not interest him, he tuned out); in career decisions (because he was getting negative feedback about his work in one area, he was contemplating resigning from a high-paying job he had held and done well at for more than 20 years); in interactions with colleagues (if they were not "in synch" with his point of view, he refused to go to lunch with them or even interact with them unless his job required it); and in relationships with friends (if they did not want to do the activities that interested him, he withdrew from the relationship). I treated all these problems simultaneously, tackling whichever one was activated when Mark came in for a session. My formulation of his case indicated that it didn't matter which domain we addressed; all provided an opportunity to address his central dysfunctional belief and his tendency to disengage.

Another example of treating multiple problems simultaneously is my work with Al on a group of behaviors (cutting himself with a razor blade, making plans to kill himself, making plans to leave town and start over somewhere else, and dissociating) that he and I labeled "extreme behaviors." I worked with Al to develop a formulation and intervention plan for all of these behaviors simultaneously. This was possible because Al and I hypothesized that all the extreme behaviors served the same function of down-regulating overwhelming intense emotions.

To help Al stop the extreme behaviors (Bs), we carried out repeated functional analyses (as described in Chapter 3) to identify the antecedents (As) and the consequences (Cs) of the Bs as they emerged. Then we carried out interventions to make changes in as many As and Bs as we could, especially interventions that would allow him to achieve the C (feelings of numbness and calm) that the Bs typically produced. Typical As were painful emotions and PTSD reexperiencing symptoms, which themselves were triggered by multiple As, including interactions with frightening people (a psychotic homeless person ranting on the street). Bs were the problem behaviors already described (self-harm, suicidality, dissociation). Al learned to increase his awareness in order to avoid triggers to painful emotions (As). (He tended to unnecessarily place himself in dangerous situations, such as interacting with homeless street people.) I taught him to change Bs by using other skills to manage powerful emotional states, especially mindfulness, problem solving, distraction, and self-soothing. These interventions simultaneously treated a group of diverse behaviors that all served the same emotion regulation functions.

Often the decision to treat multiple problems simultaneously is not made explicitly, at least not at first. Instead, the decision emerges organically from work on one problem that proves to be helpful with other problems when the patient brings them up. Sometimes, however, the gradual and implicit decision to take on multiple problems simultaneously is not a good one. Patient and therapist find they are tackling so many problems simultaneously that they don't make good progress on any. Progress monitoring at every session can identify this issue when it arises and when it does, patient and therapist can have a collaborative discussion and decide to narrow the focus to one or two problems and return to the others later to see if this strategy produces better results.

COORDINATING THE WORK OF MULTIPLE PROVIDERS

Many or even most patients who receive CBT also receive other therapies, most commonly pharmacotherapy, couple therapy, or group therapy. The cognitive-behavior therapist strives to be sure that all the therapies in the patient's treatment plan have the same or complementary goals and that the mechanisms of action of the patient's various therapies are consistent or at least not conflicting. If the other therapies that a patient is receiving conflict with CBT, treatment can fail. The group therapist, for example, might be teaching the patient to avoid situations that the individual therapist is teaching the patient to confront.

Sometimes close coordination is not necessary. For example, it may be sufficient for the cognitive-behavior therapist to ascertain that the patient who has bipolar I disorder is receiving pharmacotherapy from a competent pharmacotherapist and to monitor the patient's medication adherence. In the case of a patient who complies easily and doesn't need hospitalization or other emergency interventions, extensive collaboration with the pharmacotherapist is not needed.

In other cases, close collaboration can be helpful. I find that if one of my individual patients is also receiving couple therapy, it is sometimes helpful to collaborate closely with the couple therapy so that the two therapies are pursuing complementary goals.

When Treatments Conflict

Problems can arise if the cognitive-behavior therapist's patient is also receiving other treatment that conflicts with the CBT in some way. Common examples include the patient who is carrying out exposures to overcome fears of somatic sensations while also taking drugs to eliminate them, and the person with GAD who is working to disengage from worry behavior and who is also working in an insight-oriented therapy to follow the chain of worry thoughts to see what insights they yield.

If a conflict arises, the cognitive-behavior therapist can make an effort to contact the other provider in an effort to coordinate the two treatments. However, this strategy is not always successful. Sometimes adjunct treatment providers are unresponsive or uncollaborative. One key to solving this problem is to remember that although the therapist does not have control over the behavior of these other clinicians, the patient ultimately does. Sometimes the therapist can affect those other clinicians' behavior by being a "consultant to the patient" (Linehan, 1993a). That is, the therapist can educate patients about their formulation and treatment needs and help them take effective action to get those needs met by all the clinicians on their treatment team.

Therapists have the greatest leverage to prevent and resolve conflicts between treatment components during the pretreatment phase, as discussed in Chapter 7. At this point they can refuse to go forward with a multiple-component treatment plan in which they do not have confidence. However, even after treatment has begun, the therapist always has the option to refuse to go forward with a faulty treatment plan. I recently worked with Colleen, who, a year into therapy, acquired a second pharmacotherapist that her first pharmacotherapist did not know about. Colleen didn't want the two pharmacotherapists to know about each other. This arrangement was not in Colleen's best interest and I was not comfortable with it. However, Colleen felt quite strongly, even desperately, that she needed this arrangement.

I decided (with some consultation!) to take three tacks in my discussion of this issue with Colleen. One was to work with Colleen to obtain a collaborative conceptualization of her behavior. It did not take long to figure out that the behavior of going along with one authority while keeping secrets from the other was a strategy that Colleen had learned to survive her upbringing in a chaotic and abusive environment. A second was to point out that although Colleen's secret keeping was needed for survival in the chaos in which she grew up, it was maladaptive in her current environment. Secret keeping alienated me by putting me in the position of participating in a treatment plan I did not have confidence in. It also jeopardized my professional reputation and relationships because when the clinician who was out of the loop discovered this, she would be angry at me, and rightly so, for not collaborating with her.

Third, I let Colleen know that I was not willing to continue with her two-pharmacotherapists-who-did-not-know-about-each-other plan but I would be happy to help her think through what she wanted to do. I also let Colleen know that she needed to resolve the issue fairly soon, because if any crisis arose for her (she was prone to crises), I would need to be in touch with both of her pharmacotherapists to alert them to the situation. I also let her know that if I should happen to get a call from either of the pharmacotherapists, I would provide full information about the other pharmaco-therapist. Colleen wasn't happy but she understood my position and within a couple of weeks she discontinued her work with one of the pharmacotherapists, which solved the problem.

In another case, one of my patients, Jenine, was receiving pharmacotherapy from a psychiatrist whose pharmacotherapy treatment plan seemed idiosyncratic to me and who did not return my telephone calls when I contacted him to discuss the treatment plan. In addition, I learned from Jenine that the psychiatrist's way of assessing her response to the medications he was providing was to observe her behavior in a non-directive psychotherapy he provided. I feared that a nondirective psychotherapy was not in her best interest because it promoted a type of passivity that we were working actively to counter and because it was so costly that it undermined her treatment goal of becoming financially independent of her mother. Not surprisingly, results of progress monitoring showed that Jenine was not improving.

I used my strong relationship with her and a series of interventions I carried out over many weeks to help Jenine clean up this mess. I reviewed with Jenine the results of our progress monitoring that showed she was not making good progress. I pointed out in a very direct way to Jenine that hers was a tough case and she needed a treatment team that worked well together. I let her know that she did not have that right now because despite my efforts to collaborate with her psychiatrist, he did not return my calls. I also reviewed with her the advantages and disadvantages of her psychiatrist's strategy of monitoring medication effectiveness by providing a second psychotherapy. Following these discussions, Jenine did an excellent job of asserting herself to solve the problems in her treatment. She asked the psychiatrist to discontinue the psycho-therapy, establish an objective system for monitoring her response to medications, and collaborate with me. When he was unresponsive to her requests, she discontinued her treatment with him and accepted my referral to a psychiatrist with whom I had a good working relationship.

Complicating the therapist's efforts to effectively coordinate multiple-component treatment plans is the fact that judging whether therapies conflict or support one another is difficult. Sometimes treatment plans that appear to conflict can work together to pro-duce a good result. When the situation is not a risky one, the therapist may elect to adopt an empirical approach and collect data to find out whether two therapies that might be expected to conflict actually do. Alexa sought treatment for OCD and insisted that she wanted to maintain her long-term relationship with her psychodynamic psychothera-pist. I let her know that this would not be my recommendation or preference but that if she wanted to do it I would try it, with the understanding that if she made progress I'd be comfortable continuing the arrangement and if she did not I would want to revisit the treatment plan and likely would not want to continue with the two-therapist plan. To my surprise, Alexa made excellent progress. She moved rapidly through her exposure hier-archy and terminated her treatment with me after accomplishing her treatment goals.

However, the therapist must not agree to a risky treatment plan or one assessed as unlikely to succeed. Early in my career I treated Annette, a very ill woman who experi-enced frequent suicidal crises. Annette had two individual therapists (I was one). When Annette felt suicidal, she sometimes called me and sometimes called the other therapist. As a result, I had difficulty gaining information about the antecedents and function of Annette's suicidal behavior. In addition, the other therapist and I responded differ-ently to the suicidal behavior. Not surprisingly, Annette did not make much progress in treatment. I learned my lesson and now I simply will not agree to a treatment plan that includes two individual therapists when the patient has risky self-harming or suicidal or other risky behaviors.

To summarize, the therapist strives to coordinate and collaborate with the provid-ers of all elements of a multiple-element treatment plan. The therapist strives to ensure that the mechanisms of action of the various therapies are consistent or at least not con-flicting, using the case formulation and collecting data to test hypotheses about this, and taking careful action to address the situation when this is not the case.

STAGES OF TREATMENT

Case formulation-driven CBT occurs in stages: *pretreatment, early treatment*, and *middle treatment*, ending with *termination*. In *pretreatment*, as already described (Chapters 5, 6, and 7), the therapist obtains a formulation and diagnosis, begins to establish a thera-peutic relationship, proposes a treatment plan, and obtains the patient's agreement to it. Here we hope that what Howard, Lueger, Maling, and Martinovich (1993) called remoralization begins. In *early treatment*, the patient and therapist flesh out the formula-tion and intervention plan and tackle a first problem or problems. If things go well, the patient obtains some symptom relief and gets into a smooth working rhythm with the therapist.

In *middle treatment*, work continues on the first problems and the therapist often begins layering on interventions to address other symptoms and problems. Some of this work is what Howard et al. (1993) called remediation—that is, tackling some of the psychosocial difficulties that triggered or laid the groundwork for the acute symptom exacerbation that propelled the patient into treatment. At the *termination* of treatment, patient and therapist review what was accomplished and help the patient make plans for handling similar difficulties should they recur. After termination, some patients return for booster sessions or for help with other problems or a return of symptoms.

Patterns of Change during Treatment

Little is known about the process of change during CBT or, indeed, any psychotherapy. There is some evidence that psychotherapy typically produces more rapid change at the beginning of treatment than later (Howard, Kopta, Krause, & Orlinsky, 1986; Lambert et al., 2001; Lutz, Martinovich, & Howard, 1999). This phenomenon is often called *early gains*. This pattern appears to be common in CBT for depression (Ilardi & Craighead, 1994; Fennell & Teasdale, 1987), bulimia nervosa (Agras et al., 2000), and substance abuse (Breslin et al., 1997).

An initial early gain is typically viewed by psychotherapy researchers as part of a larger picture of gradual change (Lutz et al., 1999). Even the statistical procedures used to study psychotherapy, such as repeated measures analysis of variance, assume that change is gradual (Thomas & Persons, 2008).

Other ideas about the pattern and process of change in psychotherapy include the sudden gains hypothesis, which proposes that change is not gradual. Instead, many patients show large symptom improvements following a single critical therapy session (Tang & DeRubeis, 1999; Tang, DeRubeis, Hollon, Amsterdam, & Shelton, 2007). Sudden gains have been shown to occur in many types of therapies (Busch, Kanter, Landes, & Kohlenberg, 2006; Gaynor et al., 2003; Tang, Luborsky, & Andrusyna, 2002). However, a recent study suggests that these marked fluctuations are consistent with a gradual change process (Thomas & Persons, 2008).

Other recent ideas about patterns of change in psychotherapy include the notion that an effective therapy might include a period of dysregulation, disorganization, and worsening in the process of reorganization to arrive at a new equilibrium (A. M. Hayes et al., 2007). In fact, this notion is consistent with Foa and Kozak's (1986) account of what happens in emotional processing to overcome phobic and anxiety disorders (described in Chapter 4). Emotional processing requires first activating the fear network before it can be changed. Consistent with this notion, Foa et al. (2002) showed that some PTSD sufferers showed a temporary exacerbation of symptoms in response to imaginal exposure. Another type of worsening that can happen in early or middle treatment is the increased chaos experienced by the patient (as in the example of Jason described above) who agrees to abandon maladaptive emotion regulation strategies (e.g., of self-harm or drug abuse) but then, in the early phases of recovery, experiences painful and chaotic emotions without many adaptive coping tools.

I return to these points as I discuss the early, middle, and termination stages of therapy in some detail and illustrate them with the case of Angela.

The Early Stage of Treatment

Although devising an initial formulation and specifying the elements of the treatment plan are pretreatment tasks, it is typically not until treatment is under way that the details of the formulation and the intervention plan begin to come into clear focus. As the patient brings in specific problem situations and behaviors, the therapist fleshes out the details of the formulation, makes decisions about how to intervene, and collects data to test the effectiveness of his or her approach. When things go smoothly in early treatment, patient and therapist get in a good rhythm of working together so that by session 6 or 8 the therapy is well under way and the patient has made the early gains that are often seen in a successful treatment (see Figure 12.1).

Revising the Formulation and Intervention Plan

Sometimes as treatment gets under way, new information comes in that leads to a major shift in the formulation and intervention plan, as in the case of Al. He sought treatment for depression, anxiety, and conflict in his marriage. Al had a high-powered job as an executive in a Japanese-owned firm. The firm culture called for heavy drinking several nights a week. Al did not perceive this to be a problem, insisting that everyone he worked with did the same. Al and I had agreed on goals of improving the marriage and

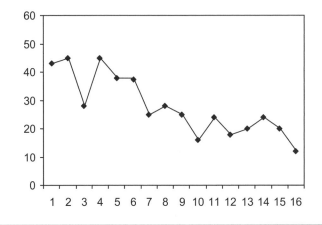

FIGURE 12.1. Plot of BDI score at each session for a patient who has a good outcome.

reducing his depression and anxiety. We had agreed to disagree about the role of alcohol. I included it on my Problem List but Al did not see it as a problem and he was unwilling to set a treatment goal of reducing his alcohol intake. However, he had agreed that treatment would include a discussion of our disagreement about the alcohol problem.

Al's highest-priority problem was the conflict in his marriage. His wife had refused couple therapy, so we were working in his individual therapy to see what we could do to improve the marriage. In an early session, Al and I carried out a behavioral chain analysis (see Chapter 3) of a spat with his wife. What stood out for me as we reviewed the chain analysis was one of the antecedents of the fight: Al had been drinking. When I pointed this out, Al opined that drinking had not been a factor in the argument. However, he agreed to collect some data to test our competing hypotheses. He agreed to record, at the end of every day, the time and amount of alcohol he drank and whether or not he and his wife had had fought. After three weeks of collecting these data, Al came to his session admitting that, much to his surprise, his log clearly showed that all but one of the recent fights with his wife had happened on nights that he had been out late drinking with his work buddies. As soon as he saw this pattern in data that he himself had collected, Al identified his drinking as a problem and began taking steps to reduce it.

Al's case illustrates the point that sometimes it is only after treatment begins that a full conceptualization and adequate treatment plan can be obtained. In Al's case, an extended collaborative hypothesis-testing process was needed to obtain a full conceptualization of how alcohol and marital conflict were related for him. That conceptualization led to a major shift in his treatment goals and our intervention plan.

Shifting the Focus of Treatment to Address the Next Set of Problems

Sometimes as the patient makes progress in handling the first set of difficulties tackled in therapy, the next set comes to the fore. The therapist uses the formulation to understand how the new problems are related to the original ones and to decide whether to shift focus onto them. To illustrate this point, let's return to the case of Angela discussed in Chapters 5, 6, and 7. To recap, she had diagnoses of PTSD and depression precipitated by an assault at work. We started her therapy by using activity scheduling to help Angela get more active and engaged in her life. She began exercising, having e-mail correspondence with colleagues at work, participating in her kids' activities, and interacting more with her husband.

As she got more active, Angela began reporting that she felt angry and was experiencing interpersonal tension and conflicts. This was not surprising. In fact, anger was one of Angela's presenting problems (see Figure 5.7). The trauma she experienced had involved an angry conflict. And Angela had told me in the first session how angry she was at her boss and colleagues. Nevertheless, based on my formulation hypothesis that disengagement and avoidance drove many of her symptoms, I had focused first on those. As she broke through her avoidance and began engaging with people and problems in her life, Angela's anger came to the fore.

As the anger came up, I shifted the therapy to focus on it for several reasons. First, it was making Angela quite uncomfortable and she wanted help with it. Second, it interfered both at work and at home. At work she felt furious and reported thoughts that her boss and colleagues should have been more supportive and had "stabbed me in the back," and at home she was angry that her husband was so unavailable and her kids so ill behaved.

Third, I speculated, based on my formulation (see Figure 5.7), that Angela's depression resulted from her handling difficult situations by withdrawing. Withdrawal allowed her to avoid the conflicts, and her anger about them, but also deprived her of the opportunity to get pleasure and joy from her relationships and her work. As a result she had become depressed (Lewinsohn & Gotlib, 1995; Martell et al., 2001). Now that Angela was beginning to reengage, the anger was back. We would need to address it or she would be under pressure to withdraw again.

Finally, anger often interferes with active problem solving. For example, Beck's cognitive model proposes that anger often results when a person responds to an interpersonal problem with the attitude "They *shouldn't* behave that way." This stance impedes problem solving. In contrast, problem solving flows out of the attitude "They *are* behaving that way. I don't like it. What can I do about it?"

Thus, my decision to shift the focus of Angela's treatment to anger was based on many factors, including a formulation hypothesis about the relationship of Angela's anger to her other symptoms and problems. My intervention plan for addressing her anger was also guided by formulation hypotheses about the anger that I developed by working with Angela to flesh out the details of the causes of her anger in particular situations. I used a Thought Record (Figure 2.3) and found that the cognitive model's formulation accounted well for some of the early situations we tackled, where her "should-y" (Ellis, 1962) thinking was much in evidence. Based on this formulation hypothesis, I asked Angela to read Chapter 7 of Burns (1999) and I also recommended McKay's book (McKay, Rogers, & McKay, 1989). Detailed assessment of situations in which she experienced anger also indicated that Angela did not have a repertoire of good interpersonal problem-solving skills, so I began doing some skills teaching, including using the DEAR MAN tool in Linehan (1993b).

In session 6 Angela and I focused on a screaming match that she had had with her husband when they were cooking dinner the previous evening. We did a Thought Record and I taught her some skills she could use to prevent a quarrel the next time a similar situation arose. As we wrapped our work on this conflict, Angela spontaneously stated, "I need to and I'm ready to take responsibility for my role in the assault at work." This was a big step forward. Its importance was reflected in an improvement in Angela's BDI scores (Figure 12.2) beginning in session 6 and solidifying in session 8.

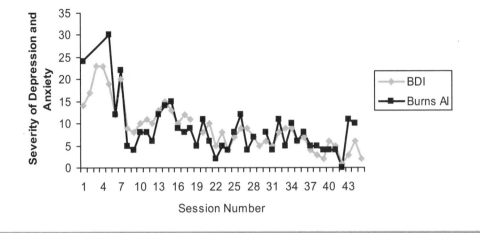

FIGURE 12.2. Severity of symptoms of depression and anxiety for Angela at each session.

To summarize, in the *early stage* of treatment, the patient and therapist work to flesh out and implement the details of the initial formulation and intervention plan. This work is sometimes a smooth continuation of work that began in pretreatment. But sometimes it requires a major change in the formulation and intervention plan, as in Al's case. And sometimes, after some early gains in response to the initial interventions, a shift in the focus of treatment when new issues come to the fore, as in Angela's case.

The Middle Stage of Treatment

When things are going well in the middle stage of treatment, the problems tackled in early treatment have been solved or are on the way to being solved. Patient and therapist have a good alliance and are working well together. The patient is doing homework assignments to practice the skills he or she is learning with less supervision and guidance than was needed in early treatment. Now the therapist often begins layering on interventions to address other disorders and symptoms, difficulties in functioning, or psychosocial stressors that precipitated the distress that brought the patient to treatment.

Often in the middle treatment stage the pace of change slows. This is typically because the patient has achieved some substantial symptom relief and there is less room for symptom change than there was at the beginning of therapy. In addition, patients often begin to work on problems that are more difficult to change. For example, they may begin working to change their job, career choice, relationship with their partner, or social isolation. Progress on these issues can proceed slowly and extend over many weeks, months, or even years.

Revising the Formulation and Intervention Plan

Sometimes in middle treatment (as in early treatment) new information comes out that leads to a change in the formulation and intervention plan. One example is the case of a patient I identified in pretreatment as having major depressive disorder and panic disorder. She only felt comfortable telling me about her PTSD symptoms (she had been raped) four months into therapy.

In Angela's case I also obtained new information in middle treatment that led to a shift in her formulation and intervention plan. Following the breakthrough in session 6 when Angela took responsibility for her role in the assault, we carried out a chain analysis of the events leading up to the assault. The chain analysis and the discussion that followed from it revealed several new pieces of information. I learned that the assault had occurred in a context of long-simmering resentment about how this client treated her and how little support she received from her boss for her work with this difficult client. More generally, I learned that Angela had a history of tolerating significant levels of resentment and unhappiness for long periods of time without being fully aware of these feelings. Because she was unaware of it, Angela did not take any steps to address her unhappiness. For example, although she felt unsupported by her boss for her work with this client, she had not taken any effective action to get help from her boss or colleagues.

Angela also had a history of interpersonal conflict and impulsivity. She had had a major blowup with a colleague the previous year that had led to an entry in her personnel record. We discussed and tied all these phenomena to her upbringing in an abusive environment in which her father frequently blew up and physically abused his children. At the same time the family maintained the fiction that family life was good and the kids had had a happy childhood.

This discussion illuminated aspects of Angela's case that I had not included in my original formulation of her case: her failure to attend to and acknowledge emotional distress, poor interpersonal problem-solving skills, impulsivity, and interpersonal conflicts. This new information led me to reformulate Angela's case using a hypothesis that deficits in emotion regulation were at the heart of her difficulties. Although I did not sit down to write out the new formulation, if I had, it would have looked like this.

Angela grew up in an abusive environment in which she learned to ignore, invalidate, and minimize her own emotional experience, especially when she was distressed. As a result of this mode of functioning and numerous stressors at home and work, she had been depressed, unhappy, and resentful in the months or even years before the assault at work without being fully aware of this fact. She also had interpersonal skills deficits and was especially poor at asking for help from others. (Angela's parents had not modeled these skills and in fact had modeled the behavior she was using—invalidating herself, suppressing emotions, and then losing control). As a result, Angela experienced periodic impulsive angry conflicts with others, both at home and work. When she found herself involved in a conflict with a client she had long felt angry at, she verbally attacked him and he responded by physically attacking her. Angela coped with the negative emotions this event provoked by minimizing and avoiding them, which promoted the development of PTSD symptoms and prevented her from resuming work. The loss of reinforcers at work and home she experienced as a result of her avoidant coping with PTSD symptoms and related stressors increased her depressive symptoms. Unemployment led to financial and marital problems.

This new formulation gave a more central role to avoidance of affect, anger, impulsivity, and interpersonal conflict than did the original formulation based on operant conditioning theory (Figure 5.7). The new formulation led to several changes in the Treatment Plan. We set a new goal of reducing interpersonal conflict and new mechanism change goals of learning to identify, validate, and acknowledge (instead of avoiding and suppressing) negative emotions and learning interpersonal skills, especially assertiveness, to ask effectively to get her needs met. This plan led to a number of new interventions that did not flow out of the earlier conditioning formulation. These included self-monitoring and other interventions to help Angela attend to, validate, identify, and make effective use of information about her emotions, and skills training to teach assertiveness skills.

Brief Symptomatic Worsening

In the middle treatment stage, as in early treatment, the case formulation can help the therapist predict some symptomatic worsening as the depressed patient (or any patient) begins approaching problems he or she previously avoided. I warned Angela that as she approached the date she had set to return to work (just before session 12), she would likely get more distressed, and she did (see Figure 12.2). I explained the formulation to her so she would understand why she felt worse, why feeling worse was progress, and that her choice was to retreat back to depression or tolerate the increased distress, learn to manage it, and push on through to the other side. Angela indicated that she was ready to do what was needed to keep moving ahead.

As she got ready to return to work, I added cognitive and behavioral strategies to help Angela cope as her anxiety and other PTSD symptoms intensified. Most of her anxiety was about how to handle interpersonal situations (e.g., how to behave with people who had "stabbed me in the back") and I intervened with skills teaching, including role plays. Shortly after returning to work, Angela had two nightmares of being chased by people who were trying to kill her. In one of them she killed her antagonist. This was a flare-up of PTSD experiencing symptoms. I addressed it with psychoeducation about PTSD, positive activity scheduling, and continued monitoring of negative emotions and work on assertiveness. I told Angela that I expected these strategies in the context of the *in vivo* exposure to the work situation to reduce her symptoms but that if reexperiencing symptoms continued, we could do some imaginal exposure. This proved unnecessary. The reexperiencing symptoms gradually died down as Angela continued going to work, monitoring her emotions, and working actively to practice assertiveness and other interpersonal skills to improve relationships with her boss and colleagues.

Conducting a Progress Review

If the middle stage of treatment is long, it is a good idea to carry out a periodic progress review. Ideally, this should happen every quarter (12 sessions or so) but certainly every 6 months (26 sessions), using the methods described in Chapter 9. I did this with Angela in session 17 in the context of preparing a progress report for her workers' compensation insurance carrier. She had not yet returned to work full time so was still receiving some benefits. Angela and I reviewed her goals. She had reached her goals of reducing depressive symptoms to a BDI of less than 10 and improving her interactions with her husband and kids. She was back to work three-quarter time but not yet full time and was able to encounter "problem people" at work with little or no distress. She had made excellent progress.

However, Angela and I agreed that more work was needed on her goal of reducing interpersonal conflicts. She was still finding herself flaring up with her husband more than she wanted and had found herself sending impulsive ill-advised e-mail messages to colleagues and clients. She also needed a bit more help feeling comfortable about returning to work full time. As we discussed her progress, Angela stated that she felt she was not advocating effectively for the specialized services her diabetic child needed. She set a new goal of improving her skills and activity in that arena.

Working on Multiple Domains Simultaneously

In the middle phase of treatment, the patient and therapist often work on the same issues repeatedly and in multiple domains. This was true in Angela's case. We worked on increasing her ability to identify and acknowledge unpleasant emotions and use them as guides to appropriate action. This included asserting herself to make requests of others and giving positive reinforcement when others treated her well. We worked on those issues in her interactions with peers and superiors at work, with her husband and children, and with her children's teachers and health care providers.

Sometimes in this phase therapy begins winding down and the therapist recommends meeting less frequently. This strategy helps patient and therapist assess whether the patient can maintain the new skills learned and the gains he achieved in therapy without regular sessions.

Termination

When things go well, treatment comes to an end when outcome monitoring, a progress review, or the patient indicates that the goals of treatment have been accomplished or when patients feel confident they can leave therapy and continue to move forward on their own to accomplish their goals. In a productive final session, patient and therapist carry out a series of tasks, including:

- Review the patient's treatment goals.
- Review the progress toward the goals. Methods for doing this are described in Chapter 9 in the section on longer-term monitoring. It is useful to review progress toward each of the patient's treatment goals.
- Review tools or ideas that were learned in therapy. It can be helpful to make a list of these in the termination session. This list provides useful feedback to the therapist and is one that the patient can pull out when problems reemerge and coping tools are needed.
- Teach the patient about the risk of relapse or the chronicity of his or her disorder.
- Discuss or make a plan for determining when the patient needs to reinstate coping or return to therapy.

In the case of a chronic disorder, the therapist will want to educate the patient about the need for ongoing use of the skills learned in therapy to keep functioning at its maximum and symptoms at their minimum. Sometimes I give patients a copy of the monitoring tools (e.g., the Mood Chart or the Burns AI) we used to track symptoms so they can use these to evaluate their status.

In the case of a patient who is at risk of relapse, a review of the events that triggered the symptoms and pushed the patient into treatment can help predict future times of vulnerability (e.g., moving, relationship rupture). For example, Suzanne learned in therapy that she was vulnerable to a manic episode at times of transition (e.g., a change in schedule) or stress. She also learned that early signs of an impending manic episode included difficulty sleeping, urges to make lots of long-distance phone calls, and paranoid thoughts about her husband wanting to harm her. At the end of therapy we reviewed the lists we had made during therapy of her times of vulnerability and early signs of mania. We also reviewed and listed all the strategies she had learned to help her cope when symptoms emerged (e.g., alert her husband to the situation and ask for his help, reduce stress, reduce activity level, and temporarily increase some of her medications). Suzanne took these lists and plans with her when she ended her treatment with me and moved to another city when her husband's job was relocated.

In Angela's final session, which was her 45th session, we carried out all of these tasks. When we reviewed her goals she reported that she had accomplished them all except that she needed to continue to practice remaining mindful of her negative emotions and using her interpersonal skills to reduce distress and interpersonal conflict. I also reminded her that dysthymia was a chronic problem and MDD a recurrent one and that she would need to continue to use coping tools to manage her mood and to remain alert for relapse. We also agreed that she needed to continue to work on her relationship with her husband.

When I asked Angela what she had learned in therapy, she reported this list:

- Figure out how I feel. Pay attention to my feelings.
- Thank my husband for the good stuff he does.
- Refocus on positives with both my husband and my kids.
- Be assertive.
- Exercise.

Angela and I agreed that she was ready to discontinue her psychotherapy but would continue her pharmacotherapy and return for a check-in session if her BDI score rose above 15 for 3 weeks in a row.

Angela's therapy was a success. Of course, success is always desirable. However, to conclude this chapter—and the book—I would like to propose that good quality care has more to do with process than outcome. That is, the most important feature of good quality care is to follow a systematic and empirical process in the context of a collaborative and caring therapeutic relationship. Following the steps represented in Figure 1.1, the therapist works with the patient to assess, diagnose, formulate, obtain informed consent, intervene, and assess again. First-line formulations and interventions are based on empirically supported therapies and theories. And the therapist uses an empirical hypothesis-testing approach to each case. Even when success is elusive, therapists using these methods can feel confident they are providing top-quality care.

References

Abramson, L. Y., Seligman, M. E. P., & Teasdale, J. (1978). Learned helplessness in humans: Critique and reformulation. *Journal of Abnormal Psychology, 87*, 49–74.

Abramson, L. Y., Metalsky, G. I., & Alloy, L. B. (1989). Hopelessness depression: A theory-based subtype of depression. *Psychological Review, 96*, 358–372.

Acocella, J. (2003, January 6). Second act. *The New Yorker*, pp. 48–61.

Addis, M. E., & Carpenter, K. M. (2000). The treatment rationale in cognitive behavioral therapy: Psychological mechanisms and clinical guidelines. *Cognitive and Behavioral Practice, 7*, 147–156.

Agras, W. S., Crow, S. J., Halmi, K. A., Mitchell, J. E., Wilson, G. T., & Kraemer, H. C. (2000). Outcome predictors for the cognitive behavior treatment of bulimia nervosa: Data from a multisite study. *American Journal of Psychiatry, 157*(8), 1302–1308.

Albano, A. M. (2003). *Modularized cognitive behavioral treatment of depression and its comorbidities in adolescents.* Paper presented at the annual meeting of the Association for Advancement of Behavior Therapy, Boston.

Alexander, F., & French, T. M. (1946). *Psychoanalytic therapy: Principles and applications.* New York: Ronald Press.

American Psychiatric Association. (2000). *Diagnostic and statistical manual of mental disorders* (4th ed., text rev.). Washington, DC: Author.

American Psychological Association. (1992). Ethical principles of psychologists and code of conduct. *American Psychologist, 47*, 1597–1611.

Arkowitz, H., & Westra, H. A. (2004). Integrating motivational interviewing and cognitive behavioral therapy in the treatment of depression and anxiety. *Journal of Cognitive Psychotherapy: An International Quarterly, 18*(4), 337–350.

Arntz, A., & Wertman, A. (1999). Treatment of childhood memories: Theory and practice. *Behaviour Reseach and Therapy, 37*, 715–740.

Bandura, A. (1977). *Social learning theory.* Englewood Cliffs, NJ: Prentice-Hall.

Barber, J. P., & DeRubeis, R. J. (1989). On second thought: Where the action is in cognitive therapy for depression. *Cognitive Therapy and Research, 13*, 441–457.

Barkham, M., Margison, F., Leach, C., Lucock, M., Mellor-Clark, J., Evans, C., et al. (2001). Service profiling and outcomes benchmarking using the CORE-OM: Toward practice-based evidence in the psychological therapies. *Journal of Consulting and Clinical Psychology, 69*, 184–196.

Barkley, R. A., & Benton, C. M. (1998). *Your defiant child: Eight steps to better behavior.* New York: Guilford Press.

Barkley, R. A., Edwards, G. H., & Robin, A. L. (1999). *Defiant teens: A clinician's manual for assessment and family intervention.* New York: Guilford Press.

Barlow, D. H. (2002). *Anxiety and its disorders: The nature and treatment of anxiety and panic* (2nd ed.). New York: Guilford Press.

Barlow, D. H., Allen, L. B., & Choate, M. L. (2002, November 14–17). *All for one and one for all: Treating anxiety and related disorders with a single, unified protocol.* Paper presented at the annual meeting of the Association for Advancement of Behavior Therapy, Reno, NV.

Barlow, D. H., & Chorpita, B. F. (1998). The development of anxiety: The role of control in the early environment. *Psychological Bulletin, 124,* 3–24.

Barlow, D. H., & Craske, M. G. (2000). *Mastery of your anxiety and panic: Client workbook for anxiety and panic.* San Antonio, TX: Graywind Publications.

Barlow, D. H., Gorman, J. M., Shear, M. K., & Woods, S. W. (2000). Cognitive-behavioral therapy, imipramine, or their combination for panic disorder. *Journal of the American Medical Association, 283*(19), 2529–2536.

Barlow, D. H., Hayes, S. C., & Nelson, R. O. (1984). *The scientist-practitioner: Research and accountability in clinical and educational settings.* New York: Pergamon Press.

Barnard, P. J., & Teasdale, J. D. (1991). Interacting cognitive subsystems: A systematic approach to cognitive-affective interaction and change. *Cognition and Emotion, 5,* 1–39.

Barrett, L. F., Gross, J., Christensen, T. C., & Benvenuto, M. (2001). Knowing what you're feeling and knowing what to do about it: Mapping the relation between emotion differentiation and emotion regulation. *Cognition and Emotion, 15,* 713–724.

Basco, M. R., & Rush, A. J. (1996). *Cognitive-behavioral therapy for bipolar disorder.* New York: Guilford Press.

Bates, A., & Clark, D. M. (1998). A new cognitive treatment for social phobia: A single-case study. *Journal of Cognitive Psychotherapy: An International Quarterly, 12*(4), 289–302.

Baxter, L. R., Schwartz, J. M., Bergman, K. S., Szuba, M. P., Guze, B. H., Mazziotta, J. C., et al. (1992). Caudate glucose metabolic rate changes with both drug and behavior therapy for obsessive–compulsive disorder. *Archives of General Psychiatry, 49,* 681–689.

Beck, A. T. (1976). *Cognitive therapy and the emotional disorders.* New York: International Universities Press.

Beck, A. T. (1983). *Cognitive theory of depression: New perspectives.* In P. J. Clayton & J. E. Barrett (Eds.), *Treatment of depression: Old controversies and new approaches* (pp. 265–288). New York: Raven Press.

Beck, A. T. (2005). The current state of cognitive therapy. *Archives of General Psychiatry, 62,* 953–959.

Beck, A. T., Brown, G., Berchick, R., Stewart, B. L., & Steer, R. A. (1990). Relationship between hopelessness and ultimate suicide: A replication with psychiatric outpatients. *American Journal of Psychiatry, 147,* 190–195.

Beck, A. T., Butler, A. C., Brown, G. K., Dahlsgaard, K. K., Newman, C. F., & Beck, J. S. (2001). Dysfunctional beliefs discriminate personality disorders. *Behaviour Research and Therapy, 39*(10), 1213–1225.

Beck, A. T., Emery, G., & Greenberg, R. L. (1985). *Anxiety disorders and phobias: A cognitive perspective.* New York: Basic Books.

Beck, A. T., Epstein, N., Brown, G., & Steer, R. (1988). An inventory for measuring clinical anxiety: Psychometric properties. *Journal of Consulting and Clinical Psychology, 56,* 893–897.

Beck, A. T., Freeman, A., Davis, D. D., & Associates. (2004). *Cognitive therapy of personality disorders* (2nd ed.). New York: Guilford Press.

Beck, A. T., Rush, J. A., Shaw, B. F., & Emery, G. (1979). *Cognitive therapy of depression.* New York: Guilford Press.

Beck, A. T., Steer, R. A., & Brown, G. K. (1996). *Manual for Beck Depression Inventory-II.* San Antonio, TX: Psychological Corporation.

Beck, A. T., Wright, F. D., Newman, C. F., & Liese, B. S. (1993). *Cognitive therapy of substance abuse.* New York: Guilford Press.

Beck, J. S. (1995). *Cognitive therapy: Basics and beyond.* New York: Guilford Press.

Beck, R., & Fernandez, E. (1998). Cognitive-behavioral therapy in the treatment of anger: A meta-analysis. *Cognitive Therapy and Research, 22,* 63–74.

Becker, C. B., & Zayfert, C. (2001). Integrating DBT-based techniques and concepts to facilitate exposure treatment for PTSD. *Cognitive and Behavioral Practice, 8,* 107–122.

Becker, C. B., Zayfert, C., & Anderson, E. (2004). A survey of psychologists' attitudes towards and utilization of exposure therapy for PTSD. *Behaviour Research and Therapy, 42,* 277–292.

Beevers, C. G., Wenzlaff, R. M., Hayes, A. M., & Scott, W. D. (1999). Depression and the ironic effects of thought suppression: Therapeutic strategies for improving mental control. *Clinical Psychology: Science and Practice, 6*(2), 133–148.

Bell, J. (2007). *Rewind, replay, repeat.* Center City, MN: Hazelden.

Bennett-Levy, J., Butler, G., Fennell, M., Hackmann, A., Mueller, M., & Westbrook, D. (Eds.). (2004). *Oxford guide to behavioural experiments in cognitive therapy.* Oxford: Oxford University Press.

Bernstein, D., & Borkovec, T. (1973). *Progressive muscle relaxation: A manual for the helping professions.* Champaign, IL: Research Press.

Bloom, M., Fischer, J., & Orme, J. G. (1995). *Evaluating practice: Guidelines for the accountable professional.* Boston: Allyn & Bacon.

Boice, R. (1983). Contingency management in writing and the appearance of creative ideas: Implications for the treatment of writing blocks. *Behaviour Research and Therapy, 21,* 537–544.

Bordin, E. (1979). The generalizability of the psychoanalytic concept of the working alliance. *Psychotherapy, 16,* 252–260.

Borkovec, T. D. (1994). The nature, functions, and origins of worry. In G. C. L. Davey & F. Tallis (Eds.), *Worrying: Perspectives on theory, assessment and treatment* (pp. 5–33). New York: Wiley.

Borkovec, T. D. (2002). Life in the future versus life in the present. *Clinical Psychology Science and Practice, 9,* 76–80.

Borkovec, T. D., Alcaine, O., & Behar, E. (2004). Avoidance theory of worry and generalized anxiety disorder. In R. G. Heimberg, C. L. Turk, & D. S. Mennin (Eds.), *Generalized anxiety disorder: Advances in research and practice.* New York: Guilford Press.

Bouton, M. E. (1988). Context and ambiguity in the extinction of emotional learning: Implications for exposure therapy. *Behaviour Research and Therapy, 26,* 137–149.

Bouton, M. E. (2002). Context, ambiguity, and unlearning: Sources of relapse after behavioral extinction. *Biological Psychiatry, 52,* 976–986.

Bouton, M. E., Mineka, S., & Barlow, D. H. (2001). A modern learning-theory perspective on the etiology of panic disorder. *Psychological Review, 108*(1), 4–32.

Bower, G. H. (1981). Mood and memory. *American Psychologist, 36,* 129–148.

Breslin, F. C., Sobell, M. B., Sobell, L. C., Buchan, G., & Cunningham, J. A. (1997). Toward a stepped care approach to treating problem drinkers: The predictive utility of within-treatment variables and therapist prognostic ratings. *Addiction, 92,* 1479–1489.

Brewin, C. R. (1989). Cognitive change processes in psychotherapy. *Psychological Review, 96*(3), 379–394.

Brewin, C. R. (2006). Understanding cognitive behaviour therapy: A retrieval competition account. *Behavioral Research and Therapy, 44,* 765–784.

Brody, J. (2000, June 20). How germ phobia can lead to illness. *New York Times,* p. D8.

Brown, T. A., Chorpita, B., & Barlow, D. H. (1998). Structural relationships among dimensions of the DSM-IV anxiety and mood disorders and dimensions of negative affect, positive affect, and autonomic arousal. *Journal of Abnormal Psychology, 107,* 179–192.

Brown, G. K., Haye, T. T., Henriques, G. R., Xie, S. X., Hollander, J. E., & Beck, A. T. (2005). Cognitive therapy for the prevention of suicide attempts: A randomized controlled trial. *Journal of the American Medical Association, 294*(5), 563–570.

Brown, M. Z., Comtois, K. A., & Linehan, M. M. (2002). Reasons for suicide attempts and nonsuicidal self-injury in women with borderline personality disorder. *Journal of Abnormal Psychology, 111,* 198–202.

Brown, T. A., DiNardo, P. A., & Barlow, D. H. (1994). *Anxiety disorders interview schedule for DSM-IV: Lifetime version (ADIS-IV-L).* Albany, NY: Graywind Publications.

Burns, D. D. (1980). *Feeling good: The new mood therapy.* New York: Morrow.

Burns, D. D. (1989a). Agenda setting: How to make therapy productive when you and your patient feel stuck. In *The Feeling Good Handbook: Using the New Mood Therapy in Everyday Life* (pp. 523–543). New York: Morrow.

Burns, D. D. (1989b). *The feeling good handbook: Using the new mood therapy in everyday life.* New York: Morrow.

Burns, D. D. (1997). *Therapist's toolkit.* Available at *www.feelinggood.com.*

Burns, D. D. (1999). *Feeling good: The new mood therapy.* New York: Morrow.

Burns, D. D., & Eidelson, R. (1998). Why are measures of depression and anxiety correlated?: I. A test of tripartite theory. *Journal of Consulting and Clinical Psychology, 60,* 441–449.

Burns, D. D., & Nolen-Hoeksema, S. (1992). Therapeutic empathy and recovery from depression in cognitive-behavioral therapy: A structural equation model. *Journal of Consulting and Clinical Psychology, 60,* 441–449.

Burns, D. D., & Persons, J. B. (1982). Hope and hopelessness: A cognitive approach. In L. E. Abt & I. R. Stuart (Eds.), *The newer therapies: A workbook* (pp. 35–57). New York: Van Nostrand Reinhold.

Busch, A. M., Kanter, J. W., Landes, S. J., & Kohlenberg, R. J. (2006). Sudden gains and outcome: A broader temporal analysis of cognitive therapy for depression. *Behavior Therapy, 37,* 61–68.

Butler, A. C., Chapman, J. E., Forman, E. M., & Beck, A. T. (2006). The empirical status of cognitive-behavioral therapy: A review of meta-analyses. *Clinical Psychology Review, 26,* 17–31.

Butler, G., Fennell, M., & Hackmann, A. (2008). *Cognitive-behavioral therapy for anxiety disorders: Mastering clinical challenges.* New York: Guilford Press.

Caire, J. B. (1991). The forbidden zone: Managing resistance in patients with obsessive–compulsive disorders. *Behavior Therapist, 14,* 75–76.

Castonguay, L. G., & Beutler, L. E. (Eds.). (2006). *Principles of therapeutic change that work.* New York: Oxford University Press.

Castonguay, L. G., Goldfried, M. R., Wiser, S., Raue, P. J., & Hayes, A. M. (1996). Predicting the effect of cognitive therapy for depressoin: A study of unique and common factors. *Journal of Consulting and Clinical Psychology, 64,* 497–504.

Cautela, J. R. (1967). Covert sensitization. *Psychological Reports, 20,* 459–468.

Chambless, D. L., Caputo, G., Bright, P., & Gallagher, R. (1984). Assessment of fear in agoraphobics: The Body Sensations Questionnaire and the Agoraphobic Cognitions Questionnaire. *Journal of Consulting and Clinical Psychology, 52,* 1090–1097.

Chambless, D. L., Caputo, G. C., Jasin, S. E., Gracely, E. J., & Williams, C. (1985). The Mobility Inventory for Agoraphobia. *Behaviour Research and Therapy, 23,* 35–44.

Chiles, J. A., & Strosahl, K. D. (1995). *The suicidal patient: Principles of assessment, treatment, and case management.* Washington, D.C.: American Psychiatric Press.

Chorpita, B. F. (2006). *Modular cognitive behavior therapy for childhood anxiety disorders.* New York: Guilford Press.

Clark, D. M. (1986). A cognitive approach to panic. *Behaviour Research and Therapy, 24,* 461–470.

Clark, D. M. (2001). A cognitive perspective on social phobia. In W. R. Crozier & L. E. Alden (Eds.), *International handbook of social anxiety: Concepts, research and interventions relating to the self* (pp. 405–430). Chichester, UK: Wiley.

Clark, D. M., & Wells, A. (1995). A cognitive model of social phobia. In R. G. Heimberg, M. R. Liebowitz, D. A. Hope, & F. R. Schneier (Eds.), *Social phobia: Diagnosis, assessment, and treatment* (pp. 69–93). New York: Guilford Press.

Clore, G. L., & Ortony, A. (2000). Cognition in emotion: Always, sometimes, or never? In R. D. Lane & L. Nadel (Eds.), *Cognitive neuroscience of emotion* (pp. 24–61). New York: Oxford University Press.

Cohen, L. H., Gunthert, K. C., Butler, A. C., O'Neill, S. C., & Tolpin, L. H. (2005). Daily affective reactivity as a prospective predictor of depressive symptoms. *Journal of Personality, 73*(6), 1–27.

Cone, J. D. (2001). *Evaluating outcomes: Empirical tools for effective practice.* Washington, DC: American Psychological Association.

Curry, J., & Reinecke, M. (2003). Modular therapy for adolescents with major depression. In M. Reinecke, F. Dattilio, & A. Freeman (Eds.), *Cognitive therapy with children and adolescents* (pp. 95–128). New York: Guilford Press.

Davidson, J., Martinez, K. A., & Thomas, C. (2006). *Validation of a new measure of functioning and satisfaction for use in outpatient clinical practice.* Chicago, IL: Association for Behavioral and Cognitive Therapies.

Davidson, J., Persons, J. B., & Tompkins, M. A. (2000). *Cognitive-behavior therapy for depression: Structure of the therapy session* [videotape]. Washington, D.C.: American Psychological Association.

Deblinger, E., Thakkar-Kolar, R., & Ryan, E. (2006). Trauma in childhood. In V. M. Follette & J. I. Ruzek (Eds.), *Cognitive-behavioral therapies for trauma* (2nd ed.). New York: Guilford Press.

Deffenbacher, J. L., & McKay, M. (1998). *Overcoming situational and general anger: Therapist protocol.* Oakland, CA: New Harbinger.

Depue, R. A., & Iacono, W. G. (1989). Neurobehavioral aspects of affective disorders. *Annual Review of Psychology, 40,* 457–492.

Derogatis, L. R. (2000). *Symptom Checklist-90—Revised.* Washington, DC: American Psychological Association.

DeRubeis, R. J., & Feeley, M. (1990). Determinants of change in cognitive therapy for depression. *Cognitive Therapy and Research, 14*(5), 469–482.

DeRubeis, R. J., Hollon, S. D., Amsterdam, J. D., Shelton, R. C., Young, P. R., Salomon, R. M., et al. (2005). Cognitive therapy vs. medication in the treatment of moderate to severe depression. *Archives of General Psychiatry, 62*(4), 409–416.

Dimburg, U., & Ohman, A. (1996). Behold the wrath: Psychophysiological responses to facial stimuli. *Motivation and Emotions, 20,* 149–182.

Dimeff, L. A., & Koerner, K. (Eds.). (2007). *Dialectical behavior therapy in clinical practice: Applications across disorders and settings.* New York: Guilford Press.

Dimidjian, S., Hollon, S. D., Dobson, K., Schmaling, K. B., Kohlenberg, R. J., Addis, M. E., et al. (2006). Randomized trial of behavioral activation, cognitive therapy, and antidepressant medication in the acute treatment of adults with major depression. *Journal of Consulting and Clinical Psychology, 74*(4), 658–670.

Dobson, K. S., & Cheung, E. (1990). Relationship between anxiety and depression: Conceptual and methodological issues. In J. D. Maser & C. R. Cloninger (Eds.), *Comorbidity of mood and anxiety disorders* (pp. 611–632). Washington, DC: American Psychiatric Press.

Dougher, M. J. (Ed.). (2000). *Clinical behavior analysis.* Reno, NV: Context Press.

Duffy, M., Gillespie, K., & Clark, D. M. (2007). Post traumatic stress disorder in the context of terrorism and other civil conflict in Northern Ireland: Randomised controlled trial. *British Medical Journal.* Available online at: *doi:10.1136/bmj.39021.846852.BE.*

Dunn, R. L., & Schwebel, A. I. (1995). Meta-analytic review of marital therapy outcome research. *Journal of Family Psychology, 9,* 58–68.

Ehlers, A., & Clark, D. M. (2000). A cognitive model of posttraumatic stress disorder. *Behaviour Research and Therapy, 38,* 319–345.

Eifert, G. H., Evans, I. M., & McKendrick, V. G. (1990). Matching treatments to client problems not diagnostic labels: A case for paradigmatic behavior therapy. *Journal of Behavior Therapy and Experimental Psychiatry, 21,* 163–172.

Ekman, P. (1992). An argument for basic emotions. *Cognition and Emotion, 6,* 169–200.

Ekman, P. (2003). *Micro Expression Training Tool DVD.* San Francisco: Mozgo Media.

Ekman, P. (2004). *Subtle Expression Training Tool DVD.* San Francisco: Mozgo Media.

Elkin, I., Shea, M. T., Watkins, J. T., Imber, S. D., Sotsky, S. M., Collins, J. F., et al. (1989). NIMH Treatment of Depression Collaborative Research Program: General effectiveness of treatments. *Archives of General Psychiatry, 46,* 971–982.

Elliott, R. (2002). Research on the effectiveness of humanistic therapies: A meta-analysis. In D. Cain & J. Seeman (Eds.), *Humanistic psychotherapies: Handbook of research and practice.* Washington, D.C.: American Psychological Association.

Ellis, A. (1962). *Reason and emotion in psychotherapy.* Secaucus, NY: Lyle Stuart.

Elstein, A. S., Shulman, L. S., & Sprafka, S. A. (1978). *Medical problem solving: An analysis of clinical reasoning.* Cambridge, MA: Harvard University Press.

Endicott, J., Nee, J., Harrison, W., & Blumenthal, R. (1993). Quality of life enjoyment and satisfaction questionnaire: A new measure. *Psychopharmacology Bulletin, 29*(2), 321–326.

Ericsson, K. A. (2006). The influence of experience and deliberate practice on the development of superior expert performance. In K. A. Ericsson, N. Charness, P. J. Feltovich, & R. R. Hoffman (Eds.), *The Cambridge handbook of expertise and expert performance* (pp. 683–703). New York: Cambridge University Press.

Fairburn, C. G., Cooper, Z., & Shafran, R. (2003). Cognitive behaviour therapy for eating disorders: A "transdiagnostic" theory and treatment. *Behaviour Research and Therapy, 41,* 509–528.

Fairburn, C. G., Kirk, J., O'Connor, M., & Cooper, P. J. (1986). A comparison of two psychological treatments for bulimia nervosa. *Behaviour Research and Therapy, 24,* 629–643.

Fennell, M. (2006). *Overcoming low self-esteem: Self-help course.* London: Robinson.

Fennell, M. J. V., & Teasdale, J. D. (1987). Cognitive therapy for depression: Individual differences and the process of change. *Cognitive Therapy and Research, 11,* 253–271.

Ferster, C. B. (1973). A functional analysis of depression. *American Psychologist, 28,* 857–870.

Finzi, E., & Wasserman, E. (2006). Treatment of depression with botulinum toxin A: A case series. *Dermatologic Surgery, 32*(5), 645–649.

First, M. B., Spitzer, R. L., Gibbon, M., & Williams, J. B. W. (2002). *Structured Clinical Interview for DSM-IV-TR Axis I Disorders, Research Version, Patent Edition* (SCID-I/P). New York: New York State Psychiatric Institute.

Foa, E. B. (2001). *Imaginal exposure* [videotape]. Clinical Grand Rounds Series. New York: Association for Advancement of Behavior Therapy.

Foa, E. B., Hembree, E., & Rothbaum, B. (2007). *Prolonged exposure therapy for PTSD: Emotional processing of traumatic experiences* [therapist guide]. New York: Oxford University Press.

Foa, E. B., Huppert, J. D., & Cahill, S. P. (2006). Emotional processing theory: An update. In B. O. Rothbaum (Ed.), *Pathological anxiety : Emotional processing in etiology and treatment* (pp. 3–24). New York: Guilford Press.

Foa, E. B., & Kozak, M. J. (1986). Emotional processing of fear: Exposure to corrective information. *Psychological Bulletin, 99,* 20–35.

Foa, E. B., & McNally, R. J. (1996). Mechanics of change in exposure therapy. In R. M. Rapee (Ed.), *Current controversies in the anxiety disorders* (pp. 329–343). New York: Guilford Press.

Foa, E. B., & Rothbaum, B. O. (1998). *Treating the trauma of rape.* New York: Guilford Press.

Foa, E. B., Steketee, G., & Rothbaum, B. O. (1989). Behavioral/cognitive conceptualizations of post-traumatic stress disorder. *Behavior Therapy, 20,* 155–176.

Foa, E. B., Steketee, G., Turner, R. M., & Fischer, S. C. (1980). Effects of imaginal exposure to feared disasters in obsessive–compulsive checkers. *Behaviour Research and Therapy, 18,* 449–455.

Foa, E. B., & Wilson, R. (1991). *Stop obsessing! How to overcome your obsessions and compulsions.* New York: Bantam.

Foa, E. B., Zoellner, L. A., Feeny, N. C., Hembree, E. A., & Alvarez-Conrad, J. (2002). Does imaginal exposure exacerbate PTSD symptoms? *Journal of Consulting and Clinical Psychology, 70,* 1022–1028.

Follette, W. C. (1996). Introduction to the special section on the development of theoretically coherent alternatives to the DSM system. *Journal of Consulting and Clinical Psychology, 64,* 1117–1119.

Foulks, E. F., Persons, J. B., & Merkel, R. L. (1986). The effect of illness beliefs on compliance in psychotherapy. *American Journal of Psychiatry, 143,* 340–344.

Frank, E. (2005). *Treating bipolar disorder: A clinician's guide to interpersonal and social rhythm therapy.* New York: Guilford Press.

Franklin, M. E., Abramowitz, J. S., Kozak, M. J., & Foa, E. B. (2000). Effectiveness of exposure and ritual prevention for obsessive–compulsive disorder: Randomized compared with nonrandomized samples. *Journal of Consulting and Clinical Psychology, 68,* 594–602.

Frederickson, B. L. (2001). The role of positive emotions in positive psychology: The broaden-and-build theory of positive emotions. *American Psychologist, 56,* 218–226.

Freeman, A. (1992). Developing treatment conceptualizations in cognitive therapy. In A. Freeman & F. Dattilio (Eds.), *Casebook of cognitive-behavior therapy* (pp. 13–23). New York: Plenum Press.

Friedman, M. A., Detweiler-Bedell, J. B., Leventhal, H. E., Horne, R., Keitner, G. I., & Miller, I. W. (2004). Combined psychotherapy and pharmacotherapy for the treatment of major depressive disorder. *Clinical Psychology: Science and Practice, 11,* 47–68.

Frost, R. O., Martin, P., Lahart, C., & Rosenblate, R. (1990). The dimensions of perfectionism. *Cognitive Therapy and Research, 14,* 449–468.

Garb, H. N. (1998). *Studying the clinician: Judgment research and psychological assessment.* Washington, D.C.: American Psychological Association.

Garcia, J., & Koelling, R. A. (1966). Relation of cue to consequence in avoidance learning. *Psychonomic Science, 4,* 123–124.

Garner, D. M., Rockert, W., Davis, R., Garner, M. V., Olmsted, M. P., & Eagle, M. (1993). Comparison of cognitive-behavioral and supportive expressive therapy for bulimia nervosa. *American Journal of Psychiatry, 150,* 37–46.

Garratt, G., Ingram, R. E., Rand, K., & Sawalani, G. (2007). Cognitive processes in cognitive therapy: Evaluation of the mechanisms of change in the treatment of depression. *Clinical Psychology: Science and Practice, 14*(3), 224–239.

Gaus, V. L. (2007). *Cognitive-behavioral therapy for adult Asperger syndrome.* New York: Guilford Press.

Gawande, A. (2007). The bell curve. In *Better: A surgeon's notes on performance* (pp. 201–230). New York: Metropolitan Books.

Gaynor, S. T., Weersing, V. R., Kolko, D. J., Birmaher, B., Heo, J., & Brent, D. A. (2003). The prevalence and impact of large sudden improvements during adolescent therapy for depression: A comparison across cognitive-behavioral, family, and supportive therapy. *Journal of Consulting and Clinical Psychology, 71,* 386–393.

Ghaderi, A. (2006). Does individualization matter? A randomized trial of standardized (focused) versus individualized (broad) cognitive behavior therapy for bulimia nervosa. *Behaviour Research and Therapy, 44,* 273–288.

Gibbs, L., & Gambrill, E. (1999). *Critical thinking for social workers: Exercises for the helping professions.* Thousand Oaks, CA: Pine Forge Press.

Giesler, R. B., Josephs, R. A., & Swann, W. B. (1996). Self-verification in clinical depression: The desire for negative evaluation. *Journal of Abnormal Psychology, 105*(3), 358–368.

Gilbert, P., & Procter, S. (2006). Compassionate mind training for people with high shame and self-criticism: Overview and pilot study of a group therapy approach. *Clinical Psychology and Psychotherapy, 13,* 353–379.

Gladwell, M. (2006, May 22). What the dog saw. *The New Yorker,* pp. 48–57.

Goldfried, M., & Davila, J. (2005). The role of relationship and technique in therapeutic change. *Psychotherapy: Theory, Research, Practice, Training, 42*(4), 421–430.

Goldfried, M. R., & Davison, G. C. (1994). *Clinical behavior therapy.* New York: Wiley.

Goldsmith, S. K., Pellmar, T. C., Kleinman, A. M., & Bunney, W. E. (Eds.). (2002). *Reducing suicide: A national imperative.* Washington, DC: National Academies Press.

Goodman, W. K., Price, L. H., Rasmussen, S. A., Mazure, C., Fleischman, R. L., Hill, C. L., et al. (1989). The Yale–Brown Obsessive–Compulsive Scale I: Development, use, and reliability. *Archives of General Psychiatry, 46,* 1006–1011.

Gotlib, I. H., & Krasnoperova, E. (1998). Biased information processing as a vulnerability factor for depression. *Behavior Therapy, 29,* 603–617.

Gray, J. A. (1973). Causal theories of personality and how to test them. In J. R. Royce (Ed.), *Contributions of multivariate analysis to psychological theory* (pp. 409–463). New York: Academic Press.

Gray, J. A. (1990). Brain systems that mediate both emotion and cognition. *Cognition and Emotion, 4,* 269–288.

Greene, B., & Blanchard, E. B. (1994). Cognitive therapy for irritable bowel syndrome. *Journal of Consulting and Clinical Psychology, 62,* 576–582.

Gross, J. J. (1998). The emerging field of emotion regulation: An integrative review. *Review of General Psychology, 2,* 271–299.

Gross, J. J., & Muñoz, R. F. (1995). Emotion regulation and mental health. *Clinical Psychology: Science and Practice, 2,* 151–164.

Grosso, F. C. (2002). *The legal and ethical corner: When a client refuses a therapeutic recommendation.* Retrieved 2005 from *www.fgrosso.com.*

Gruber, J. L., & Persons, J. B. (2008). *Handling treatment refusal in bipolar disorder.* Unpublished manuscript.

Gunthert, K. C., Cohen, L. H., Butler, A. C., & Beck, J. S. (2005). Predictive role of daily coping and affective reactivity in cognitive therapy outcome: Application of a daily process design to psychotherapy research. *Behavior Therapy, 36*(1), 77–88.

Haaga, D. A., DeRubeis, R. J., Stewart, B. L., & Beck, A. T. (1991). Relationship of intelligence with cognitive therapy outcome. *Behaviour Research and Therapy, 29,* 277–281.

Haaga, D. A., Dyck, M. J., & Ernst, D. (1991). Empirical status of cognitive therapy of depression. *Psychological Bulletin, 110,* 215–236.

Hackmann, A. (1998). Working with images in clinical psychology. In A. S. Bellack & M. Hersen (Eds.), *Comprehensive clinical psychology* (Vol. 6). New York: Pergamon Press.

Harvey, A. G., Watkins, E., Mansell, W., & Shafran, R. (2004). *Cognitive behavioural processes across psychological disorders: A transdiagnostic approach to research and treatment.* Oxford: Oxford University Press.

Hawkins, R. P. (1986). Selection of target behaviors. In R. O. Nelson & S. C. Hayes (Eds.), *Conceptual foundations of behavioral assessment* (pp. 331–385). New York: Guilford Press.

Hayes, A. M., Laurenceau, J.-P., Feldman, G., Strauss, J. L., & Cardaciotto, L. (2007). Change is not always linear: The study of nonlinear and discontinuous patterns of change in psychotherapy. *Clinical Psychology Review, 27,* 715–723.

Hayes, S. C., Luoma, J. B., Bond, F. W., Masuda, A., & Lillis, J. (2006). Acceptance and commitment therapy: Model, processes and outcomes. *Behaviour Research and Therapy, 44,* 1–25.

Hayes, S. C., Masuda, A., Bissett, R., Luoma, J., & Guerrero, L. F. (2004). DBT, FAP, and ACT: How empirically oriented are the new behavior therapy technologies? *Behavior Therapy, 35,* 35–54.

Hayes, S. C., Nelson, R. O., & Jarrett, R. B. (1987). The treatment utility of assessment: A functional approach to evaluating assessment quality. *American Psychologist, 42,* 963–974.

Hayes, S. C., Strosahl, K. D., & Wilson, K. G. (1999). *Acceptance and commitment therapy: An experiential approach to behavior change.* New York: Guilford Press.

Haynes, S. N. (1992). *Models of causality in psychopathology: Toward dynamic, synthetic, and nonlinear models of behavior disorders.* New York: Macmillan.

Haynes, S. N., Kaholokula, J. K., & Nelson, K. (1999). The idiographic application of nomothetic, empirically based treatments. *Clinical Psychology: Science and Practice, 6,* 456–461.

Haynes, S. N., Leisen, M. B., & Blaine, D. D. (1997). Design of individualized behavioral treatment programs using functional analytic clinical case models. *Psychological Assessment, 9,* 334–348.

Haynes, S. N., & O'Brien, W. H. (2000). *Principles and practice of behavioral assessment.* New York: Kluwer Academic/Plenum Publishers.

Hays, P. A., & Iwamasa, G. Y. (Eds.). (2006). *Culturally responsive cognitive-behavioral therapy: Assessment, practice, and supervision.* Washington DC: American Psychological Association.

Henggeler, S. W., Schoenwald, S. K., Borduin, C. M., Rowland, M. D., & Cunningham, P. B. (1998). *Multisystemic treatment of antisocial behavior in children and adolescents.* New York: Guilford Press.

Hersen, M. (1981). Complex problems require complex solutions. *Behavior Therapy, 12,* 15–29.

Hofmann, S. G., Meuret, A. E., Smits, J. A. J., Simon, N. M., Pollack, M. H., Eisenmenger, K., et al. (2006). Augmentation of exposure therapy with d-cycloserine for social anxiety disorder. *Archives of General Psychiatry, 63,* 298–304.

Hofmann, S. G., Moscovitch, D. A., Kim, H., & Taylor, A. N. (2004). Changes in self-perception during treatment of social phobia. *Journal of Consulting and Clinical Psychology, 72,* 588–596.

Hoge, W. (2002, July 20). British inquiry finds doctor killed 215 of his patients. *New York Times,* p. A4.

Hollon, S. D., & Beck, A. T. (2004). Cognitive and cognitive behavioral therapies. In M. J. Lambert (Ed.), *Bergin and Garfield's handbook of psychotherapy and behavior change* (pp. 447–492). New York: Wiley.

Hollon, S. D., DeRubeis, R. J., & Evans, M. D. (1987). Causal mediation of change in treatment for depression: Discriminating between nonspecificity and noncausality. *Psychological Bulletin, 102,* 139–149.

Hollon, S. D., DeRubeis, R. J., Shelton, R. C., Amsterdam, J. D., Salomon, R. M., O'Reardon, J. P., et al. (2005). Prevention of relapse following cognitive therapy vs. medications in moderate to severe depression. *Archives of General Psychiatry, 62*(4), 417–422.

Holmes, E. A., & Mathews, A. (2005). Mental imagery and emotion: A special relationship. *Emotion, 5*(4), 489–497.

Horvath, A. O., & Bedi, R. P. (2002). The alliance. In J. C. Norcross (Ed.), *Psychotherapy relationships that work* (pp. 37–69). New York: Oxford University Press.

Howard, K. I., Kopta, S. M., Krause, M. S., & Orlinsky, D. E. (1986). The dose-effect relationship in psychotherapy. *American Psychologist, 41,* 159–164.

Howard, K., Lueger, R., Maling, M., & Martinovich, Z. (1993). A phase model of psychotherapy: Causal mediation of outcome. *Journal of Consulting and Clinical Psychology, 61,* 678–685.

Howard, K. I., Moras, K., Brill, P. L., Martinovich, Z., & Lutz, W. (1996). Evaluation of psychotherapy: Efficacy, effectiveness, and patient progress. *American Psychologist, 51,* 1059–1064.

Huppert, J. D., Barlow, D. H., Gorman, J. M., Shear, M. K., & Woods, S. M. (2006). The interaction of motivation and therapist adherence predicts outcome in cognitive behavioral therapy for panic disorder: Preliminary findings. *Cognitive and Behavioral Practice, 13,* 198–204.

Ilardi, S. S., & Craighead, W. E. (1994). The role of nonspecific factors in cognitive-behavior therapy for depression. *Clinical Psychology: Science and Practice, 1,* 138–156.

Imber, S. D., Pilkonis, P. A., Sotsky, S. M., Elkin, I., Watkins, J. T., Collins, J. F., et al. (1990). Mode-specific effects among three treatments for depression. *Journal of Consulting and Clinical Psychology, 58,* 352–359.

Ingram, R. E. (1984). Toward an information-processing analysis of depression. *Cognitive Therapy and Research, 8,* 443–477.

Ingram, R. E., Miranda, J., & Segal, Z. V. (1998). *Cognitive vulnerability to depression*. New York: Guilford Press.

Iwata, B. A., Duncan, B. A., Zarcone, J. R., Lerman, D. C., & Shore, B. A. (1994). A sequential, test-control methodology for conducting functional analyses of self-injurious behavior. *Behavior Modication, 18,* 289–306.

Izard, C. (1993). Four systems for emotion activation: Cognitive and noncognitive processes. *Psychological Review, 100,* 68–90.

Jacobson, N. S., Dobson, K. S., Truax, P. A., Addis, M. E., Koerner, K., Gollan, J. K., et al. (1996). A component analysis of cognitive-behavioral treatment for depression. *Journal of Consulting and Clinical Psychology, 64,* 295–304.

Jacobson, N. S., Martell, C. R., & Dimidjian, S. (2001). Behavioral activation treatment for depression: Returning to contextual roots. *Clinical Psychology: Science and Practice, 8,* 255–270.

Jacobson, N. S., Schmaling, K. B., Holtzworth-Munroe, A., Katt, J. L., Wood, L. F., & Follette, V. M. (1989). Research-structured vs. clinically flexible versions of social learning-based marital therapy. *Behaviour Research and Therapy, 27,* 173–180.

James, W. (1884). What is an emotion? *Mind, 9,* 188–205.

Johnson, S. (2007). *The spiral into mania: How do cognition and coping drive the process?* Paper presented at the World Congress of Behavioural and Cognitive Therapies, Barcelona.

Jones, M. C. (1924). The elimination of children's fears. *Journal of Experimental Psychology, 62,* 126–137.

Karno, M. P., & Longabaugh, R. (2005). Less directiveness by therapists improves drinking outcomes of reactant clients in alcoholism treatment. *Journal of Consulting and Clinical Psychology, 73*(2), 262–267.

Kasch, K. L., Rottenberg, J., Arnow, B. A., & Gotlib, I. H. (2002). Behavioral activation and inhibition systems and the severity and course of depression. *Journal of Abnormal Psychology, 111,* 589–597.

Kazdin, A. E. (1982). *Single-case research designs: Methods for clinical and applied settings*. New York: Oxford University Press.

Kazdin, A. E. (2001). *Behavior modification in applied settings* (6th ed.). Belmont, CA: Wadsworth/ Thomson Learning.

Kearney, A. J. (2006). A primer of covert sensitization. *Cognitive and Behavioral Practice, 13,* 167–175.

Keller, M. B., McCullough, J. P., Klein, D. N., Arnow, B., Dunner, D. L., & Gelenberg, A. J. (2000). A comparison of nefazodone, the cognitive behavioral-analysis system of psychotherapy, and their combination for the treatment of chronic depression. *New England Journal of Medicine, 342,* 1462–1470.

Keltner, D., & Haidt, J. (Eds.). (2001). *Social functions of emotions*. New York: The Guilford Press.

Keltner, D., & Kring, A. M. (1998). Emotion, social function, and psychopathology. *Review of General Psychology, 2,* 320–342.

Keltner, D., Moffitt, T., & Stouthamer-Loerber, M. (1995). Facial expressions of emotion and psychopathology in adolescent boys. *Journal of Abnormal Psychology, 104,* 644–652.

Kendall, P. C., & Chambless, D. L. (1998). Empirically supported psychological treatments [special issue]. *Journal of Consulting and Clinical Psychology, 66*(1).

Kendall, P. C., Chu, B., Gifford, A., Hayes, C., & Nauta, M. (1998). Breathing life into a manual: Flexibility and creativity with manual-based treatments. *Cognitive and Behavioral Practice, 5,* 177–198.

Kendall, P. C., Kipnis, D., & Otto-Salaj, L. (1992). When clients don't progress: Influences on and explanations for lack of therapeutic progress. *Cognitive Therapy and Research, 16,* 269–281.

Kimble, M. O., Riggs, D. S., & Keane, T. M. (1998). Cognitive behavioural treatment for complicated cases of post-traumatic stress disorder. In N. Tarrier, A. Wells, & G. Haddock (Eds.), *Treating complex cases: The cognitive behavioral approach*. New York: Wiley.

Kingdon, D., & Turkington, D. (2005). *Cognitive therapy of schizophrenia*. New York: Guilford Press.

Koerner, K. (2005, March). *Individual psychotherapy in DBT* [clinical workshop]. Oakland, CA.

Koerner, K., & Dimeff, L. A. (2000). Further data on dialectical behavior therapy. *Clinical Psychology: Science and Practice, 7*(1), 104–112.

Koerner, K., & Dimeff, L. A. (2007). Overview of dialectical behavior therapy. In L. A. Dimeff & K. Koerner (Eds.), *Dialectical behavior therapy in clinical practice: Applications across disorders and settings* (pp. 1–18). New York: Guilford Press.

Koerner, K., & Linehan, M. M. (1997). Case formulation in dialectical behavior therapy for borderline personality disorder. In T. D. Eells (Ed.), *Handbook of psychotherapy case formulation* (pp. 340–367). New York: Guilford Press.

Kohlenberg, R. J., Kanter, J. W., Bolling, M. Y., Parker, C. R., & Tsai, M. (2002). Enhancing cognitive therapy for depression with functional analytic psychotherapy: Treatment guidelines and empirical findings. *Cognitive and Behavioral Practice, 9*, 213–229.

Kohlenberg, R. J., & Tsai, M. (1991). *Functional analytic psychotherapy: Creating intense and curative therapeutic relationships*. New York: Plenum Press.

Kohlenberg, R. J., & Tsai, M. (1994). Functional analytic psychotherapy: A radical behavioral approach to treatment and integration. *Journal of Psychotherapy Integration, 4*, 175–201.

Korotitsch, W. J., & Nelson-Gray, R. O. (1999). An overview of self-monitoring research in assessment and treatment. *Psychological Assessment, 11*, 415–425.

Kraus, D. R., Seligman, D. A., & Jordan, J. R. (2005). Validation of a behavioral health treatment outcome and assessment tool designed for naturalistic settings: The treatment outcome package. *Journal of Clinical Psychology, 61*, 285–314.

Kring, A. M., & Bachorowski, J. (1999). Emotions and psychopathology. *Cognition and Emotion, 13*, 575–599.

Kring, A. M., Kerr, S. L., Smith, D. A., & Neale, J. M. (1993). Flat affect in schizophrenia does not reflect diminished subjective experience of emotion. *Journal of Abnormal Psychology, 102*, 507–517.

Kring, A. M., Persons, J. B., & Thomas, C. (2007). Changes in affect during treatment for depression and anxiety. *Behaviour Research and Therapy, 45*, 1753–1764.

Kring, A. M., & Werner, K. H. (2004). Emotion regulation and psychopathology. In P. Philippot & R. S. Feldman (Eds.), *The regulation of emotion* (pp. 359–385). Mahwah, NJ: Erlbaum.

Lambert, M. J., & Barley, D. E. (2002). Research summary on the therapeutic relationship and psychotherapy outcome. In J. C. Norcross (Ed.), *Psychotherapy relationships that work: Therapist contributions and responsiveness to patients*. New York: Oxford University Press.

Lambert, M. J., Burlingame, G. M., Umphress, V. J., Hansen, N. B., Vermeersch, D. A., Clouse, G., et al. (1996). The reliability and validity of the Outcome Questionnaire. *Clinical Psychology and Psychotherapy, 3*, 106–116.

Lambert, M. J., Hansen, N. B., & Finch, A. E. (2001). Patient-focused research: Using patient outcome data to enhance treatment effects. *Journal of Consulting and Clinical Psychology, 69*, 159–172.

Lambert, M. J., Harmon, C., Slade, K., Whipple, J. L., & Hawkins, E. J. (2005). Providing feedback to psychotherapists on their patients's progress: Clinical results and practice suggestions. *Journal of Clinical Psychology, 61*, 165–174.

Lambert, M. J., Whipple, J. L., Hawkins, E. J., Vermeersch, D. A., Nielsen, S. L., & Smart, D. W. (2003). Is it time for clinicians to routinely track patient outcome?: A meta-analysis. *Clinical Psychology: Science and Practice, 10*, 288–301.

Lamoureux, B. E., Linardatos, E., Haigh, E. A. P., Fresco, D. M., Bartko, D., Logue, E., et al. (2007, November). *Screening for major depressive disorder in a primary care medical population with the Quick Inventory of Depressive Symptomatology—Self-Report*. Poster presented at the annual meeting of the Association for Behavioral and Cognitive Therapies, Philadelphia, PA.

Lang, P. J. (1979). A bio-informational theory of emotional imagery. *Psychophysiology, 16*, 495–512.

Lang, P. J. (1987). Fear and anxiety: Cognition, memory and behavior. In D. Magnusson & A. Ohman (Eds.), *Psychopathology* (pp. 148–162). New York: Academic Press.

Lang, P. J., Cuthbert, B. N., & Bradley, M. M. (1998). Measuring emotion in therapy: Imagery, activation and feeling. *Behavior Therapy, 29,* 655–674.

Latner, J. D., & Wilson, G. T. (2002). Self-monitoring and the assessment of binge eating. *Behavior Therapy, 33,* 465–477.

Latner, J. D., Wilson, G. T., Stunkard, A. J., & Jackson, M. L. (2002). Self-help and long-term behavior therapy for obesity. *Behaviour Research and Therapy, 40,* 805–812.

LeDoux, J. E. (1989). Cognitive-emotional interactions in the brain. *Cognition and Emotion, 3,* 267–289.

Levenson, R. W. (1994). Human emotion: A functional view. In P. Ekman & R. J. Davidson (Eds.), *The nature of emotion: Fundamental questions* (pp. 123–126). New York: Oxford University Press.

Levenson, R. W. (1999). The intrapersonal functions of emotion. *Cognition and Emotion, 13,* 481–504.

Levenson, R. W., Ekman, P., & Friesen, W. V. (1990). Voluntary facial action generates emotion-specific autonomic nervous system activity. *Psychophysiology, 27,* 363–384.

Lewinsohn, P. M. (1974). A behavioral approach to depression. In R. J. Friedman & M. Katz (Eds.), *The psychology of depression: Contemporary theory and research.* Oxford: Wiley.

Lewinsohn, P. M., & Gotlib, I. H. (1995). Behavioral theory and treatment of depression. In E. E. Beckham & W. R. Leber (Eds.), *Handbook of depression* (2nd ed., pp. 352–375). New York: Guilford Press.

Lewinsohn, P. M., Gotlib, I. H., & Hautzinger, M. (1998). Behavioral treatment of unipolar depression. In V. E. Caballo (Ed.), *International handbook of cognitive and behavioural treatments for psychological disorders.* Oxford: Pergamon/Elsevier Science.

Lewinsohn, P. M., Hoberman, T., & Hautzinger, M. (1985). An integrative theory of depression. In E. E. Beckham & W. R. Leher (Eds.), *Handbook of depression* (2nd ed., pp. 352–375). New York: Guilford Press.

Lieberman, D. A. (2000). *Learning: Behavior and cognition.* Belmont, CA: Wadsworth.

Linehan, M. M. (1993a). *Cognitive-behavioral treatment of borderline personality disorder.* New York: Guilford Press.

Linehan, M. M. (1993b). *Skills training manual for treating borderline personality disorder.* New York: Guilford Press.

Linehan, M. M. (2000). *Opposite action: Changing emotions you want to change* [videotape]. Seattle: Behavioral Tech, LLC.

Linehan, M. M. (2003). *Crisis survival skills: Getting through a crisis without making it worse: I. Distracting and self-soothing* [videotape]. New York: Guilford Press.

Linehan, M. M., & Korslund, K. E. (2004). *Application of dialectical behavior therapy for the suicidal "butterfly."* Paper presented at the annual meeting of the Association for Advancement of Behavior Therapy, New Orleans, LA.

Linehan, M. M., & Manning, S. (2005, October). *Emotion regulation skills for dialectical behavior therapy* [clinical workshop]. Presented by Behavioral Tech, LLC, San Francisco, CA.

Longwell, B. T., & Truax, P. (2005). The differential effects of weekly, monthly, and bimonthly administrations of the Beck Depression Inventory-II: Psychometric properties and clinical implications. *Behavior Therapy, 36,* 265–275.

Looper, K. J., & Kirmayer, L. J. (2002). Behavioral medicine approaches to somatoform disorders. *Journal of Consulting and Clinical Psychology, 70*(3), 810–827.

Luborsky, L., Barber, J., Siqueland, L., Johnson, S., Najavits, L., Franks, A., et al. (1996). The revised helping alliance questionnaire (HAq-II). *Journal of Psychotherapy Practice and Research, 5,* 260–271.

Lutz, W., Martinovich, Z., & Howard, K. I. (1999). Patient profiling: An application of random coefficient regression models to depicting the response of a patient to outpatient psychotherapy. *Journal of Consulting and Clinical Psychology, 67*, 571–577.

Malmivaara, A., Kuukasjaarvi, P., Autti-Ramo, I., Kovanen, N., & Makela, M. (2007). Effectiveness and safety of endoscopic thoracic sympathectomy for excessive sweating and facial blushing: A systematic review. *International Journal of Technology Assessment in Health Care, 23*(1), 54–62.

Mansueto, C. S., Golomb, R. G., Thomas, A. M., & Stemberger, R. M. T. (1999). A comprehensive model for behavioral treatment of trichotillomania. *Cognitive and Behavioral Practice, 6*, 23–43.

Martell, C. R., Addis, M. E., & Jacobson, N. S. (2001). *Depression in context: Strategies for guided action.* New York: Norton.

Martin, G., & Pear, J. (Eds.). (2003). *Behavior modification: What it is and how to do it* (7th ed.). Englewood Cliffs, NJ: Prentice Hall.

Mash, E. J., & Hunsley, J. (1993). Assessment considerations in the identification of failing psychotherapies: Bringing the negatives out of the darkroom. *Psychological Assessment, 5*, 292–301.

Masters, J. C., Burish, T. G., Hollon, S. D., & Rimm, D. C. (1987). *Behavior therapy: Techniques and empirical findings* (3rd ed.). Fort Worth, TX: Harcourt Brace Jovanovich.

McCrady, B. S., & Epstein, E. E. (2003). *Treating alcohol and drug problems: Individualized treatment planning and intervention.* Paper presented at the annual meeting of the Association for Advancement of Behavior Therapy, Boston, MA.

McCullough, J. P. (2000). *Treatment for chronic depression: Cognitive behavioral analysis system of psychotherapy (CBASP).* New York: Guilford Press.

McCullough, J. P. (2006). *Treating chronic depression with disciplined personal involvement.* New York: Springer.

McKay, M., Rogers, P. D., & McKay, J. (1989). *When anger hurts: Quieting the storm within.* Oakland, CA: New Harbinger Publications.

Mennin, D. S. (2004). Emotion regulation therapy for generalized anxiety disorder. *Clinical Psychology and Psychotherapy, 11*, 17–29.

Merrill, K. A., Tolbert, V. E., & Wade, W. A. (2003). Effectiveness of cognitive therapy for depression in a community mental health center: A benchmarking study. *Journal of Consulting and Clinical Psychology, 71*, 404–409.

Meyer, T. J., Miller, M. L., Metzger, R. L., & Borkovec, T. D. (1990). Development and validation of the Penn State Worry Questionnaire. *Behaviour Research and Therapy, 28*, 487–495.

Miklowitz, D. J. (2002). *The bipolar disorder survival guide: What you and your family need to know.* New York: Guilford Press.

Millan, C., & Peltier, M. J. (2006). *Cesar's way.* New York: Harmony Books.

Miller, R. S., & Leary, M. R. (1992). Social sources and interactive functions of emotion: The case of embarrassment. In M. Clark (Ed.), *Emotion and social behavior* (pp. 202–221). Beverly Hills, CA: Sage.

Miller, W. R., & Rollnick, S. (2002). *Motivational interviewing: Preparing people for change* (2nd ed.). New York: Guilford Press.

Mineka, S., Watson, D., & Clark, L. A. (1998). Comorbidity of anxiety and unipolar mood disorders. *Annual Review of Psychology, 49*, 377–412.

Miranda, J., & Persons, J. B. (1988). Dysfunctional attitudes are mood-state dependent. *Journal of Abnormal Psychology, 97*, 76–79.

Miranda, J., Persons, J. B., & Byers, C. N. (1990). Endorsement of dysfunctional beliefs depends on current mood state. *Journal of Abnormal Psychology, 99*, 237–241.

Mohr, D. C., Hart, S. L., Julian, L., Catledge, C., Honos-Webb, L., Vella, L., et al. (2005). Telephone-administered psychotherapy for depression. *Archives of General Psychiatry, 62*, 1007–1014.

Morgan, D. L., & Morgan, R. K. (2001). Single-participant research design: Bringing science to managed care. *American Psychologist, 56,* 119–127.

Morley, S., Eccleston, C., & Williams, A. (1999). Systematic review and meta-analysis of randomized controlled trials of cognitive behaviour therapy and behaviour therapy for chronic pain in adults, excluding headache. *Pain, 80,* 1–13.

Morris, R. J., & Suckerman, K. R. (1974). Therapist warmth as a factor in automated systematic desensitization. *Journal of Consulting and Clinical Psychology, 42,* 244–250.

Mowrer, O. A. (1960). *Learning theory and behavior.* New York: Wiley.

Nathan, P. E., & Gorman, J. M. (Eds.). (2002). *A guide to treatments that work* (2nd ed.). New York: Oxford University Press.

Neimeyer, R. A., & Feixas, G. (1990). The role of homework and skill acquisition in the outcome of group cognitive therapy for depression. *Behavior Therapy, 21,* 281–292.

Nelson-Gray, R. O. (2003). Treatment utility of psychological assessment. *Psychological Assessment, 15,* 521–531.

Nelson, R. O., & Hayes, S. C. (1981). Theoretical explanations for reactivity in self-monitoring. *Behavior Modification, 5*(1), 3–14.

Nelson, R. O., & Hayes, S. C. (1986). The nature of behavioral assessment. In R. O. Nelson & S. C. Hayes (Eds.), *Conceptual foundations of behavioral assessment* (pp. 3–41). New York: Guilford Press.

Newman, C. F., Leahy, R., Beck, A. T., Reilly-Harrington, N. A., & Gyulai, L. (2002). *Bipolar disorder: A cognitive therapy approach.* Washington, DC: American Psychological Association.

Nezu, A. M., Nezu, C. M., & Lombardo, E. (2004). *Cognitive-behavioral case formulation and treatment design: A problem-solving approach.* New York: Springer.

Nezu, A. M., & Perri, M. G. (1989). Social problem-solving therapy for unipolar depression: An initial dismantling investigation. *Journal of Consulting and Clinical Psychology, 57,* 408–413.

Nezu, A. M., Ronan, G. F., Meadows, E. A., & McClure, K. S. (Eds.). (2000). *Practitioner's guide to empirically based measures of depression.* New York: Kluwer Academic/Plenum Publishers.

Ogles, B. M., Lambert, M. J., & Masters, K. S. (1996). *Assessing outcome in clinical practice.* Boston: Allyn & Bacon.

Ogles, B. M., Lambert, M. J., & Sawyer, J. D. (1995). Clinical significance of the National Institute of Mental Health Treatment of Depression Collaborative Research Program Data. *Journal of Consulting and Clinical Psychology, 63,* 321–326.

Ohman, A., & Mineka, S. (2001). Fears, phobias, and preparedness: Toward an evolved module of fear and fear learning. *Psychological Review, 108,* 483–522.

Olatunji, B. O., Sawchuk, C. N., Lohr, J. M., & de Jong, P. J. (2004). Disgust domains in the prediction of contamination fear. *Behaviour Research and Therapy, 42,* 93–104.

Opdyke, D., & Rothbaum, B. O. (1998). Cognitive-behavioral treatment of impulse control disorders. In V. E. Caballo (Ed.), *International handbook of cognitive and behavioural treatments for psychological disorders* (pp. 417–439). Oxford: Pergamon/Elsevier Science.

Organista, K. C., Muñoz, R., & Gonzalez, G. (1994). Cognitive behavioral therapy for depression in low-income and minority medical outpatients: Description of a program and exploratory analyses. *Cognitive Therapy and Research, 18,* 241–259.

Orsillo, S. M., & Roemer, L. (Eds.). (2005). *Acceptance- and mindfulness-based approaches to anxiety: Conceptualization and treatment.* New York: Springer.

Otto, M. W. (2002). Learning and "unlearning" fears: Preparedness, neutral pathways, and patients. *Biological Psychiatry, 52,* 917–920.

Padesky, C. A. (1991, October 4–5). *Treating personality disorders: A cognitive approach.* (Workshop presented by the Institute for the Advancement of Human Behavior, San Francisco, CA.)

Padesky, C. A. (1993). Schema as self-prejudice. *International Cognitive Therapy Newsletter, 5–6,* 16–17.

Padesky, C. A. (1994). Schema change processes in cognitive therapy. *Clinical Psychology and Psychotherapy, 1,* 267–278.

Padesky, C. A. (1996). *Collaborative case conceptualization: A client session* [videotape]. Oakland, CA: New Harbinger Press.

Pavlov, I. P. (1927). *Conditioned reflexes* (G. V. Anrep, Trans.). Oxford: Oxford University Press.

Persons, J. B. (1986a). The advantages of studying psychological phenomena rather than psychiatric diagnoses. *American Psychologist, 41,* 1252–1260.

Persons, J. B. (1986b). Generalization of the effects of exposure treatments for phobias: A single case study. *Psychotherapy, 23,* 160–166.

Persons, J. B. (1989). *Cognitive therapy in practice: A case formulation approach.* New York: Norton.

Persons, J. B. (1990). Disputing irrational thoughts can be avoidance behavior: A case report. *Behavior Therapist, 13,* 132–133.

Persons, J. B. (1991). Psychotherapy outcome studies do not accurately represent current models of psychotherapy: A proposed remedy. *American Psychologist, 46,* 99–106.

Persons, J. B. (1993). The process of change in cognitive therapy: Acquisition of compensatory skills or schema change? *Cognitive Therapy and Research, 17,* 123–137.

Persons, J. B. (2001). Conducting effectiveness studies in the context of evidence-based clinical practice. *Clinical Psychology: Science and Practice, 8,* 168–172.

Persons, J. B. (2007). Psychotherapists collect data during routine clinical work that can contribute to knowledge about mechanisms of change in psychotherapy. *Clinical Psychology: Science and Practice, 14*(3), 244–246.

Persons, J. B., Bostrom, A., & Bertagnolli, A. (1999). Results of randomized controlled trials of cognitive therapy for depression generalize to private practice. *Cognitive Therapy and Research, 23,* 535–548.

Persons, J. B., & Burns, D. D. (1985). Mechanisms of action of cognitive therapy: The relative contributions of technical and interpersonal interventions. *Cognitive Therapy and Research, 9,* 539–551.

Persons, J. B., Burns, D. D., & Perloff, J. M. (1988). Predictors of dropout and outcome in cognitive therapy for depression in a private practice setting. *Cognitive Therapy and Research, 12,* 557–575.

Persons, J. B., Davidson, J., & Tompkins, M. A. (2001). *Essential components of cognitive-behavior therapy for depression.* Washington, DC: American Psychological Association.

Persons, J. B., & Mikami, A. Y. (2002). Strategies for handling treatment failure successfully. *Psychotherapy: Theory/Research/Practice/Training, 39,* 139–151.

Persons, J. B., & Miranda, J. (1991). Treating dysfunctional beliefs: Implications of the mood-state hypothesis. *Journal of Cognitive Psychotherapy, 5,* 15–25.

Persons, J. B., & Miranda, J. (1992). Cognitive theories of vulnerability to depression: Reconciling negative evidence. *Cognitive Therapy and Research, 16,* 485–502.

Persons, J. B., Roberts, N. A., Zalecki, C. A., & Brechwald, W. A. G. (2006). Naturalistic outcome of case formulation-driven cognitive-behavior therapy for anxious depressed outpatients. *Behaviour Research and Therapy, 44,* 1041–1051.

Peterson, D. R. (1991). Connection and disconnection of research and practice in the education of professional psychologists. *American Psychologist, 46,* 422–429.

Premack, D. (1965). Reinforcement theory. In D. Levine (Ed.), *Nebraska symposium on motivation* (pp. 123–180). Lincoln: University of Nebraska Press.

Prochaska, J. O., & DiClemente, C. C. (1986). The transtheoretical approach. In J. C. Norcross (Ed.), *Handbook of eclectic psychotherapy* (pp. 163–200). New York: Brunner/Mazel.

Prochaska, J. O., & DiClemente, C. C. (1992). The transtheoretical approach. In J. C. Norcross & M. R. Goldfried (Eds.), *Handbook of psychotherapy integration* (pp. 300–334). New York: Basic Books.

Pryor, K. (1999). *Don't shoot the dog! The new art of teaching and training.* New York: Bantam Books.

Rachman, S. J. (1977). The conditioning theory of fear acquisition: A critical examination. *Behaviour Research and Therapy, 15,* 375–387.

Rachman, S. J. (1980). Emotional processing. *Behaviour Research and Therapy, 18,* 51–60.

Rachman, S. J. (1983). The modification of agoraphobic avoidance behaviour: Some fresh possibilities. *Behaviour Research and Therapy, 21,* 567–574.

Rector, N. A., Richter, M. A., Denisoff, E., Crawford, C., Bradbury, C., Bourdeau, D., et al. (2007). *Exposure/response prevention versus CBT for refractory OCD: Follow-up effects and predictors of outcome.* Paper presented at the Association of Behavioral and Cognitive Therapies, Philadelphia, PA.

Rector, N. A., Zuroff, D. C., & Segal, Z. V. (1999). Cognitive change and the therapeutic alliance: The role of technical and nontechnical factors in cognitive therapy. *Psychotherapy, 36*(4), 320–328.

Rescorla, R. A. (1988). Pavlovian conditioning: It's not what you think it is. *American Psychologist, 43,* 151–160.

Resick, P. A., & Schnicke, M. K. (1993). *Cognitive processing therapy for rape victims: A treatment manual.* Newbury Park, CA: Sage.

Ressler, K. J., Rothbaum, B. O., Tannenbaum, L., Anderson, P., Graap, K., Zimand, E., et al. (2004). Cognitive enhancers as adjuncts to psychotherapy. *Archives of General Psychiatry, 61,* 1136–1144.

Roemer, L., & Orsillo, S. M. (2002). Expanding our conceptualization of and treatment for generalized anxiety disorder: Integrating mindfulness/acceptance-based approaches with existing cognitive-behavioral models. *Clinical Psychology: Science and Practice, 9,* 54–68.

Rosen, G. M., & Davison, G. C. (2003). Psychology should list empirically supported principles of change (ESPs) and not credential trademarked therapies or other treatment packages. *Behavior Modification, 27,* 300–312.

Rosen, J. B., & Schulkin, J. (1998). From normal fear to pathological anxiety. *Psychological Bulletin, 105,* 325–350.

Rosenthal, T., & Bandura, A. (1978). Psychological modeling: Theory and practice. In S. L. Garfield & A. E. Bergin (Eds.), *Handbook of psychotherapy and behavior change* (2nd ed.). New York: Wiley.

Rude, S. S. (1986). Relative benefits of assertion or cognitive self-control treatment for depression as a function of proficiency in each domain. *Journal of Consulting and Clinical Psychology, 54,* 390–394.

Rusch, M. D., Grunert, B. K., Mendelsohn, R. A., & Smucker, M. R. (2000). Imagery rescripting for recurrent, distressing images. *Cognitive and Behavioral Practice, 7,* 173–182.

Rush, A. J., Trivedi, M. H., Ibrahim, H. M., Carmody, T. J., Arnow, B., Klein, D. N., et al. (2003). The 16-Item Quick Inventory of Depressive Symptomatology (QIDS), Clinician Rating (QIDS-C), and Self-Report (QIDS-SR): A psychometric evaluation in patients with chronic major depression. *Biological Psychiatry, 54,* 585.

Sackett, D. L., Haynes, R. B., Guyatt, G. H., & Tugwell, P. (1991). *Clinical epidemiology: A basic science for clinical medicine.* Boston: Little, Brown.

Sackett, D. L., Richardson, W. S., Rosenberg, W., & Haynes, R. B. (1997). *Evidence-based medicine: How to practice and teach EBM.* New York: Churchill Livingstone.

Safran, J. D., Muran, J. C., Samstag, L. W., & Stevens, C. (2002). Repairing alliance ruptures. In J. C. Norcross (Ed.), *Psychotherapy relationships that work* (pp. 235–254). New York: Oxford University Press.

Salkovskis, P. M. (1989). Somatic problems. In K. Hawton, P. Salkovskis, J. Kirk, & D. Clark (Eds.), *Cognitive behavior therapy for psychiatric problems* (pp. 235–276). Oxford: Oxford Medical Publications.

Salkovskis, P. M. (1991). The importance of behaviour in the maintenance of anxiety and panic: A cognitive account. *Behavioural Psychotherapy, 19,* 6–19.

Samoilov, A., & Goldfried, M. R. (2000). Role of emotion in cognitive-behavior therapy. *Clinical Psychology: Science and Practice, 7*, 373–385.

Santiago, N. J., Klein, D. N., Vivian, D., Arnow, B. A., Blalock, J. A., Kocsis, J. H., et al. (2005). The therapeutic alliance and CBASP-specific skill acquisition in the treatment of chronic depression. *Cognitive Therapy and Research, 29*(6), 803–817.

Scheel, K. R. (2000). The empirical basis of dialectical behavior therapy: Summary, critique, and implications. *Clinical Psychology: Science and Practice, 7*, 68–86.

Scher, C. D., Ingram, R. E., & Segal, Z. V. (2005). Cognitive reactivity and vulnerability: Empirical evaluation of construct activation and cognitive diathesis in unipolar depression. *Clinical Psychology Review, 25*, 487–510.

Schmid, S. P., Freid, C. M., Hollon, S. D., & DeRubeis, R. J. (2002). *Negative affect, positive affect, and autonomic arousal over the course of treatment of major depression.* Paper presented at the annual meeting of the Association for Advancement of Behavior Therapy, Reno, NV.

Schneider, B. H., & Byrne, B. M. (1987). Individualizing social skills training for behavior-disordered children. *Journal of Consulting and Clinical Psychology, 55*, 444–445.

Schulte, D., Kunzel, R., Pepping, G., & Schulte-Bahrenberg, T. (1992). Tailor-made versus standardized therapy of phobic patients. *Advances in Behaviour Research and Therapy, 14*, 67–92.

Schut, A. J., Castonguay, L. G., & Borkovec, T. D. (2001). Compulsive checking behaviors in generalized anxiety disorder. *Journal of Clinical Psychology, 57*(6), 705–715.

Scott, J. (1998). Where there's a will . . . Cognitive therapy for people with chronic depressive disorders. In N. Tarrier, A. Wells, & G. Haddock (Eds.), *Treating complex cases: The cognitive behavioural therapy approach* (pp. 81–104). New York: Wiley.

Sederer, L. I., & Dickey, B. (Eds.). (1996). *Outcomes assessment in clinical practice.* Baltimore: Williams & Wilkins.

Segal, Z. V., Gemar, M., & Williams, S. (1999). Differential cognitive response to a mood challenge following successful cognitive therapy or pharmacotherapy for unipolar depression. *Journal of Abnormal Psychology, 108*, 3–10.

Segal, Z. V., Kennedy, S., Gemar, M., Hood, K., Pedersen, R., & Buis, T. (2006). Cognitive reactivity to sad mood provocation and the prediction of depressive relapse. *Archives of General Psychiatry, 63*, 749–755.

Segal, Z. V., Williams, M. G., & Teasdale, J. D. (2002). *Mindfulness-based cognitive therapy for depression.* New York: Guilford Press.

Seligman, M. E. P. (1971). Phobias and preparedness. *Behavior Therapy, 2*, 307–320.

Seligman, M. E. P., & Johnston, J. C. (1973). A cognitive theory of avoidance learning. In F. O. McGuigan & D. V. Lumsden (Eds.), *Contemporary approaches to conditioning and learning* (pp. 69–107). Washington, DC: V. H. Winston.

Seligman, M. E. P., Steen, T. A., Park, N., & Peterson, C. (2005). Positive psychology progress: Empirical validation of interventions. *American Psychologist, 60*, 410–421.

Shafran, R., Thordarson, D. S., & Rachman, S. (1996). Thought-action fusion in obsessive–compulsive disorder. *Journal of Anxiety Disorders, 10*, 379–391.

Sharpe, J. P., & Gilbert, D. G. (1998). Effects of repeated administration of the Beck Depression Inventory and other measures of negative mood states. *Personality and Individual Differences, 24*(4), 457–463.

Shaw, B. F., Elkin, I., Yamaguchi, J., Olmsted, M., Vallis, T. M., Dobson, K. S., et al. (1999). Therapist competence ratings in relation to clinical outcome in cognitive therapy of depression. *Journal of Consulting and Clinical Psychology, 67*(6), 837–846.

Simons, A. D., Garfield, S. L., & Murphy, G. E. (1984). The process of change in cognitive therapy and pharmacotherapy for depression. *Archives of General Psychiatry, 41*, 45–51.

Sloan, T., & Telch, M. J. (2002). The effects of safety-seeking behavior and guided threat reappraisal on fear reduction during exposure: An experimental investigation. *Behaviour Research and Therapy, 40*, 235–251.

Smith, J. E., & Meyers, R. J. (2000). CRA: The Community Reinforcement Approach for treating alcohol problems. In M. J. Dougher (Ed.), *Clinical behavior analysis*. Reno, NV: Context Press.

Smits, J. A. J., Powers, M. B., Cho, Y., & Telch, M. J. (2004). Mechanism of change in cognitive-behavioral treatment of panic disorder: Evidence for the fear of fear mediational hypothesis. *Journal of Consulting and Clinical Psychology, 72*, 646–652.

Smucker, M. R., & Niederee, J. (1995). Treating incest-related PTSD and pathogenic schemas through imaginal exposure and rescripting. *Cognitive and Behavioral Practice, 2*, 63–93.

Steketee, G. (1993). *Treatment of obsessive–compulsive disorder*. New York: Guilford Press.

Strauman, T. J., Kolden, G. G., Stromquist, V., Davis, N. K., L., Heerey, E., & Schneider, K. (2001). The effects of treatments for depression on perceived failure in self-regulation. *Cognitive Therapy and Research, 25*(6), 693–712.

Strauman, T. J., Vieth, A. Z., Merrill, K. A., Kolden, G. G., Woods, T. E., Klein, M. H., et al. (2006). Self-system therapy as an intervention for self-regulatory dysfunction in depression: A randomized comparison with cognitive therapy. *Journal of Consulting and Clinical Psychology, 74*(2), 367–376.

Strauss, J. L., Hayes, A. M., Johnson, S. L., Newman, C. F., Brown, G. K., Barber, J. P., et al. (2006). Early alliance, alliance ruptures, and symptom change in a nonrandomized trial of cognitive therapy for avoidant and obsessive–compulsive personality disorders. *Journal of Consulting and Clinical Psychology, 74*(2), 337–345.

Stricker, G., & Trierweiler, S. J. (1995). The local clinical scientist: A bridge between science and practice. *American Psychologist, 50*, 995–1002.

Stuart, R. B. (1980). *Helping couples change: A social learning approach to marital therapy*. New York: Guilford Press.

Sutherland, A. (2008). *What Shamu taught me about life, love, and marriage: Lessons for people from animals and their trainers*. New York: Random House.

Tang, T. Z., & DeRubeis, R. J. (1999). Sudden gains and critical sessions in cognitive-behavioral therapy for depression. *Journal of Consulting and Clinical Psychology, 67*(6), 894–904.

Tang, T. Z., DeRubeis, R. J., Hollon, S. D., Amsterdam, J., & Shelton, R. (2007). Sudden gains in cognitive therapy of depression and depressive relapse/recurrence. *Journal of Consulting and Clinical Psychology, 75*, 404–408.

Tang, T. Z., Luborsky, L., & Andrusyna, T. (2002). Sudden gains in recovering from depression: Are they also found in psychotherapies other than cognitive-behavioral therapy? *Journal of Consulting and Clinical Psychology, 70*, 444–447.

Tarrier, N. (Ed.). (2006). *Case formulation in cognitive behaviour therapy*. New York: Routledge.

Teasdale, J. D. (1988). Cognitive vulnerability to persistent depression. *Cognition and Emotion, 2*, 247–274.

Thomas, C. (2008, March). *Using feedback and deliberate practice to increase clinical expertise*. San Francisco: San Francisco Psychological Association.

Thomas, C., & Persons, J. B. (2008). *Do gains in psychotherapy occur suddenly after a single critical session?* Unpublished manuscript.

Tomarken, A. J., Dichter, G., Freid, C., Addington, S., & Shelton, R. C. (2004). Assessing the effects of bupropion SR on mood dimensions of depression. *Journal of Affective Disorders, 78*, 235–241.

Tompkins, M. A. (2004). *Using homework in psychotherapy*. New York: Guilford Press.

Tompkins, M. A., Persons, J. B., & Davidson, J. (2000). *Cognitive-behavior therapy for depression: Schema change methods* [videotape]. Washington, DC: American Psychological Association.

Tsao, J. C. I., Mystkowski, J., Zucker, B., & Craske, M. G. (2002). Effects of cognitive-behavioral therapy for panic disorder on comorbid conditions: Replication and extension. *Behavior Therapy, 33*, 493–509.

Turkat, I. D. (Ed.). (1985). *Behavioral case formulation*. New York: Plenum Press.

Turkat, I. D., & Brantley, P. J. (1981). On the therapeutic relationship in behavior therapy. *Behavior Therapist, 4*, 16–17.

Turkat, I. D., & Maisto, S. A. (1985). Personality disorders: Application of the experimental method to the formulation and modification of personality disorders. In D. H. Barlow (Ed.), *Clinical handbook of psychological disorders: A step-by-step treatment manual* (pp. 502–570). New York: Guilford Press.

Wampold, B. E. (2001). *The great psychotherapy debate: Models, methods, and findings.* Mahwah, NJ: Erlbaum.

Watson, D., Clark, L. A., & Tellegen, A. (1988). Development and validation of brief measures of positive and negative affect: The PANAS scales. *Journal of Personality and Social Psychology, 54,* 1063–1070.

Watson, D. L., & Tharp, R. G. (2002). *Self-directed behavior: Self-modification for personal adjustment.* Belmont, CA: Wadsworth.

Watson, D., Wiese, D., Vaidya, J., & Tellegen, A. (1999). The two general activation systems of affect: Structural findings, evolutionary considerations, and psychobiological evidence. *Journal of Personality and Social Psychology, 76,* 820–838.

Watson, J. P., & Rayner, R. (1920). Conditioned emotional reactions. *Journal of Experimental Psychology, 3,* 1–14.

Wegner, D. M. (1994). *White bears and other unwanted thoughts: Suppression, obsession, and the psychology of mental control.* New York: Guilford Press.

Wegner, D. M., Wenzlaff, R. M., & Kozak, M. J. (2004). Dream rebound: The return of suppressed thoughts in dreams. *Psychological Science, 15*(4), 232.

Weissman, A. N., & Beck, A. T. (1978). *Development and validation of the Dysfunctional Attitude Scale: A preliminary investigation.* Paper presented at the American Education Research Association Meeting, Toronto, Canada.

Wells, A. (2000). *Emotional disorders and metacognition: Innovative cognitive therapy.* Chichester, UK: Wiley.

Wells, A. (2005). Worry, intrusive thoughts, and generalized anxiety disorder: The metacognitive theory and treatment. In D. Clark (Ed.), *Intrusive thoughts in clinical disorders: Theory, research, and treatment.* New York: Guilford Press.

Wells, A., & Carter, K. (2001). Further tests of a cognitive model of generalized anxiety disorder: Metacognitions and worry in GAD, panic disorder, social phobia, depression, and nonpatients. *Behavior Therapy, 32*(1).

Wells, A., Clark, D. M., & Salkovskis, P. (1995). Social phobia: The role of in-situation safety behaviors in maintaining anxiety and negative beliefs. *Behavior Therapy, 26,* 153–161.

Wenzlaff, R. M., & Wegner, D. M. (2000). Thought suppression. *Annual Review of Psychology, 51,* 59–91.

Westen, D., & Morrison, K. (2001). A multidimensional meta-analysis of treatments for depression, panic, and generalized anxiety disorder: An empirical examination of the status of empirically supported therapies. *Journal of Consulting and Clinical Psychology, 69,* 875–899.

Wheatley, J., & Hackmann, A. (2007, July). *Imagery rescripting in Axis I disorders.* Fifth World Congress of Behavioural and Cognitive Therapies, Barcelona, Spain.

Whipple, J. L., Lambert, M. J., Vermeersch, D. A., Smart, D. W., Nielsen, S. L., & Hawkins, E. J. (2003). Improving the effects of psychotherapy: The use of early identification of treatment failure and problem solving strategies in routine practice. *Journal of Counseling Psychology, 58,* 59–68.

Whisman, M. A. (1993). Mediators and moderators of change in cognitive therapy of depression. *Psychological Bulletin, 114,* 248–265.

White, K. S., & Barlow, D. H. (2002). Panic disorder and agoraphobia. In D. H. Barlow (Ed.), *Anxiety and its disorders: The nature and treatment of anxiety and panic* (2nd ed., pp. 328–379). New York: Guilford Press.

Whittal, M. L., Agras, W. S., & Gould, R. A. (1999). Bulimia nervosa: A meta-analysis of psychological and pharmacological treatments. *Behavior Therapy, 30,* 117–135.

Wilhelm, S., & Steketee, G. S. (2006). *Cognitive therapy for obsessive–compulsive disorder: A guide for professionals.* Oakland, CA: New Harbinger.

Wilson, G. T. (1996a). Manual-based treatments: The clinical application of research findings. *Behaviour Research and Therapy, 34*(4), 295–314.

Wilson, G. T. (1996b). Treatment of bulimia nervosa: When CBT fails. *Behaviour Research and Therapy, 34*(3), 197–212.

Wilson, G. T. (2000). *Manual-based treatment in clinical practice: Future directions.* Paper presented at the annual meeting of the Association for Advancement of Behavior Therapy, New Orleans, LA.

Wolpe, J. (1958). *Psychotherapy by reciprocal inhibition.* Stanford, CA: Stanford University Press.

Woody, S. R., Detweiler-Bedell, J., Teachman, B. A., & O'Hearn, T. (2003). *Treatment planning in psychotherapy.* New York: Guilford Press.

Young, J. E. (1999). *Cognitive therapy for personality disorders: A schema-focused approach.* Sarasota, FL: Professional Resource Exchange.

Young, J. E., & Brown, G. (2001). *Young schema questionnaire: Special edition.* New York: Schema Therapy Institute.

Young, J. E., & Klosko, J. S. (1993). *Reinventing your life: How to break free from negative life patterns.* New York: Penguin.

Zajonc, R. B. (1980). Feeling and thinking: Preferences need no inferences. *American Psychologist, 35,* 151–175.

Zajonc, R. B. (1984). On the primacy of affect. *American Psychologist, 39,* 117–123.

Zayfert, C., & Becker, C. B. (2007). *Cognitive-behavioral therapy for PTSD: A case formulation approach.* New York: Guilford Press.

Zinbarg, R. E., & Barlow, D. H. (1996). Structure of anxiety and the anxiety disorders: A hierarchical model. *Journal of Abnormal Psychology, 105,* 181–193.

Zuercher-White, E. (1995). *An end to panic: Breakthrough techniques for overcoming panic disorder.* Oakland, CA: New Harbinger Press.

Index